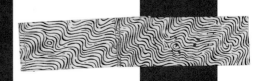

TRADITIONAL CHINESE MEDICINE CUPPING THERAPY

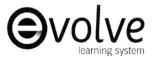

Evolve Learning Resources for Students and Lecturers.
See the instructions and PIN code panel on the inside cover for access to the web site:
http://evolve.elsevier.com/Chirali/cupping/

Think outside the book...evolve

DEDICATION

To my wife Emine, son Zihni and daughter Aliye

Senior Content Strategist: Alison Taylor
Content Development Specialist: Carole McMurray
Senior Project Manager: Beula Christopher
Designer: Christian Bilbow
Illustration Manager: Jennifer Rose
Illustrator: Ethan Danielson

TRADITIONAL CHINESE MEDICINE CUPPING THERAPY Third Edition

ILKAY ZIHNI CHIRALI MBAcC RCHM

Private Practitioner, Acupuncture and Stress Therapy Clinic, London;
Lecturer, Cupping and Traditional Chinese Medicine

Member of The Register of British Acupuncture Council
Member of The Register of Chinese Herbal Medicine
Dip. Acupuncture (Australia); Cert TCM (Australia);
Dip. Clinical Hypnosis (Australia); Dip. Chinese Herbal Medicine (England);
Cert Pathology (England); Cert Paediatric Acupuncture (England);
Cert Chinese Herbal Medicine (Nanjing, PR China);
Cert Acupuncture – Clinical (Nanjing, PR China)

With contributions by
Bruce Bentley
Mark Bovey
Hui-juan Cao
Roslyn Gibbs
Jian-ping Liu
Hossam Metwally
Kei Ngu
Pedro Paiva

Foreword by
Michael McIntyre MA, FNIMH, MRCHM, MBAcC, D.Univ.
Practicing Acupuncturist and Herbalist; Visiting Professor, Middlesex University,
London, UK

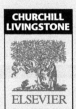

Edinburgh London New York Oxford Philadelphia St Louis Sydney Toronto 2014

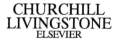

CHURCHILL
LIVINGSTONE
ELSEVIER

First edition 1999
Second edition 2007
Reprinted 2008
Third edition 2014

ISBN 978-0-7020-4352-9
ebook ISBN 978-0-7020-5834-9

British Library Cataloguing in Publication Data
A catalogue record for this book is available from the British Library

Library of Congress Cataloging in Publication Data
A catalog record for this book is available from the Library of Congress

Notices

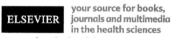

your source for books,
journals and multimedia
in the health sciences
www.elsevierhealth.com

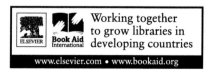

Working together
to grow libraries in
developing countries

www.elsevier.com • www.bookaid.org

The
Publisher's
policy is to use
**paper manufactured
from sustainable forests**

Printed in China

CONTENTS

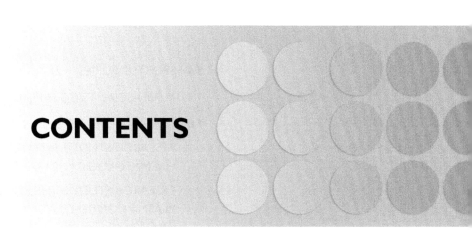

CONTRIBUTORS   vii
FOREWORD   viii
PREFACE TO THE FIRST EDITION   ix
PREFACE TO THE SECOND EDITION   xi
PREFACE TO THE THIRD EDITION   xii
ACKNOWLEDGEMENTS   xiii
GLOSSARY   xiv
ACUPUNCTURE/ACUPRESSURE POINTS   xvi

  1   HISTORY OF CUPPING THERAPY   1

  2   CUPPING'S FOLK HERITAGE: PEOPLE IN PRACTICE   17
      Bruce Bentley

  3   PART 1 CUPPING IN BUDDHIST MEDICINE   33
      Pedro Paiva

      PART 2 CUPPING IN THAILAND'S TRADITIONAL LANNA
      MEDICINE   41
      Kei Ngu

  4   BENEFITS OF CUPPING THERAPY   47

  5   PREPARING THE PATIENT FOR CUPPING TREATMENT   65

  6   COMPLEMENTARY AND ALTERNATIVE MEDICINE (CAM) THERAPIES
      THAT CAN SAFELY INTRODUCE CUPPING TO THEIR TREATMENT
      PROTOCOL   72

  7   THE CUPPING PROCEDURE   79

  8   WHAT TO EXPECT DURING AND AFTER CUPPING THERAPY   87

  9   TWELVE METHODS OF CUPPING THERAPY   91

  10 CUPPING THERAPY ON CHILDREN AND ADULTS   118

  11 COSMETIC CUPPING THERAPY   123

  12 CUPPING THERAPY IN THE TREATMENT OF COMMON
      DISORDERS   144

  13 TREATING MISCELLANEOUS DISORDERS WITH CUPPING
      THERAPY   184

14 SPORTS INJURIES   211

15 MYOFASCIAL TRIGGER POINTS CUPPING THERAPY   231

16 CUPPING THERAPY EVIDENCE-BASED RESEARCH   247

RESEARCH STUDY 1 EFFECTS OF CUPPING THERAPY ON VARIOUS
HAEMATOLOGICAL PARAMETERS   248

RESEARCH STUDY 2 THE EFFECTS OF CUPPING THERAPY ON THE
PLASMA CONCENTRATION OF INFLAMMATORY MEDIATORS   251
Ilkay Zihni Chirali, Roslyn Gibbs and Mark Bovey

RESEARCH STUDY 3 CUPPING AND MYOFASCIAL PAIN
SYNDROME   256
Hossam Metwally

RESEARCH STUDY 4 A SYSTEMATIC LITERATURE REVIEW OF CLINICAL
EVIDENCE-BASED RESEARCH   277
Hui-juan Cao and Jian-ping Liu

17 FREQUENTLY ASKED QUESTIONS AND PRECAUTIONS AND
CONTRAINDICATIONS   311

COLOUR PLATE SECTION

INDEX   315

NOTE The online materials accompanying this text include video sequences of the different cupping techniques indicated in the text by the computer mouse icon. To look at the video for a given technique, click on the relevant icon in the contents list on the website. The website is designed to be used in conjunction with the text and not as a stand-alone product.

CONTRIBUTORS

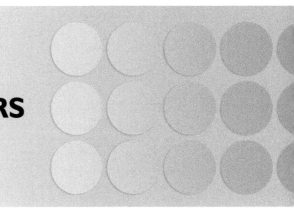

Bruce Bentley, MA, BA (Hons), BHSc
Director of Health Traditions,
    Victoria, Australia

Mark Bovey, MSc
External Examiner for MSc Acupuncture,
    Northern College of Acupuncture, North
    Yorkshire; Middlesex University, London, UK

Hui-juan Cao, PhD
Research Associate, Centre for Evidence-Based
    Chinese Medicine, Beijing University of
    Chinese Medicine, Beijing, China

Roslyn Gibbs, BSc, PhD, MBAcC
Principal Lecturer and Division Head of
    Biomedical Science, School of Pharmacy
    and Biomedical Sciences, University of
    Portsmouth, Portsmouth, UK

Jian-ping Liu, PhD, MD
Professor, Director of Centre for Evidence-
    Based Chinese Medicine, Beijing
    University of Chinese Medicine, Beijing,
    China

Hossam Metwally, MBChB, BSc.APh, MDA, MRCA (London), MSc
Chronic Pain Specialist, Diana Princess of
    Wales Hospital, North East Lincolnshire
    and Goole Hospitals; Managing Director,
    Lincs Pain Management Clinic, Grimsby,
    UK

Kei Ngu, (R. de Feitas), Dip KHa, Dip Oc, Dip TTa, Dip ATMmt, Dip OOm
Principal Teacher, Shivago Thai School of
    Traditional Thai therapy, Edinburgh and
    London, UK; Member, Union of Thai
    Traditional Medicine Society, Thailand

Pedro Paiva, Dip SAt, Dip AVm, Dip TTm, Dip OC
Principal Teacher, Shivago Thai School;
    Principal Teacher, Espaco Jivaka; Principal
    Teacher, Centro de Estudos Tibetanos;
    Lecturer, Tibetan phycology, Centro de
    Estudos Tibetanos, Lisbon, Portugal;
    Teacher, Oriental Medicine Academy,
    Edinburgh, York and London, UK

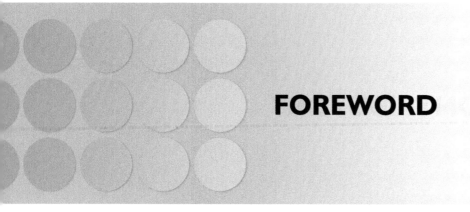

FOREWORD

In 1982, whilst studying acupuncture in a hospital in Nanjing, PRC, I encountered cupping therapy on a daily basis. The Chinese doctors with whom I worked routinely treated a variety of acute and chronic ailments – from injuries, sprains and strains to chest infections – with bamboo and glass cups. In time I too became adept at creating a therapeutic vacuum in a cupping jar by the simple expedient of burning the oxygen in the cup with a lighted piece of cotton wool safely held in forceps before quickly applying the cup to my patient. I saw firsthand the remarkable improvements this simple technique could yield, but actually I knew this already as this was not my first experience of cupping. My mother, who is Greek, had regularly used cupping on my brother, sister and me when we suffered from childhood coughs and colds. This treatment was common in Greece until relatively recently and one of the cups I still use in my practice was purchased some 40 years ago from a chemist shop in Greece.

Studying the Knight's Tale by Chaucer at school in England in the 1960s, our class came across the following passage:

But speke of palamon and of arcite.
Swelleth the brest of arcite, and the soore
Encreesseth at his herte moore and moore.
The clothered blood, for any lechecraft,
Corrupteth, and is in his bouk ylaft,
That neither veyne-blood, ne ventusynge,
Ne drynke of herbes may ben his helpynge.

The Middle English word 'ventusynge' here means cupping, coming from the French 'ventoúza' (βεντούζα) in Greek, but my English teacher looked totally nonplussed when I said that I knew all about this treatment referred to by Chaucer because my mother had applied cups to me at home when I was sick. I soon learnt not to mention my mother's cupping therapy to my English friends as discussion of it was always greeted with astonishment and I certainly did not appreciate my mother being called a witch! Ironically, today one of my most treasured possessions is the bamboo cupping jar my teacher in Nanjing presented me with when I left the hospital and I am proud to continue the ancient art of cupping therapy in my practice.

Given this, I am delighted to greet this third edition of Ilkay Chirali's excellent account of the use of cupping from ancient times till the present. Since it was first published in 1999, this has become the standard textbook for anyone interested in the history or practical uses of cupping therapy. This new expanded third edition contains valuable insights gained from consideration of traditional cupping techniques from the Middle Eastern, Jewish, Chinese, Tibetan and Thai traditions as well as practical advice about using a variety of modern cupping methods such as electromagnetic cupping and the use of rubber and silicon cups. The book also has satisfyingly informative chapters on the use of cupping in cosmetic treatment as well as on the use of this therapy for a range of common disorders such as bronchitis and allergic rhinitis, for treating sports and musculoskeletal injuries and additionally its use in myofascial therapy. Importantly in this age of evidence-based medicine, the book concludes with a survey of research into the outcomes of cupping therapy, some of which has been conducted by the author himself, which supports the launch of further more extensive outcome studies to validate this treatment. I thoroughly commend this book to anyone interested in cupping therapy – this is a most useful reference book to add to your bookshelf.

MICHAEL MCINTYRE MA, FNIMH, MRCHM, MBAcC, D.UNIV.

PREFACE TO THE FIRST EDITION

The first time I experienced cupping was as a 7-year-old child, when I had a bad cold and my mother applied cups to my back. I remember that she first rubbed my back with olive oil and, as I lay down, she applied the cups. I could feel their edges digging into my flesh. It was a strange feeling of my skin being pulled away from me! With a sensation of my back becoming increasingly warm, coupled to a rather uncomfortable feeling of a heavy blanket covering me, I lay there. Then she removed the cups, only to reapply them even more vigorously! After a few more minutes she took the cups off and rubbed me with an alcohol preparation called Zivania. She put me back to bed and covered me with blankets. Half an hour later I was drenched with sweat. My mother was pleased because there was evidence that the cold was out. The next day I was able to go and play with other boys. My cold was gone.

My grandmother, Rahmeli Ebe (see photo), who died in 1964, was a village midwife and a herbalist. Her mother, Havva Ebe, was also the village midwife, and was even more popular than my grandmother. Havva Ebe travelled on horseback while Rahmeli Ebe preferred walking to visit her patients. My great grandmother Havva Ebe died just before I was born, but we lived with Rahmeli Ebe and later on, when she was old and no longer able to travel, she stayed with us in Gazi Baf (Paphos), Cyprus, until her death in 1964. Our house was always busy with people seeking remedies for their complaints. Their payments were usually in the form of a chicken, eggs, or home-made cheese! Rahmeli Ebe used cups for almost all her expectant mothers. She was a great believer in 'removing the Cold and Wind' from the body. She regarded cold as the biggest threat to expectant mothers and their babies. She would often take her clients to the Turkish baths (Hamams) where they would spend a few hours washing and sitting in a herbal steam room, while gaining benefit from cupping before finally relaxing.

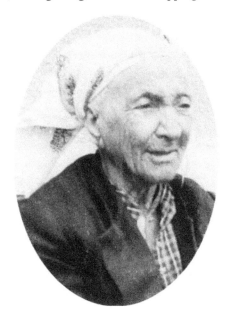

In more recent years as a Chinese medicine practitioner of acupuncture and herbal medicine, I have taken special interest in cupping and its uses. Only now can I fully appreciate what my grandmother and great grandmother, two ordinary village midwives, were trying to do! They were actually getting rid of the external pathogenic factors like Wind and Cold from the body, which could easily penetrate through the weak Wei Qi (Defensive or Protective energy) of a pregnant woman (see section on Glossary of terms at the front of the book). Not only were they concerned with the health of the expectant mother, but they were also equally concerned with the health of the newborn baby. It is an old Turkish custom that the new mother has to stay homebound for 40 days after the delivery, so that the baby is not exposed to external pathogenic factors such as Wind, Cold, Heat or air pollution. These 40 days of rest and care are thought to be enough for the child to build up his or her initial Protective/Defensive energy. The mother is also cared for, to build up her energies to a normal level again, during this invaluable convalescent period. While she is establishing a special bond between her and her child, she receives help and care from her entire family for 40 days!

In the West, however, this early care for mother and child is greatly underestimated and overlooked. It can be argued that, in the West, we now have much better sanitary and living conditions than most Eastern countries. But this relative comfort should not dismiss the most natural human need – to be taken care of – that we all need and expect from time to time, especially when our emotions and energies are running low.

Health care in the West is becoming more finance oriented, and the care for the new mothers and their babies is rapidly diminishing due to financial restraints. If the delivery goes smoothly and without any complications, the child and mother are usually discharged from hospital within a day or two.

It is also very common in the West to see mothers going out shopping with a baby just a few weeks old strapped to its pram, and sometimes turning blue from the effects of cold or wind. This clearly demonstrates that new mothers are unaware of the possible dangers of adverse weather conditions for their children or themselves.

This book is intended as a valuable manual for practitioners to use for effective cupping therapy, so that this ancient Chinese healing art and its benefits can be made known to many more practitioners in alternative therapies and also in more conventional medical practice. The sense of 'duty' to pass on my knowledge and experience has taken on a different dimension and urgency, since my studies in China during 1994. I have decided to write this book because I see a distinct lack of knowledge on the subject by many practitioners. I have also encountered a real enthusiasm from participants in my cupping workshops over the years. I am convinced that this simple, inexpensive and unsophisticated method could more frequently and effectively be put into practice.

ILKAY ZIHNI CHIRALI
LONDON 1997

PREFACE TO THE SECOND EDITION

Six years following publication of the first edition of *Cupping Therapy*, I am truly excited to encounter a massive new and growing interest in the training and application of this useful therapy. I am particularly pleased to find the general public enquiring about the treatment and its benefits.

In this edition I have decided to eliminate the word 'bruise' and replace it with 'cupping mark' as I am quite satisfied that these characteristics are not bruises but straightforward marks on the skin resulting from the cupping application.

I have added a number of explanatory drawings and pictorial illustrations in order to enhance the visual effect of the therapy itself and to simplify overall understanding for the reader. New chapters – *Sports Injuries* and *Myofascial Trigger Points Cupping Therapy* – have been added to this edition as the therapy reaches wider spheres of interest. I have also asked the publishers to move the Glossary and the Appendix (Acupuncture/Acupressure points) sections to the front of the book in order to help users (in particular non-TCM practitioners) to locate more acupuncture points quickly during the treatment.

ILKAY ZIHNI CHIRALI
2007

PREFACE TO THE THIRD EDITION

Twelve years on from the first edition and six years following the publication of the second edition of *Traditional Chinese Medicine Cupping Therapy*, we are witnessing a global increase in the practice of cupping therapy. This increase in the application of cupping therapy is particularly visible via social media networks and many cupping websites have appeared over the last few years. I am delighted to see that this increase is not restricted to TCM practitioners, but to wider healing professional bodies, as well as in the field of cosmetic medicine.

In this new edition I decided to invite contributing authors to share their cupping experiences. As a result four new chapters have been added: these are chapters on *Cupping's Folk heritage; Cupping Therapy in Buddhist Medicine; Cupping in Thailand Lanna Medicine* and an *Evidence-Based Research* chapter with contributions from authors from England and China. These are significant additions to this edition. A Frequently Asked Questions (FAQ) chapter is also included. Chapter 13, *Treating Miscellaneous Disorders with Cupping Therapy* has been extended to embrace further pathological conditions. Additionally the *Benefits of Cupping Therapy* chapter has been expanded. The herbal formulas present in the first and the second editions have been omitted from this edition. And finally, in order to enhance the visual effects of Cupping Therapy, there are many more illustrations and photographs.

O'uz Yorgancioglu, a historian, teacher, anthropologist and author to whom I am related and who comes from the same village as myself (Lemba [Çıralı] in Paphos), told me that my great-grandmother Havva Ebe (midwife and herbalist – see Preface to the 1st edition), who died 4 years prior to my birth on May 1942 when she was 111 years old, learned her midwifery skills from a Lusignan midwife who lived in the village next to ours, called Chloraga in Paphos. (The Lusignans ruled Cyprus between 1192 and 1489.) According to Yorganciogu, when the island was handed over to the British Empire by the Ottoman Turks in 1878, the British Naval commander of the Paphos fleet who sailed to Paphos port had his heavily pregnant wife on board. On the day of the arrival to the port of Paphos she went into labour. Unfortunately the baby was breached, which meant that both the mother and the baby were at risk. The captain was notified of her predicament and he decided to ask for assistance. The locals advised him that there was a renowned midwife called Havva Ebe who lived in the nearby village Lemba, which was just 2 miles away from the port! She was duly summoned to the ship where she corrected the breached baby and a successful delivery was achieved as a result. From that time on in the Paphos region my great-grandmother and her daughter Rahmeli Ebe, my grandmother, were both held in great esteem as herbalists and as midwives. On numerous occasions during my teen years my grandmother continued to receive medical boxes as 'donations' from the British colonial authorities, mostly containing first aid material, although she had no idea how to make use of them! It was my job to take the medical boxes and donate them to the local hospital in Paphos.

ILKAY ZIHNI CHIRALI
2014

ACKNOWLEDGEMENTS

I am deeply indebted to my mother Cemaliye and my father Zihni Ali, who cared for us (five sisters and two brothers) through very difficult and turbulent years in Cyprus and yet injected us with love and compassion as well as an understanding of the magic of nature.

I wish to express my gratitude to all my patients over the last 30 years, and in particular those who volunteered to be part of this project. I would like to thank also the contributing authors Bruce Bentley, Dr Hossam Metwally, Kei Ngu, Pedro Paiva, Hui-juan Cao, Jian-ping Liu, Dr Roslyn Gibbs and Mark Bovey. I also wish to thank all my teachers and interpreters of Nanjing College of Traditional Chinese Medicine (Nanjing University of Traditional Chinese Medicine), Jason Tsai, who helped to translate Chinese medical texts, the doctors and the teachers of the Chang Gung Memorial Hospital, Taipei and China Medical University Hospital, Taichung, Taiwan, for sharing their cupping experiences with me, and Dr Winder Wen-Te Chang, Gabriel Fuentes, Cooper Wei for their unwavering support while in Taiwan. My special thanks go to great practitioners and friends Julian Scott, who wrote the 1st and the 2nd edition forewords, and Michael McIntyre for writing the present one.

I would also like to thank the staff of Elsevier for their expertise and efficiency, in particular Karen Morley, Carole McMurray and Claire Wilson for their encouragement and continued support throughout this project. Finally, this edition as well as the first publication would not have been possible without the colossal help of my friend Gerald Bishop; I am, once again, deeply indebted to him.

ILKAY ZIHNI CHIRALI
2014

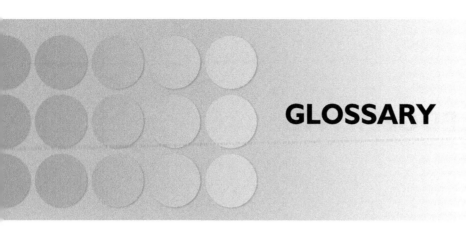

GLOSSARY

Accumulation disorder is a digestive deficiency where food is retained in the digestive system, stomach or intestines; it is commonly observed in young children and the elderly.

Accumulation (Xi-Cleft) point is where the Qi of the organ / channel accumulates; it is mostly effective in the acute stages of the disease.

Ashi (Ah Shi) point is a point that is painful when palpated.

Artery Blood vessel taking blood from the heart to the tissues of the body; **arcuate artery** = curved artery in the foot or kidney; **axillary artery** = artery leading from the subclavian artery at the armpit; **basilar artery** = artery that lies at the base of the brain; **brachial artery** = artery running down the arm from the axillary artery to the elbow, where it divides into the radial and ulnar arteries; **cerebral arteries** = main arteries taking blood into the brain; **common carotid artery** = main artery leading up each side of the lower part of the neck; **communicating arteries** = arteries that connect the blood supply from each side of the brain, forming part of the circle of Willis; **coronary arteries** = arteries that supply blood to the heart muscle; **femoral artery** = continuation of the external iliac artery, which runs down the front of the thigh and then crosses to the back; **hepatic artery** = artery that takes blood to the liver; **common iliac artery** = one of the two arteries that branch from the aorta in the abdomen and divide into the internal and external iliac arteries; **ileocolic artery** = branch of the superior mesenteric artery; **innominate artery** = largest branch from the aortic arch, which continues as the right common carotid and right subclavian arteries; **interlobar artery** = artery running towards the cortex on each side of a renal pyramid; **interlobular arteries** = arteries running to the glomeruli of the kidneys; **lingual artery** = artery that supplies the tongue; **lumbar artery** = one of four arteries that supply the back muscles and skin; **popliteal artery** = artery that branches from the femoral artery at the knee and leads into the tibial arteries; **pulmonary arteries** = arteries that take deoxygenated blood from the heart to the lungs to be oxygenated; **radial artery** = artery that branches from the brachial artery, starting at the elbow and ending in the palm of the hand; **renal arteries** = pair of arteries running from the abdominal aorta to the kidneys; **subclavian artery** = artery running from the aorta to the axillary artery in ach arm; **tibial arteries** = two arteries that run down the front and back of the lower leg; **ulnar artery** = artery that branches from the brachial artery at the elbow and joins the radial artery in the palm of the hand.

Back-Shu points are the points on the Bladder channel on the back of the body where the Qi of a particular organ converges; they are mostly used in chronic diseases.

Blood injury occurs through poor dieting and excessive demand on the body, such as overwork without having adequate rest or sleep in between, long-lasting bleeding, excessive sexual activity, and a demanding exercise regimen despite poor, ineffective recovery from a previous activity or physical injury.

Blood stasis indicates obstruction of the movement of blood in the channels.

Connecting (Luo) points are the points on main channels from which collaterals diverge to join nearby Yin–Yang (Exterior–Interior)-related channels.

Ebe: Turkish for 'midwife'.

Extraordinary points are important treatment points outside the regular 14 channels.

Front-Mu points or Alarm points are the points on the chest and abdomen where the Qi of the respective organs meet.

Identification of Patterns according to the Four Stages is mainly concerned with the febrile disorders caused by external Heat.

Identification of Patterns according to the Six Stages is more concerned with the diseases caused by external Cold progressively penetrating to deeper layers, turning into a febrile disease on the way.

Lingering pathogenic factor is a condition that is not completely cured and acts as a stepping stone for a new disease.

Moxibustion treatment using the dried leaves of *Artemisia vulgaris* (mugwort), which are rolled into a cigar-like cone and lit for their therapeutic properties.

Original Qi or Essential Qi originates from the Kidneys; it is considered the ultimate resource of the Yin- and Yang-Qi of the body.

Pathogenic factors are the six external weather factors influencing and altering the general health of the body. They are Wind, Cold, Summer Heat, Damp, Dryness and Heat.

Release the Exterior mean to get rid of the external pathogen, usually by inducing sweating or applying acupuncture, cupping or Gua Sha.

San Jiao (Triple Burner/Warmer/Energizer) is an organ (system) in charge of controlling and maintaining the proper circulation of the body fluids between the three energetic layers of the body (Upper Jiao, Middle Jiao, Lower Jiao).

Shi indicates an Excess condition.

Source (Yuan) points all 14 main channels have a Source point. This is where the Original Qi of that particular organ and channel is retained; therefore they are considered to be very effective treatment points.

Tonify means to strengthen.

Xu (Empty) indicates Deficiency.

Yang is the stronger of the two, the outside, active, the brighter side of things, hot, fire.

Yin is the weaker of the two, the inner aspect, passive, the darker side, cold, water.

ACUPUNCTURE/ ACUPRESSURE POINTS

ABBREVIATIONS

LU   Lung
LI   Large Intestine
ST   Stomach
SP   Spleen
HT   Heart
SI   Small Intestine
BL   Bladder
K   Kidney
P   Pericardium
SJ   San Jiao (Triple Warmer / Burner / Energizer – TW / TB / TE)
GB Gall Bladder
Liv Liver
Ren Ren Mai (Conception / Directing Vessel – CV / DV)
Du Du Mai (Governing Vessel – GV)

POINTS

LU-1 Zhongfu Central treasury (Front-Mu point of the Lung). Location: 'Three ribs above the breast, in the depression where the artery is felt'. Indications: Regulates the Lung-Qi, disperses the Heat in the Lung, helps with the descending action of the Lung-Qi and stops coughing.

LU-2 Yunmen Cloud gate. Location: Below the clavicle, in the depression 2 inches (5 cm) to the side of ST-13 Qihu (Qi door). Indications: Cough, asthma, pain in the chest, shoulder and arm, and fullness in the chest. This is also the point where the channel-Qi cycle begins and goes through the 12 organ channels, hence the name 'Cloud Gate'.

LU-5 Chize Cubit marsh (He / Sea, Water point). Location: 'At the centre of the elbow above the crease and at the artery'. Indications: Regulates the circulation of the Body Fluids, clears pathogenic Heat in the Lungs, clears Phlegm from the Lungs, stops coughing, sore throat, oedema and restricted movement of the elbow.

LU-6 Kongzui Collection hole (Xi-Cleft, Accumulation point). Location: 'Below LU-5, 7 cun from the wrist crease, in the depression between the two bones'. Indications: All acute Lung conditions, clears Lung Heat, stops bleeding, regulates the Lung-Qi, epigastric pain and arm pain.

LU-7 Lique Broken sequence (Connecting / Luo point, connects to the Large Intestine channel). Location: 'Above the wrist 1.5 cun, as the two hands are clasped, the point is where the forefinger of the opposite hand reaches between the two tendons'. Indications: One of the most important acupuncture points influencing the Defensive Qi, clears the Exterior of pathogens, invigorates the channels, strengthens the Lung-Qi descending action, clears nasal blockage and stops coughing.

LU-9 Taiyuan Greater abyss (Shu / Stream and Yuan / Source point). Location: 'At the pulsating vessel, at the inner extremity of the crease, behind the hand'. Indications: Ventilates and moistens the Lungs, tonifies the Lung-Qi, resolves Phlegm and stops coughing; a major point to use in cases of asthma or wheezing.

LU-10 Yuji Fish border (Ying / Spring point). Location: 'Back of the main joint of the thumb, on the inner aspect, in the centre of the vessels'. Indications: Clears Lung Heat, Wind, and induces perspiration, moistens the Lungs and stops coughing.

LI-4 Hegu Union valley (Yuan / Source point). Location: 'In the depression where the index finger and thumb bones part'. Indications: This is the major point used for pain relief; removes obstruction from the channel and releases the exterior Wind-Heat, regulates the Qi and Blood.

LI-10 Shousanli Arm three miles. Location: '2 cun below Quchi (LI-11) at the end of the muscle'. Indications: Invigorates the flow of the Qi and Blood, removes obstruction; a very important point for tonifying the upper muscles and tendons, facial paralysis, rheumatic pain in the upper extremities.

LI-11 Quchi Pool at the bend (He / Sea point). Location: 'The outer portion of the elbow at the end of the elbow crease'. Indications: Very important point for tonifying the body, clears exterior Wind and internal Heat, especially from the Blood level, therefore it is used in all hot Skin conditions such as eczema, psoriasis and itching.

LI-14 Binao Upper arm. Location: '7 cun above the elbow at the end of the muscle'. Indications: Clears the obstruction from the channels and promotes the circulation of Blood, sedates pain; often used in the treatment of painful 'Bi' syndrome.

LI-15 Jianyu Shoulder bone. Location: 'In the centre of the depression at the end of the shoulder, a hollow appears at the point when the arm is lifted'. Indications: Clears obstruction from the channels, invigorates the flow of Qi and Blood, expels external Wind, benefits the sinews; a major point when treating painful shoulder and paralysis of the arm.

LI-16 Jugu Great bone. Location: In the upper aspect of the shoulder, in the depression between the acromial extremity of the clavicle and the scapular spine. Indications: Pain and motor impairment of the upper extremities, pain in the shoulder and back.

LI-20 Yingxiang Welcome fragrance. Location: '0.5 cun to the sides of the nostrils'. Indications: Clears exterior Wind, such as in facial paralysis, dissipates Lung Heat, opens nasal obstructions, and restores the sense of smell.

ST-1 Chengqi Tear container. Location: '0.7 cun below the eye, on the vertical line of the pupil'. Indications: Clears pathogenic Wind and Heat, improves vision, lacrimation and facial paralysis.

ST-2 Sibai Four whites. Location: '1 cun below the eye, under ST-1, in the hollow of the cheekbone, level with the pupil'. Indications: Expels Wind and Heat; used in facial paralysis, trigeminal neuralgia; brightens the eyes.

ST-3 Nose Juliao Great bone-hole. Location: '0.8 cun to the sides of the nostrils, on the vertical line of the pupil'. Indications: Expels pathogenic Wind and invigorates the channel; used in facial paralysis, trigeminal neuralgia, lacrimation.

ST-4 Dicang Earth granary. Location: '0.4 cun from the corner of the mouth'. Indications: Expels Wind, opens the channels and strengthens the local muscle and tendons; used in facial paralysis, trigeminal neuralgia.

ST-6 Jiache Jawbone. Location: '0.8 cun below the ear in the depression in front of the angle of the jaw'. Indications: Expels Wind and invigorates the channels, promotes the circulation of Qi and benefits the muscles and the ligaments.

ST-7 Xiaguan Lower gate. Location: 'In the centre of the depression in front of the ear, which when the mouth is closed there is a space, and when open the space is closed'. Indications: Clears external Wind, opens the channels, benefits the ear and stops pain.

ST-12 Quepen Empty basin. Location: In the midpoint of the supraclavicular fossa, 4 cun lateral to the Ren Mai. Indications: Coughing, asthma, sore throat, and pain in the supraclavicular fossa.

ST-14 Kufang Storeroom. Location: 'In the first intercostal space, on the mammillary line'. Indications: Clears pathogenic Heat from the Lungs, stops coughing, asthma, fullness and pain in the chest.

ST-15 Wuyi Roof. Location: 'In the second intercostal space, on the mammillary line'. Indications: Cough, asthma, fullness and pain in the chest; clears pathogenic Heat from the Lungs and mastitis.

ST-18 Rugen Breast root. Location: 'In the intercostal space, one rib below the nipple'. Indications: Regulates the circulation of Qi and Blood and removes stagnation from the breast, benefits the Stomach-Qi.

ST-19 Burong Cannot contain. Location: 'On the abdomen, 6 cun superior to the umbilicus, and 2 cun either side of the midline'. Indications: Regulates the Spleen and Stomach, abdominal distension and pain, vomiting, sighing and diarrhoea.

ST-21 Liangmen Beam gate. Location: 'On the abdomen 4 cun superior to the umbilicus, and 2 cun lateral to the anterior midline'. Indications: Regulates the Stomach and Spleen, calms Rebellious Qi, and stops vomiting and gastric pain.

ST-22 Guanmen Lower gate of the Stomach. Location: 'One cun below ST-21 and 2 cun either side of the midline'. Indications: Treats diarrhoea, borborygmus, regulates the Stomach / Spleen and sedates pain.

ST-24 Huaroumen Slippery flesh gate. Location: '1 cun superior to the umbilicus, and 2 cun lateral to the anterior midline'. Indications: Regulates the gastrointestinal system, sedates the mind, dysphonia, insomnia, stiffness of the tongue, abdominal discomfort, borborygmus and diarrhoea.

ST-25 Tianshu Heavenly pillar (Front-Mu point of the Large Intestine). Location: '2 cun lateral to the centre of the umbilicus'. Indications: Regulates the Stomach and Spleen, resolves Dampness, clears Heat in the Stomach and Intestines, stops diarrhoea, vomiting and abdominal pain. A very important point when treating gastrointestinal (Excess) patterns.

ST-29 Guilai Returning. Location: 4 cun inferior to ST-25, or 2 cun lateral to Ren-3. Indications: Regulates the Lower Burner, relieves Blood stagnation, warms and benefits the uterus. A very influential point when treating gynaecological complaints.

ST-30 Qichong Surging Qi. Location: 5 cun below the umbilicus, 2 cun lateral to Qugu (Ren-2). Indications: Abdominal pain, hernia, swelling and pain of the genitalia, impotence, dysmenorrhea, infertility, and irregular menstruation. The name 'Surging Qi' reflects this point's location at the beginning of the Chong Mai (Penetrating Vessel) and its influence on the Uterus.

ST-31 Biguan Thigh joint. Location: 'Directly below the anterior superior iliac spine, in the depression on the lateral side of m. sartorius when the thigh is flexed'. Indications: Clears Wind and Damp, invigorates the channels, relieves rheumatism, treats muscular atrophy of the lower extremities, and strengthens the leg muscles.

ST-32 Futu Crouching rabbit. Location: On the line connecting the anterior superior iliac spine and lateral border of the patella, 6 cun above the laterosuperior border of the patella, in mid rectus femoris. Indications: Pain in the lumbar and iliac region, weakness of the knee, paralysis or motor impairment and pain of the lower extremities.

ST-33 Yinshi Yin market. Location: when the knee is flexed, the point is 3 cun above the upper border of the patella, on the line joining the laterosuperior border of the patella and the anterior superior iliac spine. Indications: Numbness, pain, and motor impairment of the leg and the knee.

ST-34 Liangqiu Beam hill (Xi-Cleft point). Location: '2 cun above the knee, between the two tendons'. Indications: 'Clears obstruction from the Stomach channel, invigorates the collaterals, regulating the Stomach and sedating the pain, expels Wind and Damp from the lower extremities.

ST-35 Dubi Calf's nose (also known as External Xiyan). Location: 'Ask the patient to flex the knee. The point is in the depression below the patella and lateral to the patellar ligament'. Indications: Expels Wind, invigorates the channel, reduces swelling, stops pain and soothes the knee joint. A very effective local point when dealing with knee complaints.

ST-36 Zusanli Three miles of the leg (He / Sea point). Location: '3 cun below the knee, at the outer edge of the shin-bone'. Indications: This is one of the most important acupuncture points on the body, influencing and tonifying the entire Qi and Blood. Regulates and tonifies the Stomach and Spleen, clears obstructions from the Stomach channel and has a profound effect on general health. Expels Wind and Damp and is always used in painful 'Bi' syndrome.

ST-37 Shangjuxu Upper great hollow. Location: '3 cun below the ST-36, in the depression between the tendon and bone'. Indications: This point is also known as the 'Lower combination point of the Large Intestine'; it clears Damp and Heat from the gastrointestinal system, moves the bowels, stops abdominal pain, and is especially effective in the treatment of chronic diarrhoea.

ST-39 Xianjuxu Lower great hollow (the Lower He / Sea Point of the Small Intestine). Location: 3 cun below ST-37 Shangjuxu, one finger-breath from the anterior crest of the tibia, in mid tibialis anterior. Indications: Lower abdominal pain, backache referring to the testis, mastitis, numbness and paralysis of the lower extremities.

ST-40 Fenglong Abundant bulge (Luo / Connecting point). Location: '8 cun above the outer ankle, in the depression on the outer aspect of the lower shin-bone'. Indications: Resolves Damp and Phlegm. The most important point in clearing the Phlegm from the body; clears Stomach Heat, calms asthma, dispels Wind and invigorates the channel; used in paralysis of the lower extremities.

ST-41 Jiexi Separating stream (Jing / River point). Location: 'In the centre of the ankle, 6.5 cun directly above the midpoint of the great and the second toes'. Indications: Expels Wind and stops spasm, clears Stomach Heat, calms the mind and reduces inflammation of the ankle.

ST-44 Neiting Inner court (Ying / Spring point). Location: 'In the depression on the outer aspect of the second toe'. Indications: Clears Heat from the gastrointestinal system, treats disorders of the face, bleeding gums, and conjunctivitis, regulates Qi and benefits the digestion.

SP-4 Gongsun Yellow Emperor (Luo / Connecting point). Location: '1 cun behind the base joint of the great toe'. Indications: Tonifies and regulates the Stomach and Spleen, clears Damp-Heat from the Stomach and stops bleeding, regulates menstruation owing to the connection with the Chong Mai.

SP-5 Shangqiu Shang (Sound of metal) hill (Jing / River point). Location: 'In the depression slightly in front of the point below the internal ankle'. Indications: Tonifies the Spleen and clears Dampness; the most important point for clearing Damp and reducing swelling in the lower extremities.

SP-6 Sanyinjiao Three Yin intersection. Location: '3 cun directly above the tip of the medial malleolus, on the posterior border of the tibia'. Indications: This is the meeting point of the three Yin meridians (Kidney, Liver and Spleen); it is one of the most important tonification points, tonifying the Spleen / Stomach, Kidneys, and Liver (Blood); it resolves Dampness, regulates the flow of Qi and Blood, benefits menstruation, impotence and enuresis, and stops pain.

SP-7 Lougu Leaking valley. Location: '6 cun above the inner anklebone'. Indications: Abdominal distension and pain, nausea, vomiting, pain of the lower extremities, oedema of the ankle and foot. This point is great for draining Damp from the Spleen and Stomach, also helps reducing the swelling caused by Damp.

SP-8 Daji Earth's pivot (Xi-Cleft point). Location: '5 cun below the knee, in the depression below the inner aspect of the knee'. Indications: Regulates the Uterus, removes obstruction and stops pain; a major point when treating gynaecological and lower extremity conditions; stimulates the Spleen and Stomach.

SP-9 Yinlingquan Yin mound spring (He / Sea Water point). Location: 'Below the knee, at the depression at the end of the crease when the knee is flexed'. Indications: Warms the Middle, tonifies the Spleen and expels Dampness, opens the Water passages; a major point for removing Damp from the lower extremities.

SP-10 Xuehai Sea of Blood. Location: '2.5 cun above the inner border of the kneecap, on the margin of the white muscle'. Indications: A major point for removing Blood stasis, stimulates the circulation of Blood; one of its important functions is the cooling effect on the Blood, therefore it is used in all hot skin complaints such as eczema or psoriasis.

SP-12 Chongmen Surging gate. Location: Located in the inguinal region, 3.5 cun lateral to Ren-2, and lateral to the femoral artery. SP-12 is also the 'connecting' point of the Spleen and Liver channels, and as such represents a major thoroughfare in the Qi network.

SP-15 Daheng Great horizontal. Location: 'On the abdomen 4 cun lateral to the umbilicus'. Indications: Tonifies the Spleen, promotes the peristaltic movement of the Large Intestine, improves the flow of Qi and removes excess Water from the intestines.

SP-20 Zhourong All-round flourishing. Location: In the second intercostal space, 1 cun and 6 fen below LU-1 Zhongfu, 6 cun lateral to Ren Mai. Indications: Fullness in the chest and hypochondriac region, coughing, hiccup, and upper arm pain.

HT-7 Shenmen Spirit gate (Shu / Stream and Yuan / Source point). Location: 'On the transverse crease of the wrist, in the depression at the end of the wrist bone, i.e. at the head of the ulna'. Indications: Regulates and nourishes the Heart and sedates the mind; one of the most important and used points on the Heart channel, used in all Heart deficiency syndromes, such as insomnia, anxiety, palpitations and mental depression.

SI-9 Jianzhen True shoulder. Location: 'Below the shoulder blades, between the two bones, in the indentation behind the shoulder muscle'.

Indications: Expels pathogenic Wind and invigorates the channels, sedates pain in the shoulder, scapula and arm.

SI-10 Naoshu Upper arm point. Location: When the arm is adducted, the point is directly above SI-9 Jianzhen, in the depression inferior to the scapular spine. Indications: Pain, weakness and swelling of the shoulder and arm.

SI-11 Tianzong Heavenly gathering. Location: 'In the centre of the infrascapular fossa'. Indications: Opens the channels and invigorates the collaterals, reduces swelling and stops pain; an important point when treating painful shoulder joints.

SI-12 Bingfeng Grasping the wind. Location: 'In the centre of the suprascapular fossa, directly above the point SI-11. A depression appears when the arm is lifted'. Indications: Same as SI-11 Tianzong.

SI-13 Quyuan Crooked wall. Location: On the medial extremity of the suprascapular fossa, about midway between SI-10 Naoshu and the spinous process of the second thoracic vertebrae. Indications: Pain and stiffness of the scapular region.

SI-14 Jianwaishu Outer shoulder point. Location: 'The upper border of the shoulder blade, 3 cun lateral to the midpoint of the spinous processes of T1 and T2'. Indications: Expels pathogenic Wind and moves the channels, treats stiffness of the neck and shoulders, back pain and numbness of the hand and fingers.

BL-2 Zanzhu Gathering bamboo. Location: 'In the depression at the head of the eyebrow'. Indications: Dispels Wind and Heat from the face, particularly from the eye; an important point when treating facial paralysis.

BL-10 Tianzhu Celestial pillar. Location: At the hairline on either side of the nape, in the depression on the outer face of the large tendon, 1.5 cun lateral to Du-15 Yamen. Indications: Treats all disorders of the neck and head; clears Wind and Cold, relaxes the neck muscles and tendons and invigorates the collaterals, clearing the head and improving the vision, eye pain and inflammation. Also benefits occipital headaches, shoulder and upper back pain, wry neck, cough, sore throat and asthma.

BL-11 Dashu Great shuttle. Location: '1.5 cun lateral to the lower border of the spinous process of the first thoracic vertebra'. Indications:

This is the influential point of the bones. Expels Wind, nourishes Blood, strengthens bones and the sinews, relaxes muscles and tendons; also ventilates the Lung and stops coughing.

BL-12 Fengmen Wind gate. Location: '1.5 cun either side of the spine, below the second vertebra'. Indications: Dispels the Wind and Cold or Wind-Heat, regulates the Lung-Qi and stops coughing; a very effective point when treating pathogenic Wind syndromes, Hot or Cold.

BL-13 Feishu Lung back transporting point (Back-Shu point). Location: '1.5 cun either side of the spine, below the third vertebra'. Indications: Regulates and tonifies the Lung-Qi, stops coughing and clears Heat, benefits the Nutritive and Defensive Qi.

BL-14 Jueyinshu Pericardium back transporting point (Back-Shu point). Location: '1.5 cun lateral to the lower border of the spinous process of the fourth thoracic vertebra'. Indications: Regulates the Heart-Qi, removes Liver-Qi stagnation, clears the channels and invigorates the collaterals.

BL-15 Xinshu Heart back transporting point (Back-Shu point). Location: '1.5 cun either side of the spine, below the fifth vertebra'. Indications: Nourishes the Heart Blood and calms the Spirit, sedates and relaxes the mind.

BL-17 Geshu Diaphragm back transporting point (Back-Shu point), and also the influential point of Blood). Location: '1.5 cun either side of the spine, below the seventh vertebra'. Indications: This is the influential point of the Blood, strengthens the Spleen and Stomach, regulates and tonifies the Blood, moves the Qi in the chest, therefore is an important point when treating fullness in the chest, belching or hiccups.

BL-18 Ganshu Liver back transporting point (Back-Shu point). Location: 1.5 cun lateral to Du-8 Jinsuo, at the level of the lower border of the spinous process of the ninth thoracic vertebrae. Indications: Jaundice, pain in the hypochondriac region, redness of the eye, night blindness, mental disorders, epilepsy and backache.

BL-20 Pishu Spleen back transporting point (Back-Shu point). Location: '1.5 cun either side of the spine, below the 11th thoracic vertebra'. Indications: Tonifies the Spleen and Stomach, eliminates Dampness and Phlegm, regulates and calms Rebellious Stomach-Qi; a very important point when tonifying the Qi and Blood.

BL-21 Weishu Stomach back transporting point (Back-Shu point). Location: '1.5 cun either side of the spine, below the 12th vertebra'. Indications: Strengthens the Spleen and regulates the Stomach, dispels pathogenic Damp and removes intestinal stasis, abdominal distension and pain, vomiting, anorexia, diarrhoea, borborygmus and dysentery.

BL-23 Shenshu Kidney back transporting point (Back-Shu point). Location: '1.5 cun either side of the spine, below the 14th vertebra'. Indications: One of the most important acupuncture points on the body, tonifies the Kidneys, nourishes the Yin and strengthens the Yang, benefits the brain and marrow, improves the vision; a point to be used in all back pains, sexual deficiencies, gynaecological diseases and growth problems in children.

BL-24 Qihaishu Sea of Qi. Location: '1.5 cun either side of the spine, below the 15th vertebra'. Indications: Tonifies the Kidney-Qi and the lower back, lumbago, sprain of the lower back, paralysis of the lower extremities, and removes Blood stasis.

BL-26 Guanyuanshu Origin gate back transporting point (Back-Shu point). Location: '1.5 cun either side of the spine, below the 17th vertebra'. Indications: Tonifies the back and spine, expels Wind and Cold, opens obstructions in the channel.

BL-28 Pangguangshu Bladder back transporting point (Back-Shu point). Location: '1.5 cun either side of the spine, below the 19th vertebra'. Indications: Tonifies the Original Qi, clears Heat and regulates Water metabolism in the lower parts of the body; used in all urinary Excess or Deficiency syndromes.

BL-31 to BL-34 (Biliao) Location: These points are located at the four sacral foramina and have similar properties; they all treat gynaecological disorders in women and genital disorders in men and women – leucorrhoea, prolapse of uterus and sterility in women; impotence and prostatitis in men.

BL-32 Ciliao Second bone / hole. Location: In the second posterior sacral foramen, about midway between the lower border of the posterior superior iliac spine and the Du Mai. Indications: Clears the obstruction from the channel, benefits the reproductive organs, sedates pain; therefore it is used in the treatment of dysmenorrhoea and sciatica.

BL-35 Huiyang Meeting of Yang. Location: On either side of the tip of the coccyx, 0.5 cun lateral to the Du Mai. Indications: Clearing pathogenic Heat from the Lower Jiao, pruritus vulvae, leucorrhoea, impotence, infertility, coccyx pain, chronic haemorrhoids and chronic diarrhoea. Qi from the Bladder channel and Du Mai, the two most Yang channels of the body, meet here.

BL-36 Chengfu Support. Location: In the middle of the transverse gluteal fold. Indications: Pain in the lower back and gluteal region, muscular atrophy, pain, numbness and motor impairment of the lower extremities.

BL-37 Yinmen Gate of abundance. Location: '6 cun below Cengfu (BL-36, on the buttock crease)'. Indications: Strengthens the back, relaxes the tendons and muscles of the leg and sedates pain.

BL-40 Weizhong Bend middle (He / Sea Point). Location: 'This point is at the centre of the crease at the bend of the knee'. Indications: Cools Blood Heat and is frequently used in hot skin complaints, moves the Qi in the Bladder channel and is used for painful Bi syndromes of the lower extremities.

BL-41 Fufen Attached branch. Location: Below the second vertebrae, on the inner border of the shoulder blade, 3 cun either side of the spine. Indications: Clears pathogenic Cold and Wind, strengthen the tendons and bones, pain and stiffness of the neck, shoulder and back, also good point for numbness of the neck and the arms.

BL-42 Pohu Soul / spirit door. Location: Three cun either side of the spine, below the third vertebrae. The Po (Soul) is housed in the Lung. BL-42 is located lateral to Lung Shu (BL-13) and hence is called 'Soul door'. Indications: ventilating and regulating Lung-Qi, reversing the adverse flow of Qi (feeling emotionally low and panic attacks), breathlessness, shoulder and upper back pain, stiffness of the neck, cough with phlegm and asthma.

BL-43 Gaohuangshu Below the Heart. Location: '3 cun lateral to the lower border of the spinous process of the 4th thoracic vertebra'. Indications: Tonifies the Kidney-Qi, fullness of the chest, pulmonary tuberculosis, cough and asthma.

BL-44 Shentang Spirit hall. Location: '3 cun either side of the spine, below the fifth vertebrae'. Indications: Moves the Qi in the chest, nourishes the Heart and calms the mind.

BL-45 Yixi Sighing, laughing sound. Location: On the inner side of the shoulder, 3 cun either side of the spine, below the sixth vertebrae (this point is sensitive when firmly pressed). Indications: Chest pain radiating to the back, cough, light-headedness, eye pain, asthma, epistaxis and malaria. Bl-45 also induces perspiration and clears pathogenic Lung Heat.

BL-46 Geguan Diaphragm pass. Location: In the depression 3 cun either side of the spine, below the seventh vertebra. The point is found in straight sitting posture with shoulders spread. Location: 1.5 cun lateral to the diaphragm Shu point (BL-17), and is thus called 'Diaphragm pass'. Indications: Pain and stiffness of the back, anorexia, abdominal distension, hiccups and vomiting; also strengthens the Spleen, and removes pathogenic Dampness, regulating the Stomach and resolving stasis, relaxing the muscles and tendons and invigorating the flow of Qi.

BL-49 Yishe Reflection abode. Location: Three inches either side of the spine, below the 11th vertebrae. Indications: Strengthens the Spleen, regulates Stomach and removes Dampness. Treats epigastric pain and abdominal distension, diarrhoea, borborygmus, anorexia, vomiting, nausea, jaundice, diabetes and back pain.

BL-52 Zhishi Will-power chamber. Location: '3 cun either side of the spine, below the fourteenth vertebra'. Indications: This point reinforces the actions of Shenshu (BL-23), also strengthens the will-power in depressive and emotional conditions.

BL-53 Baohuang Bladder vitals (Bladder; Womb; Uterus membrane). Location: 3 cun lateral to the Du Mai, at the level of the second sacral posterior foramen. Indications: Borborygmus, abdominal distension and pain in the lower back. BL-53 is intimately related to the urinary bladder and it is particularly effective when treating the urinary blockages.

BL-54 Zhibian Lowermost edge. Location: '3 cun either side of the spine, below the 20th vertebra'. Indications: Strengthens the lower back and the knees, removes channel obstruction and sedates pain.

BL-57 Chengshan Mountain support. Location: 'In the parting of the flesh at the lower tip of the belly of the calf'. Indications: Invigorates the channel, removes Blood stasis, relaxes the tendons and muscles and stops the pain.

BL-60 Kunlun Kunlun mountains (Jing / River point). Location: 'In the depression between the external malleolus and tendocalcaneus'. Indications: Clears Heat, strengthens the back, removes the obstruction from the channel, and is used in all painful conditions, especially pain of the Middle and Lower Jiao; some call this the 'aspirin point'.

BL-62 Shenmai Extending pulse. Location: 'In the depression 0.5 cun below the outer ankle bone between the two tendons'. Indications: Clears Wind, relaxes the tendons and muscles of the ankle.

K-1 Yongquan Rushing spring (Jing / Well point). Location: 'In the depression of the heart of the foot, in the indentation as the foot is extended'. Indications: Nourishes the Yin, revives consciousness and clears the mind.

K-3 Taixi Great ravine (Shu / Stream and Yuan / Source point). Location: '0.5 cun behind the inner ankle bone, in the depression above the heel bone where pulse can be felt'. Indications: Nourishes the Liver- and Kidney-Yin, regulates the Ren Mai and Chong Mai; therefore it is used in all gynaecological and reproductive complaints, such as infertility and impotence; one of the most important tonification points on the body.

K-7 Fuliu Returning flow. Location: 'In the depression 2 cun above the inner ankle bone'. Indications: Tonifies the Kidney-Yang and resolves Damp, therefore it is often used in oedema of the leg, ankle and foot; also regulates perspiration.

K-11 Henggu Pubic bone. Location: 5 cun below the umbilicus, on the superior border of symphysis pubis, 0.5 cun lateral to Ren-2 Qugu. Indications: Distension and pain of the lower abdomen, dysuria, enuresis, nocturnal emission, impotence, and pain of the genitalia.

K-12 Dahe Great manifestation. Location: 4 cun below the umbilicus, 0.5 cun lateral to Ren-3 Zhongji. Indications: Nocturnal emission, impotence, leucorrhea, prolapse of the uterus, and pain in the genitalia.

K-24 Lingxu Spirit burial-ground. Location: 'In the third intercostal space, 2 cun lateral to the midsternal line'. Indications: Relaxes the chest, benefits the Heart and the mind and stops coughing.

K-25 Shencang Mind storage. Location: 'In the second intercostal space, 2 cun lateral to the midsternal line'. Indications: Benefits the Lung, dissolves Phlegm, stops coughing. Calms the mind and alleviates anxiety.

P-4 Ximen Xi-Cleft gate. Location: 'Behind the palm, 5 cun from the wrist'. Indications: Clears Heat from the Nutritive and Blood levels, subdues the Heart, calms the mind, removes obstructions from the channel and stops pain.

P-6 Neiguan Inner gate (Luo / Connecting point). Location: '2 cun above the transverse crease of the wrist, between the two tendons'. Indications: Regulates the Heart-Qi and Blood, clears Heat from the Heart, calms the mind, subdues anxiety and panic attacks, maintains the proper flow of Stomach-Qi, stopping nausea and vomiting; a major point when treating emotional complaints.

SJ-4 Yangchi Yang pool (Yuan / Source point). Location: 'In the depression on the back of the wrist, in the centre of the crease'. Indications: Clears Wind and Heat, opens the collaterals, relaxes the tendons and stops pain in the arm, benefits the Stomach and the Original-Qi, transforms Damp from the Lower Burner.

SJ-5 Waiguan Outer gate (Luo / Connecting point). Location: '2 cun above the wrist crease, between the radius and ulna'. Indications: Clears Wind-Heat; a major point when treating Wind-Heat syndromes, removes channel obstructions, consequently always used when treating pain in the arm and hand; also benefits the ear.

SJ-6 Zhigou Branching ditch (Jing / River point). Location: '3 cun behind the wrist, in the depression between the two bones'. Indications: Expels Wind-Heat, especially from the skin, therefore it is often used when treating itching skin; regulates Qi of the body; an empirical point in the treatment of chronic constipation.

SJ-8 Sanyangluo Three Yang connection (the three Yang channels of the hand all pass near this point). Location: 4 cun above SJ-4 (wrist crease) between the radius and ulna. Indications: Clearing the channels, disperses pathogenic Dampness and Fire, treats sudden loss of voice, deafness, toothache, hoarseness of voice and pain in the elbow and hand.

SJ-10 Tianjing Heavenly well (He / Sea point). Location: 'The outer aspect of the elbow, and in the depression 1 cun above the elbow'. Indications: Clears Damp and Phlegm from the chest; especially beneficial when treating the lymphatic blockage of the neck in children; invigorates the Qi and relaxes the tendons and muscles of the arm and neck.

SJ-13 Naohui Upper-arm convergence. Location: On the line joining SJ-14 Jianliao and the olecranon process, on the posterior border of mid deltoid muscle. Indications: Goitre, pain in the shoulder and arm.

SJ-14 Jianliao Shoulder-bone hole. Location: Posterior and inferior to the acromion, in the depression about 1 cun posterior to LI-15 Jianyu. Indications: Pain and motor impairment of the shoulder and the upper arm.

SJ-15 Tianliao Celestial-bone hole. Location: Midway between GB-21 Jianjing, and SI-13 Quyuan, on the superior angle of the scapula. Indications: Pain in the shoulder and elbow, and stiff-neck syndrome.

SJ-17 Yifeng Wind screen. Location: 'In the depression behind the ear'. Indications: Clears Wind and Heat, removes the channel obstruction, benefits hearing, tinnitus, facial paralysis, trigeminal neuralgia and toothache.

SJ-23 Sizhukong Silk bamboo hole. Location: 'In the depression at the lateral end of the eyebrow'. Indications: Expels Wind, subdues the Liver-Yang and clear headaches and fright; an important point when treating facial paralysis and dropped eyelid.

GB-1 Tongziliao Pupil bone-hole. Location: '0.5 cun out from the outer canthus'. Indications: Clears Wind-Heat and Liver Fire; an important point when treating eye disorders or facial paralysis.

GB-14 Yangbai Yang white. Location: '1 cun above the eyebrow, on a line with the pupil'. Indications: Expels Wind-Heat and promotes the circulation of Qi; it is an important point when treating headache, pain in the eye, facial paralysis and trigeminal neuralgia.

GB-20 Fengchi Wind pool. Location: 'In the back of the ear and temple, on the hairline, between the heads of the sternocleidomastoid and trapezius muscles'. Indications: It is a major point in eliminating Wind-Heat or Wind-Cold from the head and neck; subdues the Liver-Yang and clears Heat, benefits the eyes and improves vision.

GB-21 Jianjing Shoulder well. Location: 'Midway between T1 and the acromion, at the highest point of the shoulder'. Indications: Opens obstructions and invigorates the channels, dissolves Phlegm, promotes lactation and delivery in difficult labour; a very important point when treating Wind-Cold or Wind-Heat syndromes of the neck and shoulders.

GB-25 Jingmen Capital gate (Front-Mu point of the Kidney). Location: On the lateral side of the abdomen, on the lower border of the free end of the twelfth rib. Indications: Abdominal distension, borborygmus, diarrhoea, pain in the lumbar and hypochondriac region.

GB-26 Daimai Girdle Vessel. A junction point of the Gall Bladder channel and Dai Mai (Girdling Vessel). Location: 1.8 cun below the lower rib Zangmen (Liv-13). Indications: regulates the Girdling vessel, dissipating pathogenic Heat and Dampness, clearing and invigorating the channels, regulating the menses and stopping the flow of leucorrhea, prolapsed uterus, hernia, lower abdominal pain and infertility in women.

GB-27 Wushu Fifth pivot. Location: In the lateral side of the abdomen, anterior to the superior iliac spine, 3 cun below the level of the umbilicus. Indications: Leucorrhoea, lower abdominal pain, lumbar pain, hernia and constipation.

GB-28 Weidao Linking path. Location: Anterior and inferior to the anterior superior iliac spine, 0.5 cun anterior and inferior to GB-27 Wushu. Indications: Leucorrhoea, lower abdominal pain, hernia, and prolapse of uterus.

GB-29 Femur-Juliao Squatting bone-hole. Location: 'Midway between the anterosuperior iliac spine and the greater trochanter'. Indications: Opens the obstruction from the channel and sedates pain; a very effective point when treating one-sided radiating pain to the leg.

GB-30 Huantiao Jumping circle. Location: 'In the centre of the hip joint'. Indications: A major point when treating hip and leg pains; also has a tonifying effect to the lower back, removes obstruction from the channel, relaxes muscles and tendons and stops pain; a cardinal point when treating sciatica.

GB-31 Fengshi Wind market. Location: 'Between the two ligaments on the outer side above knee, at the end of the middle finger when the hand is placed on the thigh'. Indications: Clears Wind-Heat and Wind-Cold; however, it is more effective when treating Wind-Heat in the Blood causing itchiness on the skin; it is also a major point when treating paralysis and painful legs.

GB-32 Zhongdu Central river. Location: On the lateral aspect of the thigh, 5 cun above the transverse popliteal crease, between the mid vastus lateralis and mid biceps femoris. Indications: Pain and soreness of the thigh and knee, weakness and numbness of the lower limbs.

GB-33 Xiyangguan Knee Yang joint. Location: '3 cun above Yanglingquan (GB-34) point, in the depression side of the knee'. Indications: Invigorates the collaterals, removes channel blockage, relaxes the muscles and tendons of the knee joint and stops pain.

GB-34 Yanglingquan Yang hill spring (He / Sea point). Location: '1 cun below the knee, in the depression on the outer face of the shin bone'. Indications: This is the influential point of the tendons; it is therefore one of the most important points when treating muscular weaknesses, cramps and pain, especially in the lower extremities; it promotes the smooth circulation of the Liver and Gall Bladder-Qi.

GB-39 Xuanzhong Hanging bell. Location: '3 cun above the ankle'. Indications: This is the influential point of the marrow; it is therefore used in all Blood deficiency syndromes, invigorates Qi and Blood circulation and removes obstruction from the channel; it is often used in the treatment of muscle pain due to stroke, pain and stiffness of the neck.

Liv-2 Xingjian Moving between (Ying / Spring points). Location: 'On the web of the great toe, in the depression where the pulse may be felt'. Indications: Clears Blood-Heat from the Liver, dispels Liver-Wind and subdues the Liver-Yang; it is an important point when treating Liver Excess conditions such as vertigo, dry throat, and bitter taste in the mouth, epilepsy and infantile convulsions.

Liv-3 Taichong Great surge (Shu / Stream and Yuan / Source point). Location: '1.5 to 2 cun behind the main joint of the great toe'. Indications: Promotes the smooth flow of Liver-Qi; the most important point for relieving Liver-Qi stagnation; calms the mind and is used in all emotional complaints, subdues Liver-Yang rising, therefore it is the cardinal point when treating hypertension due to Liver-Yang; it is also a major point when treating muscular spasms.

Liv-5 Ligou Woodworm canal (Luo-connecting point). Location: 5 cun above the tip of the medial malleolus, on the medial aspect and near the medial border of the tibia. Indications: retention of urine, enuresis, hernia, irregular menstruation, leucorrhoea, weakness and atrophy of the leg.

Liv-8 Quguan Spring at the bend (He / Sea point). Location: 'On the medial side of the knee joint, when the knee is bent, the point is above the medial end of the transverse popliteal crease'. Indications: Expels Damp from the Lower Jiao, invigorates the channels, regulates the flow of Qi and Blood and stops pain; therefore it is very much used in the treatment of urinary and period complaints.

Liv-9 Yinbao Yin bladder. Location: 4 cun above the medial epicondyle of Femur, between mid vastus medialis and mid sartorius. Indications: Removing Liver-Qi stagnation, regulating the Chong Mai and Ren Mai, infertility, clearing pathogenic Heat and Dampness from the Lower Jiao, benefits dysuria, enuresis, impotence, spermatorrhoea and sacral pain radiating to the lower abdomen.

Liv-11 Yinlian Yin corner. Location: 2 cun below ST-30 in the groin crease. Indications: Promotes circulation of blood, regulates the Chong Mai, treats female infertility, painful menstruation and thigh and leg pain.

Liv-12 Jimai Urgent pulse. Location: Inferior and lateral to the pubic bone, 2.5 cun lateral to the Ren Mai (Conception Vessel). Indications; Clears the channels and disperses pathogenic Cold, benefits female infertility, pain in the external genitalia, hernia, orchitis and pain in lower abdomen.

Liv-13 Zhangmen Chapter gate (Front-Mu point of the Spleen). Location: 'The outside of the pelvis, on the edge of the free ribs, at the level of the umbilicus'. Indications: Removes Liver-Qi stagnation, especially when it affects the digestive system; also invigorates the Spleen- and Stomach-Qi.

Liv-14 Qimen Cycle (one hundred years) gate. Front-Mu point of the Liver. Location: On the nipple line, two ribs below the nipple, in the 6th intercostal space. Indications: removes Liver-Qi stagnation, invigorating the flow of blood and removing stasis, strengthens the Spleen and Stomach, treats pain in the epigastric region, vomiting during pregnancy and hiccups.

Ren-3 Zhongji Central pole (Front-Mu point of the Bladder). Location: 'Directly above the pubic bone, 4 cun below the umbilicus'. Indications: Clears Damp-Heat and strengthens the Bladder; it is the main point when treating bladder complaints such as enuresis, bed-wetting, prolapse of bladder and genitalia; it also has a gentle tonifying effect on the Kidney-Yang.

Ren-4 Guanyuan Passageway of Original-Qi (Front / Mu point of the Small Intestine). Location: 'On the midline of the abdomen, 3 cun below the umbilicus'. Indications: Undoubtedly the most important tonifying point on the body, it reinforces the Original-Qi, tonifies the Kidney-Yang and nourishes the Essence, hence its significant use in the treatment of infertility, frigidity, impotence and lack of libido; also invigorates and nourishes Blood and Yin, and is therefore used in all gynaecological deficiency syndromes.

Ren-6 Qihai Sea of Qi. Location: 'On the midline of the abdomen, 1.5 cun below the umbilicus'. Indications: This is a major point for tonifying Qi and Blood and reinforcing the Essence; it is especially effective when moxa is used on this point to warm the Yang-Qi, and is a cardinal point when treating abdominal distension and pain, diarrhoea, impotence, infertility, prolapse of the bladder or uterus, anaemia and insomnia.

Ren-8 Shenque Spirit gate. Location: 'In the centre of the umbilicus'. Indications: Regulates and strengthens the Spleen and Stomach Yang-Qi, strongly tonifies and rescues collapsed Yang-Qi.

Ren-10 Xiawan Lower epigastrium. Location: 'On the midline of the abdomen, 2 cun above the umbilicus'. Indications: Tonifies the Spleen and regulates the descending action of the Stomach-Qi; also relieves stagnation of Food in the Stomach and intestines.

Ren-12 Zhongwan Middle of the epigastrium (Front-Mu point of the Stomach). Location: 'On the midline of the abdomen, 4 cun above the umbilicus'. Indications: A cardinal point when treating Stomach patterns, it regulates the Stomach-Qi and tonifies the Spleen and resolves Dampness from the digestive system; moxibustion applied to this point is particularly effective.

Ren-15 Jiuwei Dove tail (Luo / Connecting point). Location: 'Below the xiphoid process, 7 cun above the umbilicus'. Indications: Relaxes the chest (Heart, Lung and diaphragm), calms the mind, especially when treating emotional complaints, and also dissolves Phlegm and stops coughing. This point is often tender to the touch when the patient is under a great deal of emotional stress. I personally employ this point as a diagnostic tool to determine the severity of the emotional pressure upon the patient: the more tender the point, the less is the ability of the person to cope.

Ren-17 Shanzhong Middle of the chest (Front-Mu point of the Pericardium). Location: 'On the middle of the sternum, between the nipples, level with the fourth intercostal space'. Indications: Benefits the chest Qi, regulates the descending action of Lung-Qi, dissolves Phlegm and removes the obstruction from the chest, and relaxes the Heart. A very important point when treating mental and emotional conditions, it 'frees' the chest, namely the Heart and Lungs; Gua Sha applied to this point is especially effective.

Ren-20 Huagai Floral canopy. Location: 'On the midsternal line level with the first intercostal space'. Indications: Relaxes the chest and diaphragm, clears the Lungs of pathogenic Heat and stops coughing.

Ren-21 Xuanji Jade pivot. Location: 'In the depression 1 cun directly above Ren-20'. Indications: Relaxes the chest and regulates the flow of Qi, and sedates coughing.

Ren-24 Chengjiang Saliva receiver. Location: 'In the depression below the lips, in the centre of the mentolabial groove'. Indications: Expels pathogenic exterior Wind and opens the collaterals. It is an important point when treating facial paralysis with deviation of the mouth or lips.

Du-1 Changqiang (Guiwei) Long strong. Location: 'At the lower end of the spine, midway between the tip of the coccyx and the anus'. Indications: Sedates spasm and pain, dispels pathogenic Heat from the Blood level, strengthens the rectum against prolapse, tonifies Yang-Qi and strengthens the Kidney; used for rectal prolapse, diarrhoea, haemorrhoids, lumbar and sacral pain and eczema of the scrotum.

Du-2 Yaoshu Lumbar point. Location: In the coccyx region on the posterior midline at the midpoint of the sacral hiatus. Indications: Lumbar and sacral pain, atrophy of the lower extremities, haemorrhoids, epilepsy.

Du-3 Yaoyangguan Lumbar Yang gate. Location: 'Below the spinous process of the fourth lumbar vertebrae'. Indications: Tonifies the Kidney and strengthens the lower back, removes Cold and Damp, stops sacral pain; it is often used in the treatment of lower back and leg pain.

Du-4 Mingmen Life gate. Location: 'Below the spinous process of the second lumbar vertebra'. Indications: This is the most important acupuncture point for tonifying the Kidney-Yang and the Original-Qi, especially when used in conjunction with moxa; it strengthens the back and knees and nourishes the Essence, therefore it is the cardinal point when treating Kidney deficiency syndromes such as impotence, infertility, tiredness, feelings of cold, bed-wetting or dysmenorrhoea.

Du-10 Lingtai Spirit tower. Location: 'Below the sixth vertebra'. Indications: Benefits the Lungs and stops coughing, clears pathogenic Heat and detoxifies the Blood; it is therefore used in hot skin complaints such as acne, eczema or psoriasis.

Du-12 Shenzhu Body pillar. Location: 'Between the shoulder blades, below the third thoracic vertebra'. Indications: Tonifies Lung-Qi, strengthens the body, calms spasms, disperses pathogenic Heat and Wind, sedates coughing, clears the Heart and calms the Spirit.

Du-14 Dazhui Great hammer. Location: 'Above the first vertebra'. Indications: Clears Heat, expels Wind and Cold, also clears the mind and stimulates the brain. It is a major point when treating Heat patterns such as convulsions, epilepsy, hypertension, eczema, psoriasis, acne and restless mind syndrome.

Du-20 Baihui Hundred meetings. Location: 'In the hair-whorl at the centre of the vertex'. Indications: This is the meeting point of all the Yang meridians of the hand and foot with the Du Mai. Clears Heat, tonifies Yang, opens the orifices, calms the mind and strengthens the brain; it is also an empirical point when treating the prolapse of internal organs.

Du-24 Shenting Mind courtyard. Location: 'Directly above the nose, 0.5 cun within the hairline'. Indications: Calms the Heart and Spirit; used in all mental disorders and insomnia.

Du-26 Renzhong Middle of person. Location: 'Below the nose, a little above the midpoint of the philtrum'. Indications: Expels exterior Wind, therefore it is used in the treatment of facial paralysis affecting the upper lip. Revives the sensory organs and restores the unconsciousness.

EXTRA POINTS

Anmian Location: 'This point is located at the midpoint between SJ-17 and GB-20'. Indications: Calms the mind; it is an important point when treating insomnia, epilepsy, mania and hysteria; especially effective during depression or a panic attack.

Dingchuan Asthma relief. Location: '0.5 cun lateral to Du-14'. Indications: Expels exterior Wind and calms asthma; especially effective when cupping therapy is applied.

Huatuo Jiaji Location: '0.5 cun bilateral to the spinal column, between the spinous process, from C1 to S1; altogether 24 pairs of points'. Indications: The indications of these points are very similar to those of Back-Shu points, but milder in action.

Heiding Location: In the depression of the midpoint of the superior patellar border. Indications: Knee pain, weakness and paralysis of the foot and the leg.

Jianneiling (Jianqian) Inner shoulder mound. Location: 'Midway between the end of the anterior axillary fold and LI-15 Jianyu'. Indications: Expels external Wind and Cold, removes obstruction from the channel and stops pain. Very important point when treating frozen shoulder syndrome.

Shixuan Location: 'On the tips of the ten fingers, about 0.1 cun distal to the nails'. Indications: Clears Blood Heat, treats hypertension, tonsillitis, high fever, mania and infantile convulsions.

Shiqizhui Location: 'In the depression between the spinous process of L5 and S1'. Indications: Sacral pain, dysmenorrhoea and paraplegia caused by injury.

Sifeng Location: 'In the centre of the palmar aspect skin creases of the proximal interphalangeal joints of the second through fifth fingers'. Indications: Resolves Damp and promotes digestion in children; especially effective when treating Food accumulation syndrome.

Taiyang Greater Yang. Location: 'In the depression about 1 cun posterior to the midpoint between the lateral end of the eyebrow and the outer canthus'. Indications: Eliminates Wind, clears Fire. Very important point when treating one-sided headache such as migraine; also treats redness and pain in the eye.

Xiyian Knee eyes. Location: 'A pair of points in two depressions medial and lateral to the patellar ligament'. Indications: Expels Wind-Damp from the knees; it is an empirical point when treating painful or swollen knees.

Yaoyan Location: 'In the depression 4 cun bilateral to the point between the spinous process of L3 and L4'. Indications: Lumbago, diabetes and gynaecological disorders.

Yintang Location: Midway between the medial ends of the two eyebrows. Indications: Headache, nosebleed, rhinorrhoea, infantile convulsion, frontal headache, mental confusion and insomnia.

Yuyao Fish spine. Location: 'In the middle of the eyebrow'. Indications: Clears Heat, brightens the eyes and promotes clear thinking.

HISTORY OF CUPPING THERAPY

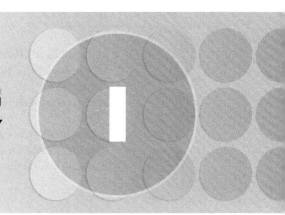

CHAPTER CONTENTS

INTRODUCTION, 1
EARLY CUPPING METHODS, 1
CUPPING IN THE WESTERN WORLD
AND THE MIDDLE EAST
(HEJAMA/HIJAMA), 4
CUPPING IN THE JEWISH TRADITION, 4
CUPPING IN THE MIDDLE EAST
AND THE MUSLIM WORLD
(HEJAMA/HIJAMA), 5

PRESENT CHALLENGES FACING THE
CONTEMPORARY MIDDLE EASTERN
CUPPING THERAPY PRACTITIONER, 6
REGULATION OF THE PRACTICE OF
CUPPING THERAPY, 7
NEW INTEREST IN CUPPING THERAPY, 7
CONTEMPORARY CUPPING
EQUIPMENT, 8
REFERENCES, 16

INTRODUCTION

Cupping as a therapeutic medium is simple, safe and at the same time quite an effective treatment tool. Cupping therapy has been in practice for several thousand years. Perhaps the simplicity of cupping in application has been a major contributing factor for the cupping underuse in modern medicine, particularly during the early 20th century where complicated medical apparatus and medications were invented and introduced to the mainstream medicinal use. The earliest written evidence was by the ancient Egyptians and also by Chinese doctors. Cupping practice, however, was not limited to the above two cultures. From east to west and north to south, many civilizations adopted cupping as part of their 'in-house' medicine and, later, integrated cupping practice as part of their mainstream medicine (Chirali, 2007).

EARLY CUPPING METHODS (FIGS 1-1 to 1-5)

Cupping therapy has been used in China and some African countries for several thousand years. At first it was applied using cattle horn and consequently was also called 'horn therapy' (see Fig. 1-3). To create a negative pressure inside the horn, the cupping practitioner used his mouth to physically suck the air out from a hole on top of the horn, thus creating a negative suction inside the horn! With the introduction of bamboo, earthenware and later on the glass cups, fire was ignited to expel the air.

As far as safety was concerned, the length of the horn would be the only protection afforded to the practitioner! This method is still employed in some rural developing countries for treating boils and carbuncles. Cupping was then used as an auxiliary method in traditional Chinese surgery. Later it was found to be effective in other diseases, and developed into a special therapeutic method.

The earliest record of cupping is in *Bo Shu* (an ancient book written on silk), which was discovered in an ancient tomb of the Han Dynasty in 1973 (Chen Bin, Dr He Chong, personal communications, 1995). Some therapeutic cupping methods were also introduced in a book by Zouhou Fang in about 28 AD (Chen Bin, Dr He Chong, personal communications, 1995). Cases of treatment of tuberculosis were recorded in Weitaimiyao in 755 AD. Three hundred years later, another ancient classic, *Susen Liang Fang*, recorded an effective cure for chronic cough and the successful treatment of poisonous snake bites using cupping therapy (Chen Bin, Dr He Chong, personal communications, 1995).

About 500 years ago, a famous surgeon called Wei Ke Zen Zong presented a detailed record of the cupping methods used in surgical practice (Chen Bin, Dr He Chong, private communications, 1995). Through several thousand years of accumulated clinical experience, the clinical applications of cupping

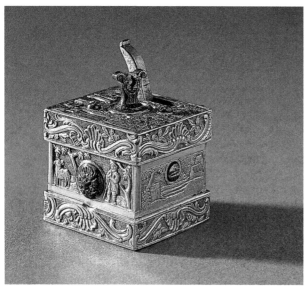

FIGURE 1-1 Scarificator with 13 lancets, 17th century, European. *(Reproduced courtesy of the British Science Museum/Science and Society Picture Library.)*

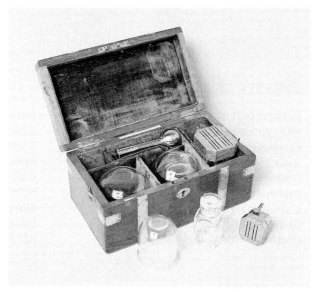

FIGURE 1-2 Cupping set, 1878. Cupping aimed to draw poisonous substances from the body and was popular from Roman times until the late 19th century. *(Reproduced courtesy of the British Science Museum/Science and Society Picture Library.)*

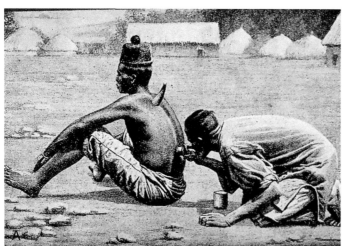

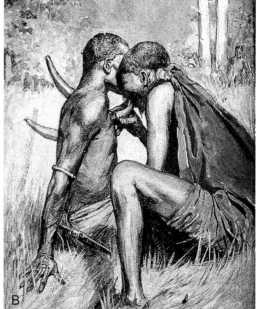

FIGURE 1-3 (A, B) An African medicine man or shaman applying the technique of cupping to a patient using animal horns; this involves drawing blood to the surface of the body. *(Wellcome Institute Library, London.)*

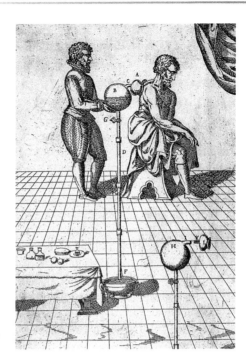

FIGURE 1-4 A surgeon applying the method of cupping to a patient. Etching by Brandini. *(Wellcome Institute Library, London.)*

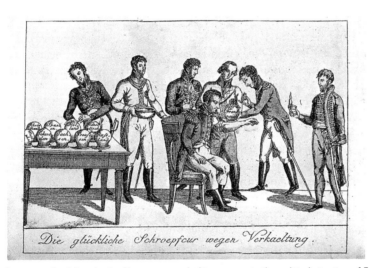

Die glückliche Schroepfcur wegen Verkaeltung.

FIGURE 1-5 One of a group of soldiers having his arm cupped; this represents the political situation of France in relation to German states in 1820. *(Wellcome Institute Library, London.)*

have become increasingly wide. During the Jin dynasty, Ge Hong (281–341 AD), in his book *A Handbook of Prescriptions for Emergencies*, first mentioned the use of animal horns as a means of draining pustules (Chirali, 2007). Zhao Xueming of the Qing dynasty (1644–1911), in his *Supplement to Outline of Herbal Pharmacopoeia*, wrote a separate chapter on the subject under the heading 'Fire-Jar Qi'. The original natural horn cup has been replaced by bamboo, ceramic or glass cups (some of my African patients report that horn cupping is still used today in rural Africa as the only way to expel poison from bites). Because cupping is widely used in Chinese folklore culture, the technique has been inherited by the modern Chinese clinical practitioner.

There is a saying in China: 'acupuncture and cupping, more than half of the ills cured.' Zhao Xue Ming, a doctor practising more than 200 years ago, compiled a book entitled *Ben Cao Gang Mu She Yi*, in which he describes in detail the history and origin of different kinds of cupping and cup shapes, functions and applications. In mainland China, the development of cupping therapy has been particularly rapid. In the 1950s the clinical efficacy of cupping was confirmed by further research in China and acupuncturists from the former Soviet Union, and was established as an official therapy practice in hospitals all over China. This issue substantially stimulated the development of further cupping research.

CUPPING IN THE WESTERN WORLD AND THE MIDDLE EAST (HEJAMA/HIJAMA)

Just how popular was cupping and to what extent was it used in the West? Were the applications and conditions similar to those in ancient China? To find an answer to these questions, I have examined a wealth of medical information and found useful data regarding cupping therapy in both ancient and contemporary clinical practice around the world. In particular, the Wellcome Institute for the History of Medicine in London has been an invaluable source.

'Cupping is an art' wrote the London cupper Samuel Bayfield in 1823, 'the value of which every one can appreciate who has had opportunities of being made acquainted with its curative power by observing its effects on the person of others, or by realising them in his own.' For thousands of years all medical authors have distinguished two forms of cupping: Dry and Wet. In Dry cupping no blood is actually removed from the body. A cup is drained of air and applied to the skin, causing the skin to tumefy (swell). In Wet cupping the process begins with Dry cupping and is followed by several incisions being made in the skin, in order to collect blood.

In 1826, the surgeon Charles Kennedy wrote:

The art of Cupping has been so well known, and the benefits arising from it so long experienced, that it is quite unnecessary to bring forward testimonials in favour of what has received not only the approbation of modern times, but also the sanction of the remotest antiquity.

Among the Egyptians, who introduced bloodletting to Greece, cupping was the usual remedy for almost every disorder, and they no doubt had received it from the more ancient nations of the East, from whom they had derived much of their knowledge. The founder of today's Royal Free and Royal Marsden Hospitals in London, surgeon William Marsden (1796–1867), also employed cuppers in his Royal Free Hospital in Gray's Inn Road, London, during the 1830s. When Dr Marsden decided to open a hospital and freely treat the poor, he enlisted surgeons and doctors who contributed their time free of charge, with the exception of a paid apothecary and a paid cupper. During my research, I was privileged to be allowed into the old medical records of the Royal Free Teaching Hospital, Hampstead, London, and to read through the 'minute ledger' of meetings. The records of the Annual General Meeting held at the Board Room of the Royal Free, 23 February, 1832, state: 'that Surgeon James Davis Lane Esq. be persuaded to continue his valuable services as Cupper to the institution'. We can safely conclude that cupping therapy was indeed used in Western hospitals from very early times, and that it was performed by highly skilled doctors and surgeons.

CUPPING IN THE JEWISH TRADITION

The Chief Rabbi of Egypt, Rabbi Moshe Ben Maimon, referred to this therapy in his medical books *Mishna Thora – Hilchot Deot*, Chapter 4 (private correspondence, Moshe Rafael Seror, the founder and principal of The College of Jewish Medicine). Most of the teaching on this chapter relates to preserving and maintaining a good, healthy mind and body:

The life (Hebr, soul) is in the blood' (Lev. Xv11.11). In the medicine of the Talmud blood plays a purely negative part. Most diseases arise in the blood. Blood is therefore not considered a remedy; but on the contrary, bleeding and cupping (that is the removal of blood) are recommended as modes of treatment.

During the Talmudic period, surgery attained a high degree of development. Venesection (phlebotomy) was extensively used on the healthy and the sick alike. Mar Samuel Yashinai went so far as to recommend its use once every 30 days. After the age of 50, venesection should be employed less frequently. Bleeding by means of cupping (the cup being called 'Karna de-ummana') is frequently mentioned.

CUPPING IN THE MIDDLE EAST AND THE MUSLIM WORLD (HEJAMA/HIJAMA)

It was a rare occasion when I came across detailed and systematic information regarding cupping therapy outside TCM practice. 'Hejama' or 'Hijama', as it is known in the Arabic world – which also translates 'to restore to basic size' or 'to diminish in volume' – has been quite extensively practised by Muslim nations throughout history. The Prophet Mohammed, peace be upon him (pbuh), is reported to have been a fervent user and advocate of cupping therapy (Hejama). In the book *Healing with the Medicine of the Prophet* written by Imam Ibn Qayyim Al-Jauziyah in 2003, an eminent scholar of Hadith (sayings of the Prophet Mohammed – pbuh) who lived in Damascus (1292–1350), cupping therapy is prescribed for many illnesses. It was reported that the Prophet said:

Cupping and puncturing the veins are your best remedies.' This Hadith is directed at people of Hijaz and warm areas in general, for their blood is delicate and circulates closer to the surface of the skin, while the pores on their skin are wide and their strength weakened (i.e. during summer). Puncturing of each of the veins usually has a special benefit. For instance, puncturing the basilic vein (the large vein running on the inner side of the upper arm) is useful against the heat of the liver and spleen and various blood-related tumours in these two organs. It is also useful for tumours of the lungs, arterial pulsation, pleurisy and all blood-related diseases of vein in the lower part of the knee to the hip. Further, puncturing of the median vein helps against the various swellings that appear throughout the entire body, especially when the swelling is blood-related, and contains spoiled blood in general. In addition, puncturing of the arm's vein helps against the ailments in the head and neck that result from excessive amounts of blood or from septic blood. Puncturing of the jugular vein helps against the ailments of the spleen, asthma, thoracic cavity and forehead pain. Cupping the upper section of the back helps against the aches of the shoulder and the throat. Further, cupping the two jugular veins helps against the ailments of the head, face, teeth, ears, eyes, nose and throat, if these ailments were caused by excessive presence of blood, soiled blood or both. The Messenger of Allah used to apply cupping on the two jugular veins and the upper part of the back.

Abu Dawud, *Healing with the Medicine of the Prophet*, p. 21.

It was not only cupping therapy in general that was advised, but also the benefits of such therapy and the locations of cups to be applied, depending on the condition of the patient as well as the correct timing of such therapy according to the lunar date. The author of *Al-Qanun (Fi'l-Tibb)* (see also notes below), Ibn-Sina (Avicenna, 1025) said:

Cupping is not preferred in the beginning of the month, because the body's various conditions will not be agitated then, nor is it preferred in the end of the month, because by then the conditions would have decreased. Cupping is preferred in the middle of the month when the substances (of the constitution or condition) accumulate and become agitated.

In different Hadith he stated: 'the messenger of Allah used to have cupping on the jugular veins and upper part of the back on the seventeenth, nineteenth or twenty first day of the month', the most beneficial time of the day being 2–3 hours after taking a bath. Dietary recommendations were also given, including fasting a day before the cupping, total avoidance of milk and milk products during the days of cupping, and plenty of green, leafy vegetables and tomatoes during and after the treatment. Advice was also given to the practitioner: 'refrain from cupping treatment on full stomach.' In separate Hadith he added: 'there is a cure provided in three substances – a drink of honey, a cut with a knife for cupping and cauterizing by fire. I forbid my Ummah [Muslim Nation] from cauterizing by fire.'

In a separate book, *Islamic Medical Wisdom – The Tibb al-A'imma*, Imam Ali ibn Abu Talib (translated by Ispahany and Newman) (2007), there are descriptions of cupping therapy benefits, effectiveness, when to apply cups, best cupping periods in a month, which parts of the body to cup, foods to have and those to avoid during the cupping sessions and observing the blood (thickness and colour) inside the cup once exuded.

Although cupping therapy was regarded as 'very effective', it was also considered 'quite dangerous' in unskilled hands. Diseases were also categorized as Hot, Cold, Wet and Dry types. While warm honey was given to Cold conditions, cupping therapy was administered for Hot (febrile)

Box 1.1   'DO'S AND DON'TS' OF CUPPING THERAPY

Dry cupping: 'Dry-Cupping produces Heat' (p. 239).

Wet cupping: is considered as 'cooling' because it is considered to 'remove heat from the body' (p. 239).

Nursing mothers: for scanty milk 'apply gentle Dry-Cupping under the breasts' (p. 364).

Excessive menstrual bleeding: apply 'Dry-Cupping to the breasts, because the blood tends to travel towards its related organ' (p. 465).

Wet cupping: is contraindicated when there is a blood deficiency 'vacuousness' (p. 475).

Do not always bleed: 'it may prove sufficient to *draw the material away* without actually evacuating!' (p. 480).

To warm the skin: 'apply Dry-Cupping ' (pp. 481, 495).

Tightness and pain under the hypochondrium: 'apply Dry-Cupping with Fire to the stomach-region' (p. 504).

Avoid bleeding cupping: during fever that is accompanied by 'wasting' (p. 521).

Best time for cupping therapy: 'the second and third hours' after getting up are 'the best hours for cupping'. 'Some authorities advise against applying cupping-glasses at the beginning of the lunar months because the humours are then not yet on the move or in a state of agitation; also against applying them at the end of the lunar month, because at that period (of the cycle) the humours are less plentiful. The proper time (according to them) is the middle of the month (when the humours are in state of agitation) and during time when the moonlight is increasing (when the humours are on the increase). During that period the brain is increasing in size within the skull, and the river water is rising in tidal rivers' (p. 522).

After bathing: 'wait an hour before cupping' (p. 522).

Infants: 'one should not begin to apply cupping to infants until they are in their third year' (p. 523).

Stomach pain: 'to allay pain, apply over the umbilicus; cupping relieves violent colic and flatulent distension of the abdomen and the uterine pain due to movement of the menstrual fluid, especially in young women' (p. 523).

Elderly: 'it is altogether contraindicated after the sixtieth year' (p. 523). When one considers the average human age was about 50 years, when the book *Canon of Medicine* was written in 1025 AD, anyone lucky enough to reach the age of sixty years old was indeed considered a 'great old man'!

Page references above are to the original text.
Al-Qanun Fi'l-Tibb, Canon of Medicine (1025).

---

conditions. It goes on to say: 'the heat of the fever is a breath of the Hell fire; cool it with water'. Here, we can clearly see some similarities with TCM aetiology where excessive heat is considered a 'pathogenic factor' that has to be cooled or removed from the body. (See Box 1.1 for 'do's and don'ts'.)

PRESENT CHALLENGES FACING THE CONTEMPORARY MIDDLE EASTERN CUPPING THERAPY PRACTITIONER

In April 2010, I was invited to Riyadh, Kingdom of Saudi Arabia (KSA) by the Ministry of Health Director of the National Centre of Complementary and Alternative Medicine KSA, to discuss the training and application of cupping therapy in the Kingdom, with a further goal of legislation.

This invitation was a direct result of the earlier decision taken by the Council of Ministers approving the setting up of a National Centre for Alternative and Complementary Medicine in the Kingdom. Similar regulations are also considered in the United Arab Emirates (UAE). The Centre will serve as a national referral authority on alternative and complementary medicine (ACM). It will be directly linked to the Minister of Health and it can seek the help of foreign ACM specialists.

The purpose of my visit was to discuss the training and the practice of cupping therapy (Hejama) in the Kingdom of Saudi Arabia. My visit lasted 7 days, mostly with the team of doctors headed by the CAM Director at the Health Ministry in Riyadh.

The practice of cupping therapy (Hejama) is currently banned (2013) and the practice is illegal. Despite this ban, cupping therapy, and especially Wet (bleeding) cupping, is widely practised as a 'traditional Muslim medicine' mostly by non-medical lay persons at some prominent clinics as well as back streets of many cities throughout the Kingdom. This trend presents a worrying situation for the health authorities in the Kingdom as well as the rest of the Arabic world.

At the end of my visit, the team managed to put together a protocol called 'Cupping therapy practice and a training protocol', which will be suitable for the medical and the non-medical staff such as the paramedics and nurses.

REGULATION OF THE PRACTICE OF CUPPING THERAPY

At present and during the preparation of this latest edition, cupping therapy in Europe and the United States of America is practised by a wide range of practitioners. This includes medical doctors, acupuncture practitioners, massage therapists, physiotherapists and even some beauty therapists. There is no single 'cupping regulatory' body or authority. However, as mentioned below, in some countries such as Britain and the USA there are individual registers of practitioners trained in the cupping therapy.

Many complementary and alternative medicine (CAM) practitioners in the West practise under their own professional register. In European countries, these registers generally operate under the 'self-regulation' principle, maintaining up-to-date registers of their members, monitoring safe practice and dealing with public enquiries and complaints. In the USA, most CAM practices are state regulated and registered by each individual state.

Professional Indemnity Insurance

When considering insurance issues, we find that professional insurance companies consider cupping therapy as an integral part of the traditional Chinese medicine (TCM) protocol, similar to moxibustion or Gua Sha treatments. If the cupping therapist has been professionally trained and is registered with a professional body, he or she then notifies the relevant insurance company of the training and requires the inclusion of cupping in their policy cover. This can be under the heading of traditional Chinese medicine, physiotherapist, massage therapist, sport injury therapist or beauty therapist. They can expect to be insured under the existing cover and can legally practise.

NEW INTEREST IN CUPPING THERAPY

Many Cupping therapy practitioners in the West consider the year 2005 to be the 'cupping therapy year'! For several months following Friday, 9 July 2005, cupping therapy was the subject of worldwide media attention. This was entirely due to Oscar-winning actress Gwyneth Paltrow, who decided to reveal her newly acquired cupping therapy marks at a film festival in New York by wearing a low-cut dress that revealed the circular marks across her back and shoulders. Newspapers, radio stations and TV networks in the USA and across Europe gave extensive coverage to cupping therapy and speculated wildly about why she was having this treatment! Some cynical comments were made but in general it has been a positive and informative approach. This helped to stimulate a healthy public debate in natural health and complementary medicine circles, simultaneously encouraging many TCM practitioners who were previously reluctant to apply this method of treatment to study further and improve their cupping skills. Social networks like YouTube and Facebook now contain hundreds of cupping sites (some good and some not so good!).

Today, as more people seek complementary and alternative therapies to deal with their health problems, therapies such as acupuncture, cupping, herbal medicine, aromatherapy, reflexology, chiropractic, osteopathy, homoeopathy, Tui Na and massage have become popular. Public awareness and education have also changed, from seeing these as 'quack' remedies to more respectable alternative treatments. In both America and Europe the education of the complementary therapist has taken on a new meaning. Here in the West, most acupuncture schools and colleges offer 3–4-year 'accredited' acupuncture courses, with optional studies in China. Many alternative therapy organizations have set up self-regulatory bodies, ensuring high educational standards and at the same time seeking better understanding and recognition by the health system and the general public.

Fortunately, most acupuncture school curricula in the West do now include reasonable teaching time for cupping therapy. Consequently, in the last 15 years since my first book was published in late 1999, I have been invited to teach cupping therapy through various TCM schools and private lectures in England, Germany, Norway, Saudi Arabia, Sweden, Denmark, Holland, Turkey, Czech Republic, Canada and Switzerland. I was also quite humbled when I was asked to present a cupping paper to the students and the practitioners of TCM in Taichung and Taipei, Taiwan. The first presentation was at the China Medical University hospital in Taichung and the final presentation to the Chang Gung Memorial Hospital, Taipei. Both the students and the doctors were impressed

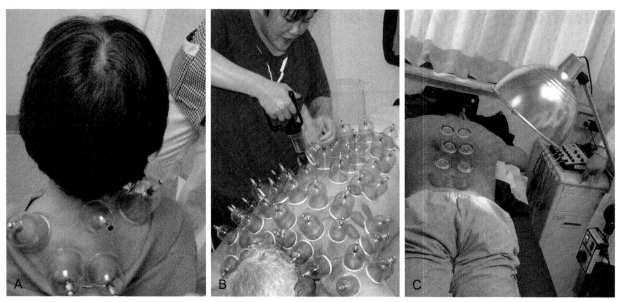

FIGURE 1-6 (A–C) Cupping therapy in Taiwanese clinics.

by the variety of cupping therapies offered in my lectures. I am also very pleased to see a genuine enthusiasm towards cupping therapy practice among the new generation of TCM practitioners as well as the contemporary massage therapists and physiotherapists. In parallel with this newly found interest, quite a number of websites are also offering online cupping therapy information. It is estimated that over 100 000 acupuncture practitioners today work outside China, practising Chinese medicine as a whole. It is clear that cupping therapy taught and used properly on its own, or alongside various tactile therapies, can positively influence and speed up the body's natural healing process (Fig. 1-6).

CONTEMPORARY CUPPING EQUIPMENT

Much of the cupping equipment used and sold today in the East as well as in the West is made of fire-resistant tough glass or clear Perspex material. Earthenware and bamboo cups are still used in developing countries. In the West, however, the use of earthenware and bamboo cups is now discontinued, or limited perhaps to an emergency situation where no other cupping equipment is available. Bamboo cups have now been replaced by clear Perspex cupping sets in most Chinese hospitals and clinics. In recent years many versions of electrical or mechanized cupping apparatus have also been introduced. Most of the new generation and elaborate vacuum cups are designed for use in the acupuncture clinics, sports clinics, beauty salons and health spas particularly during body toning, weight loss or cellulite reduction programmes. The manually operated valve cupping set (pistol-handle) is the most popular version among the Western practitioners who prefer not to employ fire during the cupping sessions (see 'Pistol-handle valve cups').

Electromagnetic Cupping Apparatus

In China the use of electric cupping apparatus involves the patient incurring additional cost. In addition, the electric cupping machine itself is expensive, bulky and impractical as far as mobility is concerned. These machines are heavy, and are consequently mounted on a portable table so that they can be taken to the nearest bed and positioned next to the patient. In Chinese TCM hospitals almost every acupuncture department has an electric cupping machine (Fig. 1-7). The cup is attached to the machine through an umbilical suction cord. At the same time, if necessary, a separate cable can be fitted to activate an electromagnetic probe inside the cup. Suction strength and duration can be adjusted and controlled electronically by the operator. The use of electromagnetic stimulation during a cupping treatment is a new experience for me; therefore I am unable to comment on the therapeutic efficacy of such a technique. According to some doctors who use such devices regularly, electromagnetic stimulation increases the

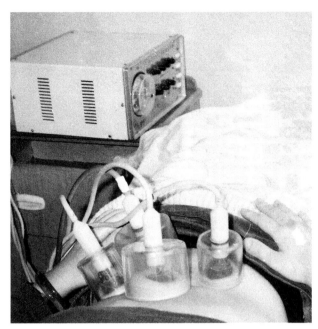

FIGURE 1-7 Electromagnetic cupping apparatus.

therapeutic effectiveness of cupping, especially when applied to joints, including the knees and elbows. One of the drawbacks of this rather sophisticated machine is that the cups cannot be sterilized as often and as efficiently as plain glass cups.

Portable Cupping Pumps

These are smaller, portable versions of mechanical cupping machines, powered by small petrol engines or batteries. They are heavy to carry around, especially when visiting patients; they are also very noisy to operate and difficult to clean. In my first book I introduced portable cupping pumps as 'easy to carry around'; however, I changed my opinion when I discovered that the average weight of these machines is around 5 kg – not so practical for a busy practitioner doing visiting rounds!

During the writing of the present edition I have also seen various electrically operated cupping machines, which have come to the market in recent years particularly from the European sources. However, most of these new machines are aimed at the cosmetic sector, in particular for toning up the skin as part of 'weight loss' programmes.

Screw-Top Cups

A more modest and rather inexpensive cupping set has an adjustable screw-threaded handle located on top of the cup and attached to a piston-like suction pump inside the cup (Fig. 1-8). The cups are made of clear Perspex material. The level of suction required is obtained by turning the handle anticlockwise and allowing the piston ring inside the cup to touch the patient's skin. The handle is then turned clockwise in order to pull the piston upwards, thereby creating a negative pressure inside the cup. Using this method, cupping treatment can be carried out in almost any environment, as neither electricity nor fire is needed. However, again a sufficient degree of sterilization cannot be achieved as the cups are lined with a fine lubricant in order to facilitate the movement of the piston. This version is the least used of the cupping sets in the clinics.

Pistol-Handle Valve Cups

This type of cup is usually made of toughened glass or clear Perspex material (Fig. 1-9) and has a valve attached to its top. So far I have seen two varieties of this cupping apparatus: one has a pump, which resembles a bicycle pump, and the other is the pistol-handle type. The operator places the cup in the desired position, inserts the pump into the valve and then proceeds to pump air out of the cup, creating suction. The strength of suction can be adjusted from the valve, which is positioned at the top of the cup. With this method the operator has absolute control over the vacuum, in particular when sensitive and small areas such facial points or a boil needs to be cupped.

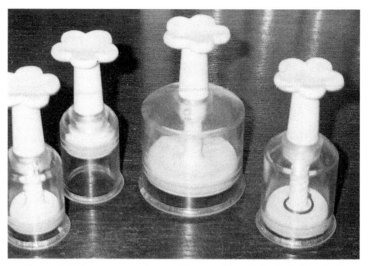

FIGURE 1-8 Screw-top cupping set. *(Courtesy of Acu-Medic Co. Ltd, London.)*

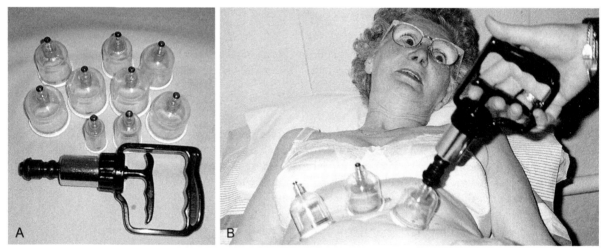

FIGURE 1-9 (A, B) Valve cupping set. *(Courtesy of Harmony Acupuncture Supplies Ltd, London.)*

The following technique is my own suggestion regarding the degree of suction control of the pistol-handle unit.

Light cupping method = one complete pull of the pistol handle.
Medium cupping method = two complete pulls of the handle.
Strong cupping method = three complete pulls of the handle.

Proper sterilization presents no problem, and the cupping sets are relatively inexpensive and easy to obtain.

Pistol-handle valve cups have become very popular with Western practitioners in recent years, largely due to the safety aspect of this particular set, where no fire of any kind is required during the application. The position of the patient is also irrelevant as the valve cups can be employed while the patient is either sitting up in a chair or lying down on the treatment couch.

Problems often encountered with pistol-handle valve cups are as follows:

1. **Not being able to create a good suction or the pistol handle feels tight when pulled:** The most frequent cause of this malfunction is a sticky valve. To remedy this problem, check to see whether the valve is moving freely from its base; if not, pull it by hand so that the valve is moving freely from its glass base when the suction is applied.

2. **Cups falling out shortly after the application:**
   a. Check and make sure that the cups are not cracked or the edges broken (sometimes the cup develops a hairline crack, which is not always visible).
   b. Apply oil liberally to the cupping location if treating hairy or dry skin conditions.
   c. Check the seal and the valve for foreign substances and remove if any.
3. **Vacuum handle not pulling:**
   a. Check the gun barrel for dirt and clear all foreign substances.
   b. Lubricate the gun if dry.

Cups with Squeeze Rubber Tops

These cups are made with a hollow rubber handle attached to the top (Fig. 1-10). The operator simply squeezes the rubber handle and places the cup on the desired point. When the rubber handle is released, a vacuum is created. A major disadvantage of these cups is that only a limited amount of air can be drawn out of the cup, and therefore the suction obtainable remains limited to light and medium strength.

When treating children under the age of 7 years this method is preferable, as there is no fire or machinery involved, and it is the only type of cupping method that parents can easily and safely be taught for use on their children at home.

Magnetic Squeeze Rubber Cups

These are operated exactly the same way as the cups above. However, these cups are attributed extra benefits owing to the magnetic field created by the magnet, which is fixed on the inside to the upper part of the cup (Fig. 1-11).

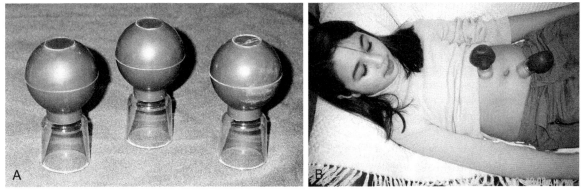

FIGURE 1-10 (A, B) Rubber-top cupping set.

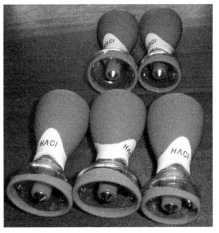

FIGURE 1-11 Magnetic cupping set.

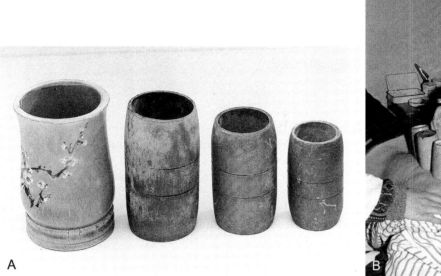
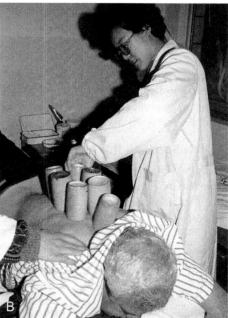

FIGURE 1-12 (A, B) Bamboo cupping set. Used in ancient times and today.

Bamboo Cups

Without doubt cups made of bamboo (Fig. 1-12) are the most commonly used in China today. Bamboo is easily available, inexpensive and extremely light to carry, and the cups are durable and last for years. There are a few disadvantages, however. First, the edges of the bamboo cups are very sharp compared with glass cups, and dig into the flesh. For this reason, I personally refrain from using bamboo cups on my Western patients, as the concept of pain in Western patients is very different from that of the Chinese. For the Chinese patient, the discomfort caused by the bamboo cup is quite acceptable. A second disadvantage is that the operator is unable to see inside the cup to monitor the strength of suction and avoid blistering. Thirdly, adequate sterilization cannot be achieved as the bamboo is very porous and absorbent, and a strong suction may draw blood or body fluids into the fibres of the cup. In a busy clinic, for example, there would therefore be a greater risk of cross-infection. For personal use in the home, however, bamboo cups are very safe.

During my studies in the Nanjing University of Traditional Chinese Medicine and the First Affiliated Hospital, Nanjing, I was allowed to visit and participate in the work of various departments such as the children's clinic, Tui Na (Chinese therapeutic massage), herbal medicine and acupuncture. Most of these departments use cupping therapy extensively alongside their main treatment modalities. For the reasons mentioned above, the most favoured medium used in all these departments was the bamboo cups.

Glass Cups

Before glass cups were introduced, earthenware and china cups were used for many hundreds of years. In fact, my grandmother Rahmeli Ebe often used large earthenware vessels resembling water jugs to treat her patients. Because of the obvious disadvantages of earthenware cups (expensive, easily broken and very heavy to handle or carry), glass cups (Fig. 1-13) were introduced soon after the invention of glass itself (around 2500 BC, by the Egyptians). The drawings on the entrance of one of the tombs in Luxor, Egypt, clearly show a cupping set, most probably made of glass, among other medical instruments (Fig. 1-14). The edges of glass cups are thicker and smoother than those of bamboo cups. They are also available in different sizes.

It is often difficult to purchase a set of glass cups all the same size: wholesalers and retailers often prefer to sell them in sets of three, all varying in size, so that large numbers of the less popular sizes do not remain in their stock!

Glass cups are the type most favoured by Western practitioners. From a practical point of view the advantage of the glass cupping set is its transparency, which enables the practitioner to observe and

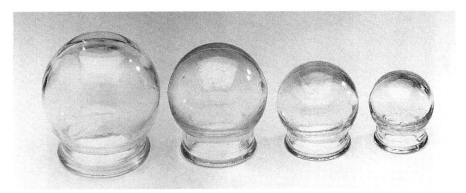

FIGURE 1-13 Glass cupping set. Used in ancient times and today.

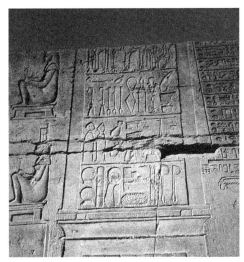

FIGURE 1-14 Drawings on the entrance to an Egyptian tomb, Luxor. *(Courtesy of Mrs J. Shilton, London.)*

monitor the strength of suction and the treatment time. Glass cups are also easier and faster to use and more suitable to sterilize. For the reasons given above I prefer the use of glass cups in my clinics. There appears to be only one disadvantage: if dropped, glass cups break very easily and are expensive to replace.

Rubber Cups

In late 1999, I was introduced to a new cupping set that is made completely of a natural rubber material (Fig. 1-15). The cups are corrugated in shape and, when the air is pushed out, a rather strong suction is obtained. The cups give a good strength of suction and are versatile in their application.

Because of the nature of the rubber material, these cups are expensive and cannot be boiled or sterilized in a strong cleaning solution as the rubber becomes soft, edges wear thin and are unable to hold onto the skin. It can be used in a busy clinic when new. Otherwise, they are only recommended for personal use. Most massage oils used during the treatment also damage the rubber, which reduces its effectiveness.

When new, the smooth surface of the mouth of the rubber cup makes it ideal for treating children as well as the Moving cupping technique on adults. Rubber cups can safely be used on the face, stomach, legs and other tender parts of the body.

Silicon Cups

In early 2011, I was invited to Vancouver, Canada as part of the Canadian Oriental Medicine Symposium for a lecture and a 'cupping therapy workshop'. There I was introduced to silicon cupping sets. Silicon cups are more resistant to any damage from oil or sterilizing liquid. The edges of the silicon cups are smoother, they are lighter in weight than rubber cups and I am also assured that they last much longer owing to the toughness of the silicon material. Silicon cups are particularly suitable during cosmetic cupping sessions, especially for cellulite treatment on the thighs and for a facial rejuvenation programme (Fig. 1-16).

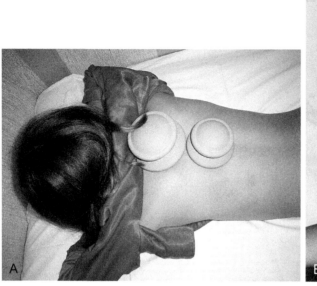
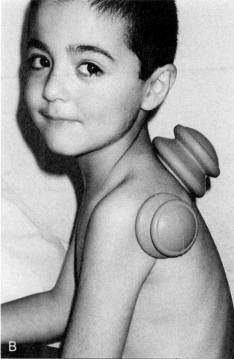

FIGURE 1-15 (A, B) Rubber cups are well tolerated, especially by children.

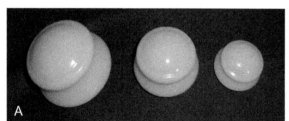
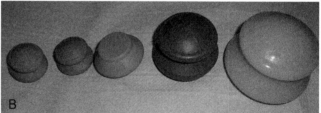

FIGURE 1-16 (A, B) Silicon cups.

Disposable Cupping Sets

These are the most recent innovation in the cupping arsenal! The most truly innovative and practical cupping set I have seen in recent years is the disposable cupping unit. Apart from the suction pump, the entire cups are once-use only and disposable. Some manufacturers, however, produce the entire cupping unit as a disposable unit. Disposable cups are most suitable for 'Wet cupping' (Hejama, Bleeding method), where the used cups can be disposed of immediately after use. This type of cupping equipment is quite reasonable to purchase and therefore affordable in terms of disposal. The cups are made of clear durable plastic material (Fig. 1-17).

Two-In-One Cupping Set with Electrical Stimulation

This new version of cupping set is designed to provide electric stimulation simultaneously with conventional cupping therapy. The electrical stimulation during treatment is similar to transcutaneous electrical nerve stimulation (TENS) stimulation. According to the manufacturer's prospectus, it 'provides cupping therapy and allows stimulation by TENS unit simultaneously, thus enhances the effect for both suction and electric stimulation treatments'. The application instructions are as follows:

For Cupping Application Only

1. Apply a thin layer of moisturizer or lotion to the skin or treatment area before operation.
2. Place the vacuum cup on the treatment area; it is recommended to use at least two cups per treatment.

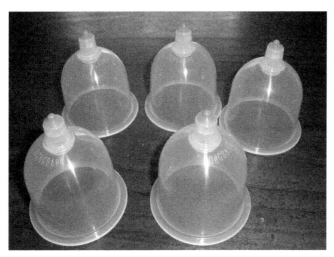

FIGURE 1-17 Disposable cupping set.

3. Use your thumb to press the top of the vacuum cup and release; the cup will stay on the skin or treatment area firmly. Press the top of the cup firmly to create a strong force, and mild pressure for less force. Adjust the suction strength according to your diagnosis.
4. When treatment is completed, squeeze the cup on both sides and the cup can be lifted up easily from the treatment area.
5. After treatment, clean the cups with soapy water and sterilizing liquid.

.For Simultaneous Cupping and Electrical Stimulation

1. Attach the cups as described above.
2. Attach the pin lead wire to the vacuum cup. Use two cups at the same time for positive and negative poles.
3. Connect the pin lead wire to the TENS unit for electric stimulation.
4. Adjust output intensity and pulse rate/width of the TENS unit according to your treatment protocol.
5. Now the cupping and TENS therapy is applied simultaneously.
6. When treatment is completed, turn off the TENS unit. Squeeze the cup on both sides and remove the cup from the treatment area.
7. Clean and sterilize the used cups as described above.

Contraindications and Precautions Regarding the Unit

This two-in-one unit is not recommended for pregnant women and persons with any form of cardiac history, in particular persons fitted with a heart pacemaker (Fig. 1-18).

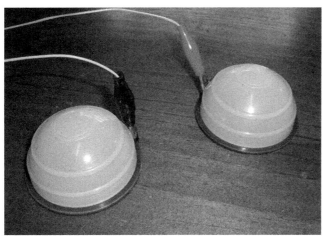

FIGURE 1-18 Two-in-one cupping set.

REFERENCES

Al-Jauziyah, I.-Q., 2003. Healing with the Medicine of the Prophet (trans Jalal Abual Rub). Dar-us-Salam Publications, Houston, USA.

Bakhtiar, L., 1999. The Canon of Medicine (Avicenna) (al-Qanun Fi'l tibb) Abu Ali al-Husayn ibn Abd Allah ibn Sina (trans Cameron Gruner and Mazar H. Shah). Great Books of the Islamic World, Chicago, USA.

Bayfield, S., 1823. A Treatise on Practical Cupping. E. Cox & Sons, London, pp. 60–62.

Chirali, I., 2007. Traditional Chinese Medicine Cupping Therapy, second ed. Churchill Livingstone, Edinburgh, UK.

Imam Ali ibn Abu Talib, 2007. In: Newman, A.J. (Ed.), Islamic Medical Wisdom – The Tibb al-A'imma (B. Ispahany, Trans.). Ansarian Publications, Qum, Iran.

Kennedy, C., 1826. An Essay on Cupping. Jackson, London, UK.

CUPPING'S FOLK HERITAGE: PEOPLE IN PRACTICE

Bruce Bentley

2

CHAPTER CONTENTS

INTRODUCTION, 17

THE VERY EARLY ROOTS OF CUPPING, 18

CUPPING AS A FOLK MEDICAL PRACTICE, 19

THE ABSENCE OF FOLK CUPPING PRACTICE
FROM SCHOLARLY WRITINGS, 21

WOMEN AS DOMESTIC CUPPERS, 22

WIND AND CUPPING, 27

ENDNOTES, 31

REFERENCES, 32

INTRODUCTION

If we were to follow the lead of traditional medical histories, and engage in what the sociologist Thomas McKeown (1970: 342) described as the chronological re-telling of the 'great men and the great movements', we would be ushered past an important stratum of cupping's social and cultural history and remain disengaged from its long and uninterrupted practice as a folk medical therapy.

I aim to redress this imbalance, by briefly exploring cupping's roots in both super-naturalistic and naturalistic medical traditions and also account for what constitutes a folk medical practice. I discuss some of the reasons why folk medicine and its practitioners have been conspicuously absent from the conservative body of historical discourse, and why the hierarchy of professional practitioners has discredited them. I focus on gender representation and give credit to those unheralded lay therapists, particularly women, who have woven the fabric of cupping's ongoing practice by passing it down in the home from generation to generation. I investigate the correlation between pain and illness in relation to Wind, and the reasons why cupping makes sense as a rational therapeutic response. Finally I present two folk cupping treatments and instructions for their practice. Along the way we will also glimpse some of the social nuances that mix and gel cupping's cross-cultural mosaic.

This chapter is based on archival research, as well as information gathered from primary contact interviews and informal conversations with cuppers (the early-19th-century name given to those who cup) in Australia and throughout Asia, Europe and North Africa. To source the fieldwork information in Europe for example, I went to towns and villages where I thought cupping was probably still being practised. Previously in Australia, I had spoken to people who had emigrated from Europe during the last half century who continue cupping their family members, albeit with curtains drawn, and got to understand that my best chances of discovering what I was looking for was in those communities that were less economically developed and had maintained links with the same traditional healing ways that their ancestors had passed on. I also found that, like the personal transmission of skills and know-how in the past, the ideal way of learning cupping in the domestic setting continues to be based on face-to-face contact, observing, asking, listening and supervised practice.

My thanks therefore go to all those home-grown cuppers who shared their knowledge and practices, as well as those scholars who gave me their time and encouragement, not least the great and sadly missed Roy Porter at the Wellcome Institute for the History of Medicine in London in 1998.

To avoid any confusion, I use the word 'cupping' to denote what has often been historically referred to in Western medical literature as 'dry' cupping, as opposed to 'wet' cupping. In China the term cupping is readily identified with dry cupping, whereas in the Islamic medical tradition as a rule it is synonymous with wet cupping; so there needs to be clarification and a line drawn between the two, especially when it comes to diagnosis and practice. Dry cupping is the act of placing a cupping vessel on an intact skin surface, whereas wet cupping requires a light incision to be made in the skin before a cup is applied over the incision to draw out a quantity of blood. The latter is a mild form of bloodletting, in contrast to the non-invasive dry form known as *ventosa* in Italian, *ventouse* in French and *vendouses* in modern Greek; all from the Latin root *ventus* or wind, and signifying a vacuum-based method of extracting and eliminating Wind as a pathogenic influence from the body. Celsus, the Greco-Roman encyclopaedist of the 2nd century AD makes this distinction clear in his *De Medicina* (Of Medicine): 'if the skin upon which the cup is to be stuck is cut beforehand with a scalpel, the cup extracts blood; when the skin is intact wind' (Spencer, 1953: 167).

Over the past few decades cupping has enjoyed a resurgence. This follows a period of discreditation and fall-out from orthodox medical practice since around the 1880s, which can be attributed to its lack of fit with modern scientific theories of illness causation and treatment methods rather than its lack of therapeutic efficacy. Furthermore, 'it represented a method that had been firmly established within the humoural paradigm of health care – a tradition that the medical fraternity clearly wanted to dismiss into the background of the past' (Bentley, 1996:i).[1] Cupping is now being practised by a diverse range of alternative or non-biomedical practitioners in the West to treat a host of different clinical syndromes: from treatments based on traditional Chinese medicine to clear stagnation, to remove climatic pathogens and to tonify deficiency[2] using glass cups and flame, to newly developed applications using flexible silicone cupping instruments to treat myofascial syndromes based on modern soft tissue perspectives (Bentley, 2013).[3]

THE VERY EARLY ROOTS OF CUPPING

Prehistoric humans began their attempts to heal by following their natural impulses and employed simple techniques such as rubbing the skin, blowing on inflamed areas and oral suction, which was the ancient precursor to using instruments designed for the task. One of the valuable applications for sucking was to withdraw stings and other noxious intrusions from the body that if left unattended could have drastic consequences. Can you remember as a child sucking your finger or thumb after it had been hit or jammed in a door to help relieve the pain? This simple act is also a form of cupping, being the application of vacuum to the skin surface for a therapeutic effect. The following are examples of people whose experiences would otherwise go untold, who are using cupping either in the form of oral suction or with a vessel to effectively alleviate various health concerns.

 CASE 2-1

Following a cupping class I taught many years ago, where I mentioned that sucking was employed in ancient times to remove toxins from insect stings, one of my students decided to try it out for himself. He kept bees as a hobby and whenever he was stung, usually on his hand, in his own words it would 'immediately swell up to twice its normal size and remain sore for the next few hours'. The next time he was stung, he immediately began sucking at the site and instantly tasted a hint of sweetness from the residues of the sting. After a couple of minutes sucking and spitting out at regular intervals he was delighted to discover his hand, for the first time, never reacted with any swelling or pain.

 CASE 2-2

A Chinese medicine colleague practising in the United States informed me that a patient of hers had witnessed her father, a lobster fisherman from a Portuguese-American fishing community in New England, Massachusetts, using cups to pull out embedded lobster spikes and infectious matter from the tissues. 'It was a messy affair, pulling out the bloodied spikes, but it worked really well,' she stated. Similarly, one person who lives in rural Victoria, Australia, told me that 'mum used to pull splinters out by cupping', and in Sicily in 1998 an elderly man said that during World War II cupping was used to extract small pieces of shrapnel from bomb blasts that had lodged in the flesh.

Historical examples of vacuum being used to extract object intrusions are included in the works of the celebrated Persian physician Ibn Sina (Avicenna) of the 10th century AD. He wrote that immediately after an engorged leech had fallen from where it had been applied for a healing purpose, 'the place should be sucked by cupping it, in order to extract some of the blood at the spot and thereby get rid of the toxic substances left in the wound' (Gruner, 1930: 514). Susruta, the renowned physician of classical Indian medicine, also recommended that a hollow cow horn[4] be used to extract the penetration of an insect from the ear, as well as being one of the best ways to go about removing salya (or pieces of arrow) and other debris from sharp weapons lodged in the body (Mukhopadhyaya, 1913: 150).

Besides expelling hostile natural penetrations and purulent exudates with oral suction, early humankind also developed complex beliefs about serious illness being brought about by supernatural forces. These could be caused to enter into the body from beyond the realm of the ordinary world by entities such as evil spirits, angry ghosts or disgruntled ancestors, or inflicted upon a person by the possessor of extraordinary powers such as the 'evil eye'. Together with esoteric mediations, sucking at the skin surface to draw out and expel these malevolent influences became the primary physical intervention of the shaman, in an enormously significant medical way of thinking that remains active throughout many parts of the world today. In his ground-breaking work on shamanism, the French scholar Mircea Eliade (1989: 256) declared suction to be a 'classic method of cure', while A. P. Elkin (1994: 41) in his book written in the 1930s titled *Aboriginal Men of High Degree* refers to sucking as 'the means by which the doctor exercises his magical and psychic power and extracts and casts away the badness'.

A very different model of healing emerged during the golden era of the Greek enlightenment with the works attributed to Hippocrates and his followers, which were mostly written from the mid 5th century BC to the first half of the 4th century. Often referred to as the 'father of Western medicine', Hippocrates (or those who are now identified as the Hippocratic writers) were the first to primarily eschew the belief that illness was due to supernatural causes. Instead they concentrated on understanding sickness being caused by factors of natural origin such as adverse weather, geographic locations, incorrect diet, unsettled emotions and insufficient rest or exercise. Known for their dedication to safe and gentle curing, the Hippocratic writers included a number of recommendations for cupping among the 60-odd volumes that make up the Hippocratic Corpus. These physicians used fashionable bronze cups, instead of dried gourds (*cucurbita*) into which a small opening was made so the lips could be applied to draw air out and form a vacuum (Turk and Allen, 1983: 128). There can be no doubt that gourds were preferred as cups by rural folk who could grow their own.

When we incorporate the broad arena of social life into medical history, we realise that professional and scholarly medical treatments were available only to the small elite of any given society, the tip of the social pyramid who could afford their services. The overwhelming majority of regular people were required to use their own know-how to heal themselves, their kinfolk and their communal brethren. In early Greek Minoan and Mycenaean medicine during the 2nd millennium BC, Arnott (2004: 162) is convinced that: 'as in other areas of the Aegean, outside the world of the palace, the population largely fended for themselves, and the tradition of self-help would have existed. Domestic medicine would have provided one area of activity.' In the same vein, during Greco-Roman times, 'the tradition of self-help in medicine must have always been strong, particularly in the countryside, although it appears infrequently in literary sources' (Nutton, 1998: 17), and Unschuld (1979: 51) is certain that 'the history of high medicine in China was never the medicine of 90 per cent of the population'.

Given its sufficiently uncomplicated apparatus and no-frills rationale and methodology, cupping has never been the exclusive practice of any cultural group, social level or therapeutic convention. Moreover, it has proved itself to be remarkably utilitarian in straddling the hurdles of divergent explanatory paradigms and folkloric customs with their varying interpretations about what causes us to feel ill. Wherever people have lived, the practice of applying vacuum to the skin surface has been an elemental course of therapeutic intervention in some way, shape or form.

CUPPING AS A FOLK MEDICAL PRACTICE

The term 'folk medicine' describes a broad range of therapeutic approaches created and performed by people who are not formally trained. According to Leininger (1976: 32) they have 'often provided health care to people for many years and long before a professional health system entered their culture'. Even today, although it may seem that modern medicine accounts for most of the medicine practised throughout the world, according to the World Health Organization (Bannerman et al, 1983: 11), 'in many countries, 80 per cent or more of the population living in rural areas are cared for by traditional practitioners and birth attendants'. These practices have lasted from antiquity until the present day because they embody the social and cultural mores of the communities they represent, and are practical common sense responses to pain and illness that have been found to work.

Unfortunately however, very little has been written about folk medicine, and precious little about cupping being performed by lay people. The fact of the matter is, the more we look socially downwards, the vaguer we become about how people cared for themselves. One reason for this is, up until recently most people in Europe and other parts of the world had next to no opportunity to learn to read and write. Even if a regular person happened to be a scribe, it is understandable that writing about what was already being successfully handed on from one generation to the next would seem superfluous.

There are differing opinions among medical sinologists about the likelihood of Chinese common folk performing cupping in ancient times. The first textual record of cupping, that we know of, is found in the Mawangdui medical manuscripts. These scripts, dated around 168 BC, are a treasure trove of information on treatments and health enhancement practices. Cupping makes a rather unflattering cameo as a preliminary treatment method for haemorrhoids – 'either large ones like a zao [jujube] and small ones like a zao [jujube] pit'. The treatment protocol advises to apply a small horn to it, for the time it takes to cook two dou (a unit of quantity) of rice. Then 'bind it with a small cord and cut it open with a knife' (Harper, 1998: 271). In his commentary, Donald Harper concludes that whether using instruments fashioned from animal horns or otherwise, cupping was adopted much less frequently in ancient China than it was in Greco-Roman medical culture around the same era. He argues that the omission of cupping from other early Chinese medical writings, as well as the lack of information given to a cup's construction and its mode of application, only adds further weight to this deduction. Yet the Chinese researcher Ma Jinxing reaches the opposite conclusion from the same evidence. He interprets the lack of details as 'a sign that cupping was already commonly practised and did not require explanation' (Harper, 1998: 271).

As far back as living memory can link us with the past, folk cures including cupping have been an indelible part of common life in China. During my time studying cupping at the Shanghai University of Traditional Chinese Medicine in 1996, my chief instructor Dr Zhou Ling said: 'cupping was passed on to the cities from the experience of the countryside. It is very practical. Country people use it especially for treating pain.' In fact Mr Wang Ruzheng, aged 80 years, who is a martial arts expert and former tuina practitioner at the Guan An Meng Chinese Medical Hospital in Beijing, China, seemed amused by the notion that professional medicine until recent times was ever within the means of the greater proportion of the Chinese population. Instead he was adamant that 'they cared for themselves, and cupping was one of the most common ways of doing that'.

The Vietnamese people as well are avid users of folk medical practices and provide an excellent study group, both in their ancestral homeland and in those parts of the world where they have migrated. They are noted for their independence and high degree of self-sufficiency, and their use of folk therapies is characteristic of these cultural traits. During the day, and especially of a night-time in Ho Chi Minh City, it is easy to find cupping specialists practising on sidewalks. Other practitioners offering cupping, gua sha[5] (cao gio in Vietnamese) and massage services can also be found riding their bicycles down the side streets and announcing themselves by shaking a stick with a row of soft drink bottle tops loosely attached to the end. In neighboring Cambodia, street-cupping is also readily available (Fig. 2-1).

In 2002, when I conducted a research project funded by the Department of Human Services (Victoria) titled 'Folk Medical Practices in the Vietnamese Community', in Melbourne, Australia, I found that cupping was one of the most popular treatments performed in Vietnamese homes. Yet it has never been detailed in writing because, as one informant explained, 'there's no need; people already know how to do it.'

Other examples of the way cupping belongs to everyday life include a female Lithuanian cupper who informed me, 'you can find a set of cupping glasses in every kitchen', and in Fiji in 2001, I questioned the locals about cupping and they said they kept a look-out for small irregular oblong-shaped coconuts

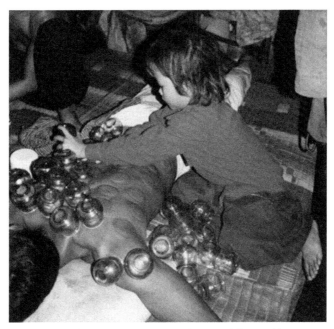

FIGURE 2-1 A young boy helps his father (partially seen squatting in the upper left corner) by removing cups at the end of treatment. This photo was taken at around 9 pm, in the plaza outside the central train station in Phnom Penh, Cambodia. About eight or nine other practitioners had also set up their regular nightly practice. *Photo courtesy: Bruce Bentley.*

to use as cupping vessels. In fact, every community I have encountered has a heritage of cupping. The following points sum up the way that most people connect and interact with cupping as a folk therapy:

- The majority of illness and pain treated by cupping is due to external climatic influences penetrating the body through the skin surface.
- The vacuum effect of cupping has the ability to draw and expel these from the body.
- The marks produced from the treatment are regarded as proof that cupping has been effective and the cause of the illness or pain has been eliminated.
- People report that they quickly recover and are satisfied with the treatment.

The most convincing way to comprehend just how long cupping has been around as a folk medical practice is by historical interpretation and the anecdotal antiquity of its practice performed by families and tribes around the world. When I ask the question 'Who taught you?' most cuppers answer it was either their mother or grandmother, who in turn was instructed by her grandmother, and back it goes. We should have no doubt that this scenario has gone on for millennia. If we follow a time line beginning with sucking, back in primordial prehistory, then shift to the earliest civilisations and onwards, for the vast majority of people there was virtually no contact with elite medicine. Instead, people dealt with illness in their own ways and through their own initiatives. Essential folk medical legacies were handed on to the next generation. It is a straightforward bow to draw and conclude that cupping has been a constant in a *big* social story.

THE ABSENCE OF FOLK CUPPING PRACTICE FROM SCHOLARLY WRITINGS

There are three telling reasons why the folk practice of cupping is absent from traditional historical discourse. First, 'old style scholarship' (which Porter & Weir [1987: 1] describe as 'whiggish') overwhelmingly had professional medicine at centre stage and was 'basically "in house", written largely by doctors about doctors for doctors, and explicitly or implicitly it sang the praises of medical progress' (Porter & Weir, 1987: 1). In tandem with this bias towards professional medicine, 'academics have traditionally made "learned medicine" or "scientific medicine" their study', rather than give equal weight to the investigation of traditional folk medicine. If folk practices ever did rate a mention in historical or academic texts, it was invariably in pejorative terms, with the inference that it was unworthy of any serious consideration.

Secondly, folk medicine has always been relegated to the lowest rung of healing by the hierarchy of professionals. The first time I observed cupping performed was in 1976, when a man was treating a friend in a shop in Tamsui, a small city on the north coast of Taiwan. When I discussed this with my teachers at the Chinese Acupuncture Hospital in Taipei, one of the doctors dismissed it as 'just folk medicine'. Professionals typically see others engaging in therapy as an encroachment on their turf. Roy Porter (1997) believes they have always sought to discredit health folklore and practices to secure medical dominance and the largest possible financial slice of the medical pie. During the Medieval period in Europe, the pecking order of healers went like this: 'physicians looked down upon the surgeons, so the surgeons of higher education, who in the Middle Ages could be counted on the fingers, looked down upon the barbers' (Garrison, 1913: 115). In turn the barbers, who performed simpler surgical procedures including wet cupping, were certain to have thought the same about cupping when it was performed by lay persons instead of by them. It all got too much for the renowned physician, alchemist and reformer of therapeutics known as Paracelsus (1493–1541), who declared, to the horror of his scholarly colleagues, that he got more learning from common folk, country healers, wise-women and gypsies than he ever did from sitting in any lecture hall! (Griggs, 1981).

Thirdly, even if a physician were available and affordable, it would seem strange that an ordinary person who was already acquainted with cupping would feel the need for professional services when the same help could be obtained free from family and other members of the local community. The following two examples illustrate this. The town of Devin in the Rhodope Mountains in Southern Bulgaria, is blessed with natural hot springs and there is a spa centre where people can receive massage and hydrotherapy. One local told me, 'they don't do cupping at the sanatorium because in these parts, it is a family tradition and you can always find someone who does it.' Again in Kalambaka, a small town at the foothills of Meteora in central Greece, Dr Konstantinos Matazanas, a 71-year-old general practitioner keen on cupping, said that he did not do it in his practice because 'in every household there is at least one person who can help'. He instead advises his patients: 'tell your mother or grandmother to do it for you'.

Although my personal contact with many cuppers has established that women are more likely to be performing cupping than men, to think there is a strict gender divide would be unfair and fail to acknowledge the genuine interest and care that some men also lend to home and community-based cupping practice. One of my stock questions whenever I talk to either a female or male cupper goes: 'is cupping practised by both women and men?' The reply in every instance has been an emphatic 'yes'. What's more, those women did not suggest that men doing cupping was anything out of the ordinary. In the same spirit, every cupper I have ever met enjoys being able to practise and care for others. It is a joy to find this egalitarianism, despite the influence that overt and subtle ways of socialization play in determining role compliance, choices and decision making.

To say that medicine begins at home is no overstatement in anyone's life. It is therefore important to bring the role that women have and continue to play as cuppers in the domestic setting into focus.

WOMEN AS DOMESTIC CUPPERS

If folk medicine has been poorly represented in old-style histories of medicine, then women as healers in the domestic setting have been virtually invisible. Thankfully however, this has been confronted and addressed by some researchers over recent decades. One of the first was Arthur Kleinman (1980: 306), the noted psychiatrist and anthropologist whose work inspired further studies into the cross-cultural and social dynamics of folk medical practice. From his ethnographic research conducted in Taiwan during the 1970s he explained, 'it may appear strange to some to consider the family as a "practitioner" ... but considering that "73 percent of all sickness episodes" ... are treated solely in the context of the family, there is nothing all that strange about looking upon the family as practitioner. Indeed, in most societies it would appear to be by far the most active form of clinical practice.' Further studies identify mothers and grandmothers as the most important health care providers of lay healing (Finerman, 1989: 25) and, 'most sources estimate 70 percent to 95 percent of all health care is domestic – not professional – and women provide nearly 95 percent of all domestic care' (Clark, 1998: 159).

Some other contemporary scholars, mostly women, have shown a great deal of interest in examining women in informal healing roles, and have drawn the curtains aside to expose their importance as healers in the home, and sometimes extending into their local community (Fig. 2-2, Fig. 2-3, Fig. 2-4). During my informal research from 1976 until 1981 in Taiwan, I discovered that, besides cupping family members, some women also open up their home to assist others. For instance, on the

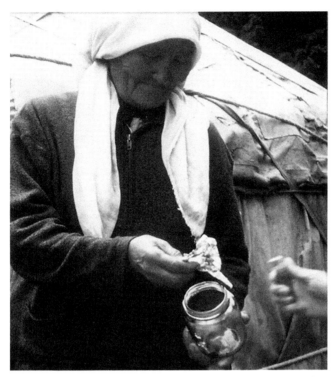

FIGURE 2-2 A Uighur woman gets a 'hand' to light the paper, which she drops into a jar to cup her son's tight shoulder. She stands in front of her family yurt, which follows the yearly graze of her goats through the districts around Tian Shan (Heavenly Lake) in Xingjiang Provence, far north-western China. *Photo courtesy: Bruce Bentley.*

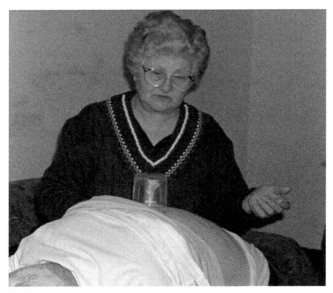

FIGURE 2-3 Inside her house in the medieval village of Erice, Sicily, Mrs Paola Povounello demonstrates her method of applying a regular drinking glass as a cupping vessel to her husband's back. She first cut a small square piece of cloth and placed a bronze coin in the centre. Bronze is understood to convey heat into the body. She then drew the four corners of the cloth together and twisted them down level with the coin. Paola then tightly wrapped a length of cotton thread around the twisted cloth to hold it together to form a wick, which she dipped in olive oil, and placed it base downwards on the site where she intended to cup. The wick was lit and the cup was placed over the flame. I have observed this way of preparing a wick on numerous occasions in Italy and occasionally in Greece. *Photo courtesy: Bruce Bentley.*

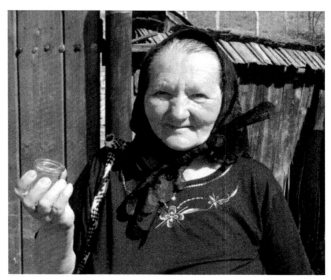

FIGURE 2-4 Maria Perta, a village woman from Botiza in Northern Transylvania, Romania, holding one of her cups. Her mother taught her and she helps the other women in her village with their health concerns. She said, 'when we're in the fields and the cold wind blows, it causes muscular and rheumatic pains.' *Photo courtesy: Bruce Bentley.*

outskirts of Taipei near the mountains where I lived, there was an elderly woman who treated people in our neighbourhood with cupping. She also happened to be the first person I had encountered who boiled bamboo cups in herbal preparations and applied them to injuries. I went to her to be treated a number of times and had excellent results. Another woman, Mrs Hyro Glykokalamos aged 55 years, learnt cupping from her grandmother when she was eight years old growing up in the small village of Kabos Vion, Sparta, in Southern Greece. Now a Melbourne resident, she informed me that 'everybody' did cupping as a household therapy in Sparta, and remembered there was one old woman 'who lived till she was more than 100, who used to attract people from all over the district. She practised cupping, bone-setting and used special herbal ointments.' She added: 'those women who have a special talent and interest in areas such as cupping are often recognized by the community and become busy practitioners.' In Bulgaria, in a small town called Shiroka Laka, I had the good fortune to study with one such woman. Petra Peevska is the current holder of a family cupping legacy that goes back 'further than any of us can remember'. She laughed and explained to me through the help of an interpreter, 'that's the same thing that I was told by my grandmother who heard the same from hers'. Petra's long family lineage of skilled cuppers has been highly respected by the folks in her village for generations. I observed in her work a similar quality found in all expert cuppers – she concentrates with a keen eye full of depth and intention.

According to those women who cup their family members and friends, cupping is a therapy perfectly suited to home practice. First, the materials required are basic and ready at hand. Secondly the practice is time efficient, relatively undemanding and as one person in Vietnam put it 'can nearly always be performed by at least one person in any family, and if not then by a neighbour – and it costs nothing'. Thirdly, cupping can empower householders with a sense of privacy and independence, as well as fostering a feeling of sharing, trust and togetherness.

Cupping at home also means it can be employed as a preventative measure or at the first sign of discomfort without the patient having to leave the home. In folk medical thinking, it is always better to deal with the possibility rather than the outcome. For rural families especially, when one person is waylaid with illness, the rest of the family is greatly affected because everyone is needed to help out with the daily workload and chores. In villages throughout Vietnam, China and Cambodia, I have often heard of farmers getting cupped by their children when they come home from a hard day in the field. There is nothing romantic about planting rice for instance. It is a hard grind being bent over all day. 'I like getting cupped before dinner,' said one female rice farmer, 'then afterwards, I feel relaxed and enjoy the rest of my evening. I always ask my children to do the cupping for me when my back aches and my muscles feel stiff. I also think it is very good when the weather changes quickly and I can catch a cold or some other sickness. I also like it when I feel tired. It takes the tiredness away.'

The sooner an illness or discomfort is treated, the better the chances of success. To leave treatment until a later time can allow a problem to develop and penetrate deeper into the body. Mr George Christou, aged 77 years, from Povla in north-eastern Greece said: 'when I was a boy, every time grandma heard me sneeze, she would say, "you've got a cold, come here and I'll do the *vendouses* for you".'

Also, and possibly most importantly, performing cupping in the home is understood as a safeguard. When I was learning from Petra Peevska in Bulgaria, she instructed: 'cupping should always be done after dinner. It is important not to venture outdoors and have contact with the cold or wind. Either go to bed or stay warm in front of the fire.' This was made plain as well during my six-week research trip to Greece in 2013. It was out of the question to expect a person to perform cupping at any time other than in the evening, when the receiver could stay indoors and keep warm and protected. Some Greek informants, including Mrs Melpomeni Christou from southern Greece, explained that when sick 'the skin pores are naturally more open because of fever. It is essential that open skin pores have no contact with the cold and wind'. Likewise, Dr Trung Thin, director of the Institute of Traditional Medicine of Ho Chi Minh City, said that traditional community clinics deal mostly with herbal medicine because 'people stay indoors and get cupping treatment from family members'. The Buddhist abbot the Venerable Thich Phuoc Tan, who accompanied me as my translator during my second research trip to Vietnam in 2000, also explained, 'Vietnamese people understand that getting a diagnosis of *gio* (Wind) means you are better off inside the home, otherwise to go outside means you are liable to be struck by Wind again and get far worse'. Cuppers also insist against showering or bathing for at least a few hours after treatment, and the majority caution not to bathe for 24 hours in order for the skin pores to fully adjust back to normal and re-establish their natural capacity to protect against any invasive climatic influences. *For cuppers who work in a clinic the message is:* make certain your patient has plenty of clothes to wear when they leave your office. Be vigilant about covering any region that has been treated, especially during windy, cold weather. Wrapping a scarf around the neck after the back of the neck or the upper back has been treated is essential. It is better not to treat someone, regardless of how appropriate and beneficial you believe cupping him or her to be, if afterwards they go outside and allow Cold, Wind, Damp or Heat to enter into the body via those warmed, open and vulnerable skin pores where the cups have been.

The thought of home-based treatment may conjure up the belief that folk-cupping deals only with superficial or simple health concerns. The following case demonstrates otherwise. A Polish woman explained that not long after the end of World War II, when drugs and modern treatments were unavailable, her mother used cupping to treat a relative in their home who had pneumonia. She explained the details to me in a solemn tone and stressed that during the critical period of her illness, 'every care was taken in case her condition deteriorated. It was life or death,' she assured me. Bedding was mounted on top of the large iron stove in the kitchen, where the patient slept and received treatment. 'We kept the stove burning constantly, so it was the warmest room in the house.' During the three days of treatment, strict protocol was observed. 'My mother and I stayed in the same room with our cousin at all times. No-one else was permitted to enter the room because the door was not allowed to be opened in case the slightest waft of cold air came in and made her worse.' She then stood up and re-enacted how they were even required to move about, and walked in extreme slow motion so as not to disturb the calm of the atmosphere. They also paid infinite attention to how they took off the cups. 'First of all, some other warm material is kept over the area being cupped. When we took the cups off, we had to slide our hand under the covering and carefully remove each one in a very gentle way so there was no hiss as the air inside was released, otherwise the Wind could sneak in. Our hand immediately covered the site as the cup was slowly removed, and gentle circular massage was performed to warm and close the skin pores.' Her cousin made a good recovery.

Historically, as mentioned before, there are few written records of women performing cupping. Fortunately however, a lively illustration from an early 14th-century illuminated manuscript depicts a woman who appears to be alternating two large cupping vessels to a man's backside, possibly to treat sciatica or to draw a boil (Fig. 2-5). From the position of her grip on the attached cup, she seems about to release it to make way for a second fast-approaching cup to be placed on the same location. This alternating method, simply done by applying one cup, taking it off and immediately reapplying it in a

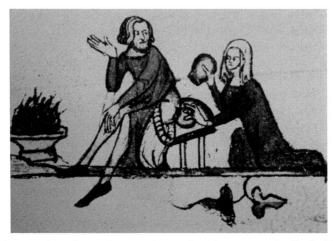

FIGURE 2-5 A medieval woman alternating two large cupping vessels to the treatment site. To the left, there is a fire burning in a large vase, made conclusive by the artist with the speckled effect given to the flying embers. *(Reproduced courtesy of the Wellcome Institute Library, The Wellcome Trust, London.)*

succession of applications is known as 'flash cupping' in modern-day Chinese practice, and in Greek folk-cupping it is the popular way of decongesting phlegm from lung tissue and withdrawing climatic pathogens.[6]

Some of the most fascinating writings on cupping can be found in *Causes and Cures* (*Causae et Curae*) by the canonized saint Hildegard of Bingen (1098–1179). It is remarkable that this text has survived, and it has recently been brought to light by Victoria Sweet (2006) in her excellent book *Rooted in the Earth, Rooted in the Sky: Hildegard of Bingen and Premodern Medicine*. Hildegard was not a formally trained physician, although she did receive medical instruction from monk infirmarians and her education within the monastery allowed her to study medical texts. Her independence, learning and determination had her in a league of her own at a time in Southern Germany that was fraught with social upheaval, intellectual persecution, suspicion and book burnings, making it a difficult and dangerous time for an interesting man, and decidedly so for a very interesting woman. In the estimation of her contemporary interpreters, her practice is considered folk medical (Sweet, 2006; Whaley, 2011), and as Pinto (1973: 513) explains, she took to 'ministering not only to nuns in her monastery, but also to lay people', and adopted their local folklore and oral traditions as well. From *Causes and Cure* she advises, 'if someone has pain in his eyes or ears, or even in his whole body, put a horn (cornu) or a ventosa on his neck and back. If he has a pain in his chest, put ventosas on the scapula: for pain in the side put them on the opposite arm and wrist. For thigh pain, on the legs, for pain in the legs, between the buttocks and on the back of the knees. Leave the ventosas or the horns on for about a quarter of an hour, so that the blood comes to the surface' [as a cupping mark] (Sweet, 2006: 88).

Hildegard also recommended cupping (including the option of other treatment methods) to relieve the effects of certain humoral[7] imbalances brought about by Wind. Indeed she highlights Wind as an illness causation factor with the kind of depth rarely written about outside the writings of the Hippocratic authors and the Yellow Emperor on Chinese medicine some thousand and more years earlier. In her medical theory and practice, she has the body (microcosm) as being permeable to the outside world (macrocosm), and she knew that Wind was an elemental life force that not only circulated internally within the body as a normal physiological constituent, but also as an exogenous factor that could enter into the microcosmic interior through the orifices and the skin pores and tilt the delicate humoural balance in health and cause a pathological process due to Wind excess. One of the chief reasons why cupping continues to remain popular as a folk practice and attracts modern day therapists is because it effectively withdraws climatic pathogenic factors from both the superficial and deeper levels of the body. Hildegard understood the action of cupping as able to play a vital role in the exquisitely holistic healing process that harmonises the interchange of oneself with nature and the universe and vice versa.

But what exactly is this 'Wind' that Hildegard and so many others talk so confidently about in relation to illness and cupping?

WIND AND CUPPING

In modern times, many people describe themselves as 'feeling under the weather' when their health is compromised. Yet the weather is given a limited role in the biomedical aetiology of illness, apart from states such as hypothermia and other types of critical conditions related to extreme climatic exposure. There is, however, a growing number of progressive medical doctors, especially in Europe, who have named their emerging clinical discipline 'biometeorology'. They are convinced that the weather is much more important to our health and wellbeing than solely our thermal comfort. This view has been shared throughout history by countless millions of people. Might this have influenced the building of the first construction, a stone windbreak, by the proto human species known as *Homo habilus* in the Olduvai Gorge in Tanzania 1.9 million years ago?

The connections made between the role that the weather, and in particular the wind, plays on human health has been prominent in all the world's scholarly traditional medical systems including traditional Chinese, Galenic, Unani, Islamic and Ayurvedic medicine. In the world's first medical manuscript, known as *The Edwin Smith Surgical Papyrus*, written in Egypt between 3000 and 2500 BC, we find information that has been deciphered to mean 'winds carrying disease', along with incantations to exorcize the 'wind of the pest' (Breasted, 1930: 473). But it is in the *Hippocratic Corpus* and *The Yellow Emperor's Classic of Internal Medicine* (*Huang Di Nei Jing Su Wen*) from China that its significance is fully elaborated. In the opening statement of 'Airs, Waters, Places' for example, the Hippocratic writer recommends to prospective medical students that they should become fully acquainted with the seasons and the impact of the weather on health before proceeding further with their studies (Jones, 1923: 71). Moreover, when Paulus of Aegineta, the Greco-Roman physician and medical encyclopaedist of the 7th century AD, came to examine what the Hippocratic physicians had written about the weather and its medical machinations he concluded:

Hippocrates gives many interesting observations on the effect of climate, and the state of the atmosphere, in influencing the health; but they are delivered so much in detail, that my limits do not admit of my entering into a full exposition of them.

(Adams, 1846: 64)

In *The Yellow Emperor's Classic of Internal Medicine*, written during the second century BC in the form of a question and answer exchange between the Yellow Emperor (Huang Di) and his medical mentor, the Daoist monk Qi Bo, there are also copious and even dramatic declarations made about the weather, and in particular about Wind. Among his disclosures, Qi Bo assured Huang Di: 'pathogenic wind is the root of all evil' (Ni, 1995: 10), and 'pathogenic Wind heads the six pathogenic factors. It is often called the leader of the rebellion' (Ni, 1995: 78).

One contemporary scholar who deserves applause for breaking the silence of 20th-century historians about the significance of Wind in classical medical literature is Shigehisa Kuriyama. In his chapter 'Wind and Self', he correctly states that people in ancient times were convinced that Wind had a diabolical influence on their health, but considers that in contemporary life, 'we rarely think of Wind, now, when we think of illness' (1999: 233). In my view, however, many people nowadays *do* think about Wind and, even more profoundly, feel and experience its impact on their health and wellbeing – although unfortunately they are often taught to doubt their own experience in the biomedical consultation. To get a glimpse into the directly felt associations between Wind and suffering, consider the many people who are adamant they must endure heightened rheumatic pains when there is a change in the weather. It is common to hear that such pain is experienced most noticeably when they are exposed to cold or hot Wind. One can also question people affected by Bell's (facial) palsy if, in the days before the onset of their condition, they were exposed to windy circumstances. Similarly, ask any primary school teacher about the behaviour of their young students on a windy day, or consider how many weather-sensitive individuals react emotionally and feel anxious during blustery conditions. Likewise office workers who work below a cold air conditioning vent frequently report having a tight, painful neck and shoulders and headaches. Perhaps you have had the experience of sitting in the firing line of hot air blasting from a overhead fan heater and end up with a 'thick' head, with headache, a sore throat, red eyes and fatigue? Many country folk in Australia say that the same happens from being out in the hot wind. Frequently also one finds that a person who wakes up in the morning with an acutely painful wry neck (torticollis) has been exposed to a draft of Cold Wind while sleeping. The chances are that all these people suffering all these different problems will agree that wind, in some form or another, had an undeniable effect on their condition. Yet such cases are sadly lacking in medical literature, unless one is reading about the aetiologies of these conditions from a Chinese medicine text. From the Chinese perspective, wry neck for example, is a severe painful contracture of the muscles on one side of the neck that results from direct exposure to a focused current of wind, which may be entering through an open window or door. This is especially likely to occur during the night-time when the protective energy (Wei Qi), which circulates throughout the surface of the body during waking hours, internalizes within the body's deeper regions during sleep and renders the surface more vulnerable to Wind attack at night. Mr Thang Le, a Vietnamese man who was my teacher in the Buddhist wandering monk medical tradition explained to me why this condition is so painful:

Wind allowed to pass through a narrow opening is 'poisonous' because it is compressed and pierces the flesh like a dagger. Its impact is funnelled and focused, as if adjusting the nozzle of a hose to concentrate its intensity.

You will note that the preceding conditions are mostly concentrated in the upper part of the body. This is characteristic of Wind, being a Yang, elevated, lofty environmental element that mostly affects the uppermost Yang regions (head and thorax) of the body, unlike Damp in contrast, which is Yin, heavy and hence tends to sink into the lower body regions. It is also well understood that Wind attacks the body's outermost levels including the skin pores, muscles and tendons, as well as the Lungs, being the most external and uppermost of the internal organs thus making it the cause for many respiratory ailments. In Tunis, Tunisia, Jamel Saadi Yakoub, a remarkable and inspiring herbalist asserted: 'wind enters the skin pores, eyes and ears and the head. Cupping takes the Cold and Hot, Wind and Damp from the "texture of the skin", the muscle and the bone'.

But the familiarity and endurance of the weather, and in particular Wind, as a lurking menace to health, can be most thoroughly agreed upon as an illness causation factor in folk-based healing practices where rural people in particular have such an intimate relationship with their natural environment. In Asian cultures, the issue of Wind is an inherited way of thinking that is validated consistently through straightforward personal experience. On the other side of the world, in the Mayan communities of Chiapas and Guatemala in Central America, Wind is considered to have just as strong a causal influence on health as it does for the Chinese. In fact, the practice of cupping is known as the 'capturing of the Winds' (García et al, 1999: 165). For people, the experience of Wind causing illness and pain is confirmed when the withdrawing ability of the cupping process brings about a cure.

From my own personal time spent in practice in Australia, I could fill up a book with comments from people from all walks of life about the weather either bringing on an acute condition or exacerbating an existing chronic one. When I was in practice in Taiwan, consultations would often have patients ascribing Wind (*feng*) as the culprit for their aches and pains, and in rural Thailand, scarcely any problem is not blamed on Wind ('*Pen lom*' in Thai, meaning 'caused by the Wind').

How can we know when exogenous Wind is present in the body? In Asian communities, a myriad of both physical and psychological ills are ascribed to Wind. *The Yellow Emperor's Classic of Internal Medicine* (Ni, 1995: 158) explains, 'once it [the Wind] penetrates the body, its dynamic is dynamic and changeable, and it has many pathological manifestations. But the cause [of illness] is always the same: pathogenic Wind attacking the body'. The presence of Wind can be inferred from the symptoms it produces. The characteristic outcomes of Wind penetration includes pain that moves and wanders – making its location unpredictable – just like the inability of wind to be pinned down in the natural world. Conditions such as aching and pain, itchiness, swellings, jerks and spasms, loss of balance and feinting, paralysis, and asocial behaviour are all defined and manifested by the presence of Wind. These ideas are embedded within the mainstream Chinese psyche, with the majority of the population being very careful about exposure to Wind and drafts; in fact, they take active measures to avoid it. It is interesting to note that in folk medical practice in the East, Wind is spoken of as the most pernicious of the meteorological pathogens, whereas in Europe and the Middle East it is Cold first, with Wind coming a close second.

Having spent such time clarifying the perils of Wind, it is only fitting to present two folk medical cupping treatments which feature the 'blanket cupping method'[8] (Fig. 2-6) aimed at getting rid of it.

CASE 2-3 Petra Peevska's Eliminate Wind and Cold Treatment (from Shiroka Laka, Bulgaria)

The Setting. Shiraka Laka is a small and secluded town in the Rhodope Mountains, a range extending along the southern Bulgarian border with Greece. I decided to go into this remote region after hearing that, even during the 40 years of the Communist era, the state had strategically opted to leave the entire area and its people alone, in exchange for information about outsiders attempting to flee across the border. In a lengthy conversation with Emmanuel Moutafor from the Department of Modern Greek Philology at the University of Sophia, he declared the people and culture throughout the Rhodope Mountains to be, 'a goldfield for the cultural anthropologist at the end of the 20th century'.

When I arrived by bus, I discovered there were no hotels to stay, so I introduced myself in the town square by smiling and raising a glass cupping-vessel in the hope that someone would figure out what I was interested in. Remarkably enough, one of the villagers sent for a woman named Maria Groudeva, whose friend was a well-known local cupper. We walked down the cobble stone path in the cold misty rain to her stone house with its mossy slate roof. Inside a fire made everything glad and toasty and warmed the old pagan masks, still worn for annual pre-Christian festivities, hanging on the wall. That evening Maria invited her friend Petra Peevska and a young man who spoke excellent English to dinner. We all stayed up until the early hours of the next morning, chatting, practising and exchanging ideas about cupping.

The following practice is one of Petra's favourites. She uses it to treat respiratory ailments such as common cold and influenza, and pain throughout the back. I asked Petra her opinion on why people catch common cold. She replied, 'often people don't dress warmly enough and make things worse by going outside without drying themselves properly after bathing. Especially their hair – this is no good. When it falls on the back of the neck it gets cold – and especially if cold wind blows, a cold is on its way. Also people staying in drafts easily catch colds. Drafts tighten the muscles too and cause them to ache.' Her treatment for this dilemma is divided into five stages. Petra performed the following practice on Maria, who told me that she had suffered bad shoulder and upper back pain for months until she had received treatment from Petra. She said 'Now I feel much better, but one more treatment won't go astray!'

TREATMENT

1. **Footbath:** Have the patient seated with their feet in a tub of hot salty water. This quickly warms the entire body and encourages sweating, which has the benefit of releasing both Wind and Cold. The water was kept hot by checking the temperature and adding to it when necessary. Having the skin pores dilated and the dynamic of the sweat pushing outwards adds to the deeper drawing power of the cups.

2. **Palpation:** While her patient's feet were bathing in the hot water and the body was warming up, Petra spent the next couple of minutes feeling throughout Maria's back for any irregularities, such as noticeable places of either hot or cold and tight or flaccid musculature. Palpation is the most essential guide to high-level cupping practice. It determines the appropriate suction level to use to harmonize each individual's presenting signs and symptoms.

3. **Cupping:** In preparation, Petra had lined her glass cups along the hearth of the open fire to warm them up. While Maria's feet remained in the hot tub of water, she began to apply about 20 cups, from the upper region of the back down to the bottom of the rib cage. The cups, which were around the size of a medium-sized Chinese cup, were applied bilaterally in linear sequences, from the shoulders down to the lower thoracic region, around T10–T11. She left the lumbar region free of cups because she said, 'it can make people feel tired if you put cups there. This is what my grandmother told me.' Petra did not cup over the spine. Instead she placed the first bilateral line of five cups lateral to the vertebral bodies and evenly spaced apart with about an inch (2.54 cm) of separation. The second row of four cups per side began at the supraspinous region and the third line had cups placed along the intercostal sides. She then covered Maria with a blanket for 15 minutes. (I call this method of covering the back with many cups the 'blanket cupping method'.)

4. **Massage:** Once Petra had removed the cups, she patted her patient's back and neck dry with a towel. She then performed a light five-minute massage to relax the skin where the cups had been.

5. **Liniment:** Petra then briskly rubbed a mixture of iodine and alcohol throughout the entire cupped region, 'to keep the body warm for a long time and to close the skin pores so no more sweating takes place. Too much sweating makes the body tired', she said.

After cupping treatment, Petra always insists that her patient remain indoors in a warm room, and to keep the body covered with plenty of blankets when sleeping. Note:

• Treatment should be performed as soon as symptoms begin.
• It is advised to treat the common cold with this method only up to and including day three. Treatment can be carried out on all days.
• For the treatment of muscular injuries and general discomfort, this practice can be performed anytime.

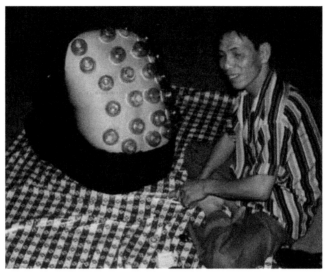

FIGURE 2-6 Dung Mat Zao and the Blanket Cupping technique. *Photo courtesy: Bruce Bentley.*

CASE 2-4   Cupping out the Wind in Vietnam (Street practice in Ho Chi Minh City)

The Setting. Off the curb at a busy intersection in Ho Chi Minh City in 2000, I came across Dung Mat Xao, a young man in his 20s using certain cupping methods I had not seen before. I have since used this treatment many times in clinic and regard it as one of the most effective I know. In Vietnam, 'catching the Wind' or being 'struck by the Wind' (*trung gio*) is the everyday reason ascribed for a plethora of illnesses and aches and pains. This treatment aims to remove Wind. I have named Mr Dung's opening practice the 'swiping off the Wind method' because, for indigenous cuppers, the family practice they were taught is simply called 'cupping'. This treatment schedule, like Petra's, is based on the principal of first eliminating Wind from the surface before progressing to deeper levels. By doing so they both ensure the most successful result.

THE PRACTICE

Stage One. The 'swiping off the Wind method'[9] is achieved by rapidly swiping a cup down alternate surface lines of the back to withdraw the frontline of recent external pathogenic attack (Fig. 2-7A). Special attention is paid to the vertical line known in Chinese medicine as the medial conduit of the Bladder meridian. From an anatomical perspective, this course-way accords closely to the midline of the erector spinae muscles running from the upper back (besides T1 or T2), all the way down to the sacrum. Mr Dung said it is 'the important first stage in ridding the body of Wind'. He said, 'it opens the surface and stimulates the Blood.' While his patient sat cross-legged on a grass mat with his back fully exposed, Mr Dung swiped a cup down the back without oil. This he pointed out had 'an effect similar to performing *cao gio* [pronounced 'gow yor' in Vietnamese, meaning gua sha (see endnote 5)] because it rubs and stimulates the skin'. When there is stagnation due to pathogenic factors lingering within this superficial defensive margin, the empirical evidence of their withdrawal is made clear by a strong red longitudinal mark that appears where the cup has been drawn. These markings, I might add, are far more robust and vibrant than if the

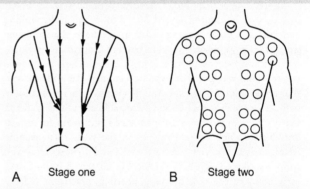

A   Stage one   B   Stage two

FIGURE 2-7 (A) The three course-ways of the 'swiping off the Wind method': Mr Dung said the reason why the two bilateral lines converge parallel with the lower ribs is because this soft and unprotected area below can often be very sensitive. (B) Mr Dung's blanket cupping method: all in all he used 36 cups to cover the entire region from the shoulders down to the hips. (Those cups missing from view in this diagram are located in a line down the sides of the ribs throughout the intercostal region.) *Courtesy: Bruce Bentley.*

same process were performed on someone who did not have any illness or pain. The 'swiping off the Wind method' should be performed only three times and quite lightly for weaker people, and up to nine times in a more robust manner for strong-bodied people. The strength of the person is always more important than the strength of the treatment.

To make this practice easier for the practitioner and more acceptable for the patient in the West, it is advised to smear a sufficient amount of oil over the region before swiping with the cup. Although not as strong as originally performed by Mr Dung, it does have a broader application because only people with a robust constitution should receive his Vietnamese way of going about it.

Be sure that all prospective lines are well lubricated; check by drawing the pad of your index finger down these surfaces. A flame is then thrust inside a cup and withdrawn, with the cup

CASE 2-4 **Cupping out the Wind in Vietnam (Continued)**

suspended above the target site momentarily before application. Allowing a small amount of time to pass enables you measure how strong you want the suction of the cup to be so it will not affix too tightly to the skin surface. The cup is therefore not allowed to remain stationary, but upon touchdown is swiftly drawn from high up on the upper back down to the sacral region. Repeat the process along these alternate lines throughout the broad expanse of the back. Do each pass with enough gusto so the cup audibly 'pops' off at the finish of each swipe to decisively release the gathered-up Wind from inside the cup.

From a traditional Chinese medical perspective, swiping a cup down the back draws Qi and Blood to the area, invigorating it and at the same time to draw out pathogenic influences such as Wind and Cold. Concurrently this mobilises the defensive (Wei) Qi, which resides as an active mesh barrier within the skin and between muscles to protect against Wind, and Wind-assisted pathogens entering the body such as Cold and Heat. Swiping cupping down the Bladder meridian pathways also withdraws pathogenic obstruction from the most externally circulating channel and from the Tai Yang (first or initial) stage of the six divisions of pathogenic progress into the body. This action stops the externally lodged pathogen from progressing from the surface into deeper and more critical internal levels.

The rapid-fire action of swiping also engenders heat, speed and drawing out and lifting off (suction) – which are all dynamic Yang attributes that collectively have the synergistic effect of boosting the body's own defensive capabilities of dislodging and venting any superficial pathogens (especially Wind) from the most superficial (*biao*) level.

Stage Two. Mr Dung then applied cups throughout the entire back, in the same way that Petra did in Treatment One, except that he included the lumbar region (Fig. 2-6 and Fig. 2-7B). He left all the cups on for approximately 10 minutes.

He explained at length to place the first three cups precisely over specific acupoints. These are:

- One cup over the space between C7 and T1, over the point Dazui (Du-14)
- Two cups (bilaterally) one and a half cun lateral to the intervertebral space between T2 and T3, over the point Fengmen (meaning 'Wind door' in Chinese acupuncture).

Cupping these points, according to scholarly Sino-Vietnamese medicine (known as the northern school of traditional Vietnamese medicine) is also noted to effectively withdraw Wind.

Stage Three. Mr Dung removed the cups and asked his patient if they felt itchy at any location where the cups had been. Itchiness is traditionally recognised to be a definitive indicator of Wind. His patient described one position on his upper back, which happened to precisely correspond with a dark circular mark produced by a cup. In Vietnamese folk practice, cupping marks are typically an indication that Wind has been successfully brought to the skin surface. It then passes through the skin and disperses back into the atmosphere. Mr Dung then proceeded to cup over the itch with the flash cupping method, which in this case, required the cup to be applied with a fairly strong vacuum level and then removed within a second or two. This he repeated another three times and enquired whether there was still any itch. His patient declared that he could feel it shifting laterally beyond where it had been previously cupped and so, like a hound after a rabbit, Mr Dung went after the passage of the itch by flash cupping its ongoing pathway until it had been completely resolved. This deserves to be called the 'chasing the Wind method'.

ENDNOTES

1. For a critique on the discreditation of cupping in the West beginning around the 1880s, refer to the 1996 MA Thesis 'Cupping as Therapeutic Technology', Latrobe University, Melbourne, Australia.
2. To learn about using cups to draw out Coldness and tonify weakness due to chronic injury, refer to the essay 'Cupping Deficiency' (Bentley, 2011).
3. In collaboration with Shirley Gabriel, an Australian massage therapist, we have developed a broad range of new cupping practices, made possible with silicone cupping vessels, to rectify myofascial integrity. We call this 'Modern Cupping'.
4. In China, cupping or *ba huoguan* was first known as *jiaofa*, meaning 'horn method', because hollow animals horns were commonly used as cupping vessels.
5. For more information read my essay 'Gua Sha: Smoothly scraping out the Sha' (Bentley, 2010).
6. In the essay 'Explorations of cupping in Greece' (Bentley, 2012), there are descriptions of two Greek cupping practices that remove pathogenic Cold.
7. The term 'humours' describes the four cardinal fluids (Blood, Phlegm, Yellow Bile and Black Blood) considered to be the essential constituents of the body. From the time of Hippocrates through to the 19th century this medical theory, based on the principal that health was maintained or restored when each was in harmony and balance with the others, dominated the Western medical tradition.
8. The 'Blanket cupping method' is where many cups are placed over a body part, be it the back or legs or chest. It has been explained to me that it is important to cup so extensively because Wind is devious and unpredictable and not bound by any pattern. It can move anywhere. Its presence will always show according to the mark produced. Some practitioners barely allow a skerrick of flesh to go uncupped. In Cambodia I counted 68 cups on one person's back. This method is widely practised from Lithuania through to Vietnam.
9. Video footage of the 'swiping off the Wind method' can be seen at www.healthtraditons.com.au.

REFERENCES

Adams, F., 1846. The Seven Books of Paulus Aegineta, vol. 1, Book 1. C & J Adlard, London.

Arnott, R., 2004. Minoan and Mycenaean medicine and its Near Eastern contacts. In: Horstmanshoff, H.F.J., Stol, M. (Eds.), Magic and Rationality in Ancient Near Eastern and Greco-Roman Medicine. Brill, Leiden.

Bannerman, R.H., Burton, J., Wen-Chieh, Ch'en, 1983. Traditional Medicine Coverage: A Reader for Health Administrators and Practitioners. World Health Organization, Geneva

Bentley, B., 1996. Cupping as Therapeutic Technology. Master of Arts (in Health Studies) thesis. Latrobe University, Victoria, Australia.

Bentley, B., 2010. Gua Sha: Smoothly scraping out the Sha. The Lantern 4 (2), 4–9. Online. Available: www.healthtraditions.com.au.

Bentley, B., 2011. Cupping Deficiency. The Lantern 8 (2), 15–27. Online. Available: www.healthtraditions.com.au.

Bentley, B., 2012. Explorations of cupping in Greece. The Lantern 10 (1), 18–22. Online. Available: www.healthtraditions.com.au.

Bentley, B., 2013. Mending the fascia with Modern Cupping. The Lantern 10 (3), 4–21. Online. Available: www.healthtraditons.com.au.

Breasted, J.H., 1930. The Edwin Smith surgical papyrus. vol. 1. University of Chicago Press, Illinois.

Clark, L., 1998. Gender and generation in poor woman's household health production experiences. In: Brown, P. (Ed.), Understanding and Applying Medical Anthropology. Mayfield Publishing, Mountain View CA, pp. 158–168 (Chapter 17).

Eliade, M., 1989. Shamanism: Archaic Techniques of Ecstasy. Arkana Penguin, London.

Elkin, A.P., 1994. Aboriginal Men of High Degree: Initiation and Sorcery in the World's Oldest Tradition. Inner Traditions, Rochester.

Finerman, R., 1989. The forgotten healers: women as family healers in an Andean Indian Community. In: McClain, C.S. (Ed.), Women as Healers: Cross Cultural Perspectives. Rutgers University Press, New Brunswick NJ, pp. 122–134.

García, H., Sierra, A., Balám, G., 1999. Wind in the Blood: Mayan Healing and Chinese Medicine. (J. Conant, Trans.) North Atlantic Books, Berkeley CA.

Garrison, F.H., 1913. An Introduction to the History of Medicine. W. B. Saunders, Philadelphia.

Griggs, B., 1981. Green Pharmacy: A History of Herbal Medicine. Jill Norman & Hobson, London.

Gruner, O.C., 1930. A Treatise on The Cannon of Medicine of Avicenna. Luzac, London.

Harper, D., 1998. Early Chinese Medical Literature: The Mawangdui Medical Manuscripts. Kegan Paul, London.

Jones, W.H.S., 1923. Hippocrates. vol. II. William Heinemann, London.

Kleinman, A., 1980. Patients and Healers in the Context of Culture: An Exploration of the Borderland Between Anthropology, Medicine, and Psychiatry. Comparative Studies of Health Systems and Health Care, No 3. University of California Press, Berkeley.

Kuriyama, S., 1999. The Expressiveness of the Body and the Divergence of Greek and Chinese Medicine. Zone Books, New York.

Leininger, M., 1976. Towards conceptualization of transcultural health care systems: concepts and a model. J. Transcult. Nurs. 4, 2.

McKeown, T., 1970. A sociological approach to the history of medicine. Med. Hist. 14 (4), 342–351.

Mukhopadhyaya, G., 1913. The Surgical Instruments of the Hindus. vol. 1. Calcutta University Press, Calcutta.

Ni, M., 1995. The Yellow Emperor's Classic of Medicine. Shambhala, Boston.

Nutton, V., 1998. Healers in the medical market place: towards a social history of Greco-Roman medicine. In: Wear, A. (Ed.), Medicine in Society: Historical Essays. Cambridge University Press, Cambridge, UK.

Pinto, L.B., 1973. The folk practice of gynecology and obstetrics in the middle ages. Bull. Hist. Med. 47, 155–523.

Porter, R., 1997. The Greatest Benefit to Mankind: A Medical History from Antiquity to the Present. Harper Collins, London.

Porter, R., Weir, A. (Eds.), 1987. Problems and Methods in the History of Medicine. Wellcome Institute Series in the History of Medicine, Croom Helm, London.

Spencer, W.G., 1953. Celsus De Medicina Book II. The Loeb Classical Library. vol. 11. William Heinemann, London pp. 1–5.

Sweet, V., 2006. Rooted in the Earth, Rooted in the Sky: Hildegard of Bingen and Premodern Medicine. Routledge, New York.

Turk, J.L., Allen, E., 1983. Bleeding and cupping. Ann. R. Coll. Surg. Engl. 65 (2), 128–133.

Unschuld, P.U., 1979. Medicine in China: A History of Ideas. University of California Press, Berkeley CA.

Whaley, L., 2011. Women and the Practice of Medical Care in Early Modern Europe, 1400-1800. Palgrave MacMillan, Basingstoke, Hants.

CUPPING IN BUDDHIST MEDICINE

3

CHAPTER CONTENTS

WHAT IS BUDDHIST MEDICINE?, 33
INTRODUCTION TO THE PRINCIPLES OF
BUDDHIST MEDICINE, 34
DISTURBANCE AND IMBALANCE OF
ELEMENTS, 35
A COMPLEMENTARY THERAPY: CUPPING
IN BUDDHIST MEDICINE, 36

INTRODUCTION TO CUPPING IN
TRADITIONAL LANNA MEDICINE, 41
THE WIND ELEMENT EXPLANATION IN
TLM, 43
APPLICATIONS OF THAI CUPPING
THERAPY, 44
ACKNOWLEDGEMENTS, 46

3-1 *Cupping in Buddhist Medicine*

Pedro Paiva

WHAT IS BUDDHIST MEDICINE?

Buddhist medicine is the natural result of the Buddha's teaching on freeing beings from existential suffering through the realization of ultimate truth. Buddhahood is a state of mind in which the individual has attained perfect freedom from the compulsive pull of changeable emotional states and thoughts, and manifests perfect wisdom and compassion. This compassion is expressed in a practical wisdom that provides relief and treatment not only for the ultimate suffering of existence but also for the relative sufferings of physical and mental illness.

Both Buddhist healers and patients can draw, through their religious tradition, on about 2600 years' worth of empirical knowledge on the prevention and healing of illness. In India, Buddhist medicine (known as Cikitsāvidya or Bodhicikitsā) originating in the teachings of the Buddha naturally became included in the canonical Buddhist scriptures, particularly in the *Tripiṭaka* but also in other texts and commentaries. It forms a corpus of transcultural wisdom that has adapted to the various sociocultural conditions without losing its timeless essence – like Buddhism itself, which many scholars call 'the earliest world religion'. Buddhist medicine has been disseminated along with the Buddhist religion through countries lying on the Silk Road, and through sea routes across Asia, always expressing a vision of the body, illness and healing that is wider than a materialistic one. Buddhist understanding about the relative nature of these body processes has thus transcended all cultural and religious boundaries, and influenced such vast and diverse territories as India, Sri Lanka, Thailand, Burma, Tibet, Korea, China and Japan. However, it was in China that it formally assumed the designation of Buddhist medicine – Fojiao Yixue – to distinguish it from the already existing Chinese traditional medicine (TCM).

Despite the adaptation of Buddhist medicine to diverse cultures, there are common core aspects. These comprise the root vision of Buddhist doctrine: illness as one of the four general unavoidable sufferings of conditioned existence (the others being birth, ageing and death), and illumination as the only definite cure for all these. The five 'components' of the human body naturally bear the potential for human suffering; of these, the aggregate of form / body is compounded by four elements that antagonize each other, and from which illness naturally stems. Karma is the principle of cause and effect (not 'destiny'), which is the main cause of illness, and Kleshas, or conflicting emotions, are one of the main causes of humour imbalance. Both medical and therapeutic actions are inseparable from Buddhism spiritual practice.

INTRODUCTION TO THE PRINCIPLES OF BUDDHIST MEDICINE

According to the Buddhist vision, which is the theoretical basis of Buddhist medicine, the universe is composed of the aggregation of subatomic particles that bear the qualities and functions of the great four elements: Earth, Water, Fire and Wind. These four interact in and with a fifth basic element, Space, and from this all aspects of the universe emerge, including phenomenal content and living beings.

From the medical point of view, three energies arising from this are especially meaningful: Wind, Fire and Water. These elements not only assemble to form the body, but also express the qualities of the mind. At death, these elements disassemble once more. During their life, the relation of individuals with these elements determines the quality of their experiences, as follows:

Wind creates and manages a vast number of functions. The best examples are breathing, inner energy flow, and circulation as expressed by blood circulation, the circulation of impulses through the nervous system, the arising of thoughts in the mind, and the transport of substances through the digestive system and the excreting organs. In the mind, it expresses itself as desire and attachment, and also conditions the individual's view of the material world. It manages memory, presence, sensory perception and speech. It also controls the opening and closing of bodily orifices.

Fire functions as the discriminative intellectual function of the mind, and originates and controls metabolism, hepatic function, eyesight, heart, gall bladder and skin. Most particularly, it regenerates the body and blood components. In the mind, the energy of Fire manifests as aggression, hate, anger, but also as zest and courage.

Water creates the physical principle by which energy is manifested in various functions. It relates to the lubrication processes in our body, and is also concerned with will and good memory, amongst other things. In the mind, Water is expressed as ignorance or lack of understanding, but also as mental stability and sensory satisfaction, and it is also related to taste experience and sleep quality.

Individual Typification

Individuals will differ in their psychosomatic constitutions according to the predominance of the above energies, as follows:

Individuals with Wind Predominance

Such individuals tend to be thin, with little physical strength and unhealthy complexions. They tend to walk with a slight crouch and are subject to many desires. When walking or moving, their joints can crack noisily. These people talk a lot and can be quite stern. They sleep little and cold weather does not agree with them. They enjoy singing and dancing. Their vitality is low, their life expectancy short and their metabolism is variable.

Individuals with Fire Predominance

These people tend to have a yellowish complexion and frequently feel hunger and thirst. Their physical strength is moderate, and they have a great tendency to sweat. They tend to be intellectually sharp and full of pride, are often entrepreneurs but can be uncaring. Their vitality and life expectancy are average. Their metabolism is strong and their bodily temperature is higher than normal.

Individuals with Water Predominance

The physical constitution of these individuals is robust, they are large and have great physical strength. Mentally their temperament tends to be easy-going and devoid of malice, they are good-humoured and have a relaxed nature. They tend to walk bending slightly backwards. They tolerate hunger and thirst well, and sleep deeply. They enjoy a long life expectancy, and often have a low body temperature and slow metabolism.

Most individuals are a mix of two or more of the above constitutions, however, single types being rare. A balanced combination of the three types is the most favourable condition for individuals, both physically and emotionally.

DISTURBANCE AND IMBALANCE OF ELEMENTS

A disturbance in any or in the combination of the elements results in disease. Disturbance can arise from eating behaviours or from environmental factors that, from their own component elements, act to disturb the characteristics of the body's elements. This results in disease in diverse ways, depending on the acute or chronic nature of the problem. Also, all illnesses must be seen as individual based on a patient's particular background.

Causes of Disease

The causes for disease are of three types: predictable causes, causes arising from daily habits, and unpredictable causes. According to Yogin Suklavastra's classic presentation, these are as follows:

Predictable Causes

- Basic elemental causes, from the effects of either their single energies or in combination with other elements
- Environmental variations caused by the change of season
- Age: infancy, childhood, young adulthood, maturity and old age
- Time of day
- Astrological conditions
- Conditions related to the location.

Daily Habits

- Eating and drinking habits
- Sleeping habits
- Work and exercise habits
- Posture: sitting, standing, walking, lying down
- Temperature extremes
- Emotional tendencies
- Repression of natural impulses.

Unpredictable Causes

- Accidents
- Poisoning
- Ghosts, spirit and demonic attacks
- Human aggression, thugs and guns
- Black magic.

Given that health depends on a balance of elements and energies, and their harmonic interaction, it follows naturally that disturbing and destabilizing conditions may cause various diseases to develop, such as an imbalance of constitutional energies arising from bad nutrition, negative emotions, bad conduct, trauma, attack by spirits, etc. Thus several types of imbalance may arise: deficiency or excess of elements, or 'conflict' between them. According to the Master Dharmaraja Ratna Akash, the causes are summarized as follows:

Wind diseases can result, for example, from eating too much light food, raw food, and generally little nourishing food, but also from lack of proper sleep, working on an empty stomach, too much sexual activity, exposure to cold and wind, intense intellectual activity, excessive talking; from sadness, worrying and mental obsession, among others.

Fire diseases can result for example from an excess of spicy and oily food, excess of alcohol, and excessive exertion at work and physical exercise, but also from afternoon naps, exposure to dry and hot environments, etc.

Water diseases can result from excess sugar in the diet, but also from too much oily, heavy and cold food. They can also arise from none or little physical exercise, and from sleeping during the day. Cold and wet environments are particularly destabilizing to mindsets characterized by apathy and passivity, as are also eating vitality-lacking food, such as fast food and milk products, and also lengthy intervals between meals.

Symptoms of Imbalance

Some symptoms of elemental imbalance are listed by the Buddhist Yogin Vajrabodhi as:

For Wind, visible and recognizable inquietude, jitters, reduction in the function of sensory organs, trembling, frequent need to stretch the limbs, frequent yawning. Also pain on the hips, waist and joints, and shifting pains. Nausea and retching. All these symptoms are aggravated by an empty stomach.
For Fire, a bitter taste in the mouth is a telling sign, and also hypothermia, sharp pains on the upper part of the body and headache. All the symptoms are aggravated after digestion is completed.
For Water, lack of appetite and difficult digestions can be observed, as also vomiting, heaviness after meals, burping, fatigue and apathy, and a generalized feeling of cold. All symptoms are aggravated after meals.

Additional symptoms of imbalance of these elements in the body can be observed by tongue, wrist and urine diagnosis.

Treatment Approaches

Once the nature of the imbalance or illness is diagnosed, it can be treated through multiple approaches: dietary changes, behavioural changes, appropriate medication and the use of external therapies, one of which is cupping.

A COMPLEMENTARY THERAPY: CUPPING IN BUDDHIST MEDICINE

The practice of cupping was widespread in the ancient world and so it became included in Buddhist medicine. In Tibet, Thailand and other countries, heated cups made of copper, horn, glass and bamboo were used to ease both chronic and acute located pain. Cupping has been used since antiquity in Eastern naturopathy to increase the blood circulation in the back and shoulders, to relax tense and stressed muscles, and to ease chronic pain throughout the body.

There is historical evidence in old Tibetan and Chinese texts that cupping has been practised in both countries for 3500 years. Since then, Buddhist medicine has maintained that cupping can help unblock the channels that carry the vital energy (Qi), thus contributing to rejuvenation, revitalization and regeneration of worn and tired bodily tissues.

The cupping technique generally consists of holding a naked flame under the cup and then immediately pressing the heated cup on the part of the body to be treated (though there are many other traditional cupping methods). The vacuum created by the flame inside the cup exerts a suction on the skin and body tissues directly underneath, and creates a powerful lifting action of both tissues and skin. This lifting action causes an increase in the blood circulation in the treated area and an activation of the lymphatic system, thus allowing the elimination of dangerous toxins such as carcinogens in that area. Due to the action on the deep tissues, it also constitutes a powerful method of deep massage.

Traditionally, copper or glass cups are used. Copper is said to have absorption properties that help negative energy to exit the body, and silver and brass are said to share those properties, though glass cups are most used nowadays. The technique extracts impurities and brings blood to the skin, and is known as *Dry cupping*. *Wet cupping* involves cutting the cupping marks to allow the practitioner to extract impure or stagnated blood.

Modern methods must be also mentioned, such as those using plastic cups that rely on a valve and hand pump for suction. These allow the therapists, specially beginners, better control over suction intensity, as well as monitoring of the skin reaction and the overall therapeutic process. Nevertheless, we must not ignore the fact that particular cup materials can add to the effects of the therapy, as can various oils used as lubricant on the areas to be treated. As for the duration of the cupping, this will depend mainly on the state of the patient's health. All these procedures rebalance the humors and restore health.

Uses for Cupping Therapy

- When there is a perceived sensation of 'blockage', in either a physical or emotional sense
- Rigidity, tension and blocking of the neck, chest and breathing tract due to excessive mucus
- Energy stagnation
- Relief of musculoskeletal rigidity, tension and pain
- Digestive problems
- Blood circulation problems
- Diverse conditions related to humoral imbalance:
  - Pain and swelling
  - Respiratory disorders
  - Skin conditions such as boils, eczema
  - Facial paralysis
  - Common colds.

Since the technical aspects of cupping in Buddhist medicine are quite similar to those described elsewhere in this book by Ilkay Chirali and by Kei Ngu (who in Part 2 of this chapter describes cupping in traditional Thai medicine, a variant of Buddhist medicine adapted to Thai culture, tradition and climate), I have not burdened the reader with a repetition of similar content here.

As Buddhist medicine is essentially an oral tradition that relies on apprenticeship, it is difficult to discuss at length the diagnostic methods (namely those that use the cupping marks themselves), the energy lines and points according to Buddhist tradition, and the characteristics of the oils, plants and other therapeutic aids used in Buddhist medicine. I therefore simply present a handful of case studies below, and recommend all those who are truly interested in learning to learn more to seek an apprenticeship with a teacher of Buddhist medicine, and I would be pleased to suggest qualified masters in this medical lineage.

Case Studies

CASE 3-1 Female Patient Aged 34 (Fatigue and Mental Issues)

Condition. Fatigue, mental agitation and depression

Medication. None

Pulse Observation. Preponderance (big) of Wind element, weak and irregular.

Background. The patient works in the accounts department of the local municipality. The responsibility entailed and the competition experienced in the workplace cause great mental agitation and emotional and physical stress. The ongoing economic recession has recently led to reductions in the workforce, causing anxiety about career and job dissatisfaction. The patient's partner is in an unstable work situation, leading to worries at home and relationship problems. The patient is very thin and has sleep problems.

Diagnosis. Imbalance of Wind element causing the mental disquietude, depression and insomnia. Wind element is also perturbing Fire element.

Objective of Treatment. Overall rebalancing of elements and stabilization of Wind element.

Treatment. Dietary change to rebalance elements. Breathing exercises to calm the mind. Application of compresses with medicinal herbs, namely nutmeg, on the body points that control the inner Wind to calm the anxiety and mental agitation, and address the restlessness and insomnia. The patient has also used a phytotherapic tonic.

Cupping therapy was applied with Flash cupping and Light cupping in 10-minute sessions.

Moxibustion therapy was used on the Wind control points in the cervical spine and thoracic areas.

Massage therapy was used with oils to calm the Wind element and enhance Water element without an effect on Fire element.

Results. The patient felt less tense and physically more relaxed after the first session, but her insomnia continued. After five sessions, improvement in sleep quality and reduction in restlessness were observed, and the patient showed more acceptance of her work situation and a more relaxed attitude in her relationship. She was then changed to a monthly session maintenance routine, and was advised to start a regular meditation practice so as to handle her emotional issues better, without either suppressing or compulsively acting on her thoughts and emotions.

CASE 3-2 Female Patient Aged 26 (Cervical Pain and Immobility)

Condition. Cervical spine trauma in a car accident

Medication. Cervical collar, anti-inflammatory and analgesic medication.

Observations and Background. Neck immobility, strong muscular tension in the cervical area, and headaches. The patient had been given a recovery prognosis of 6 to 9 months, which led to professional issues as the patient is a personal trainer.

Diagnosis. Blocking and stagnation of Wind and Blood on the cervical area due to backlash trauma. Inflammation of muscles and tendons caused by the hyper-stretching. Blocking, tension and stagnation of the meridians and stress causing the headaches.

Objectives of Treatment. Tension and muscular rigidity relief. Dealing with the inflammatory condition. Unblocking Blood stagnation and re-establishing Wind flow in the meridians.

Treatment. Massage therapy was used on reflex and relaxing points with anti-inflammatory oils. Also vibratory massage techniques were used on the meridians.

Cupping therapy was applied on the trigger points of the affected area.

Results. Immediate relief of headache after the first session. After six sessions, spaced regularly three times a week, the patient was able to leave off the cervical collar, except when driving. Total recovery in $2\frac{1}{2}$ months.

CASE 3-3 Male Patient Aged 68 (Shoulder lesion)

Condition. Lesion on shoulder, pain and arm mobility issues.

Medication. None.

Observation and Background. The patient is a dentist and the lesion on the shoulder had been caused by the many repetitive small-amplitude movements he employed in his professional work.

Diagnosis. Blocking, stagnation and inflammation. Tendinitis.

Objectives of Treatment. Relief of tension and muscular rigidity. Addressing the inflammatory condition, unblocking Blood stagnation and re-establishing Wind flow in the meridians.

Treatment. Massage therapy was used with anti-inflammatory oils.

Cupping therapy was applied to reflex points on the shoulder, and also locally on the affected area (Fig. 3-1).

Treatment was in four sessions, with a 1-day interval between each.

Results. Mobility partially recovered after the first session, and pain was felt partially only in the extension and abduction movements of the shoulder. After the third session the immobility and pain disappeared and the treatment was discontinued because the patient had completely recovered.

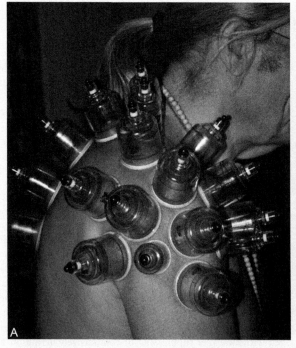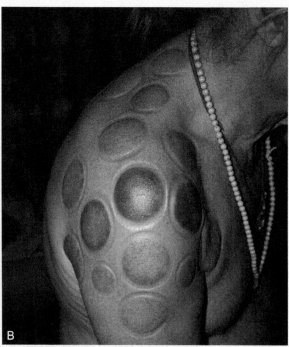

FIGURE 3-1 (A) Treatment of shoulder pain; (B) result after treatment.

CASE 3-4 Male Patient Aged 80 (Shoulder lesion)

Condition. Shoulder lesion, pain and immobility after a fall.

Medication. Anti-inflammatory and analgesic medication.

Observation and Background. After the fall, the patient had received hospital treatment, which comprised anti-inflammatory and analgesic medication, application of ice and balms, and physiotherapy massage. After 3 months without recovery, the patient attended our clinic, complaining of pain, inability to move the arm and sleep problems due to muscular sensitivity.

Diagnosis. Blocking and stagnation of Wind and Blood on the trauma area on the shoulder. Inflammation of the muscle and the tendon. Blocking, tension and stagnation of meridians down the arm reaching the hand.

Objectives of Treatment. Relief of pain and muscular rigidity. Addressing the inflammatory condition, unblocking Blood stagnation and re-establishing Wind flow in the meridians.

Treatment. Massage therapy was applied on the reflex and relaxing points using anti-inflammatory oils.

Moxibustion therapy was applied on the reflex points of shoulder, elbow and forearm.

Cupping therapy applied on the reflex points of shoulder, and also locally on the affected area.

Treatment was in five sessions with 48-hour intervals between each.

Results. After the first session, there was partial reduction of pain and the flexion and extension shoulder movements were recovered, the sole remaining difficulty being in the horizontal abduction and adduction movements. Between the second and third sessions the pain disappeared and the patient was able to sleep without discomfort. He regained the amplitude of the remaining shoulder movements. At the conclusion of the treatment the patient felt fully recovered.

CASE 3-5 Female Patient Aged 37 (Sacral pain)

Condition. Lumbago.

Observation and Background. Severe pain affecting also the sacral area. The patient attempts to stand up rather crookedly, but cannot maintain an upright position due to backlash pain in the lumbar area. The patient is suffering from functional incapacity, since she works in catering and spends many hours daily standing on high-heeled shoes. She also suffers from longstanding work-related stress.

Diagnosis. Blocking and stagnation of Wind and Blood on the lumbar region of trauma. Inflammation of muscles and tendons due to repetitive effort and incorrect posture. Blocking, tension and stagnation in the adjacent meridians.

Objectives of Treatment. Relief of pain and muscular rigidity. Addressing the inflammatory condition, unblocking Blood stagnation and re-establishing Wind flow in the meridians.

Treatment. Massage therapy was applied along the spinal column and on the reflex and relaxing points, with anti-inflammatory oils.

Cupping therapy was applied on the affected area, gluteal muscles and on the leg (Fig. 3-2, Fig. 3-3).

Treatment was in five sessions, the first three taking place consecutively and the last two with a 48-hour interval.

Results. After the first session, the patient regained a vertical posture and also the ability to walk unaided; she also reported reduction in her pain. After the second and third sessions, she recovered full mobility, though reported some of the pain was still present. After the third session, the patient was able to resume her job, with limitations. At the completion of the treatment, she felt completely recovered from her lumbar area to the top of her head.

CASE 3-5

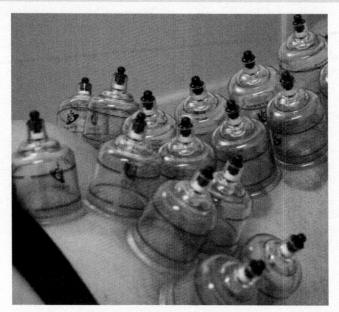

FIGURE 3-2 Treatment of lumbago pain.

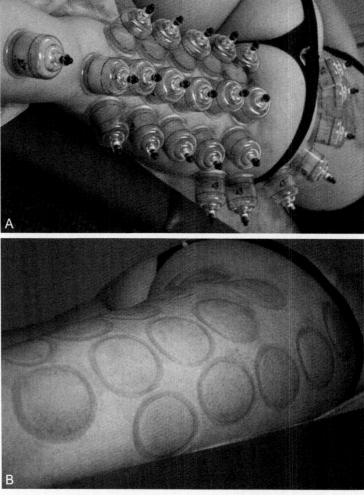

FIGURE 3-3 (A) Treatment of sciatica pain; (B) result after treatment.

3-2 *Cupping in Thailand's Traditional Lanna Medicine*

Kei Ngu

INTRODUCTION TO CUPPING IN TRADITIONAL LANNA MEDICINE

What is Traditional Lanna Medicine?

Traditional Thai medicine (TTM) and traditional Lanna medicine (TLM) are two separate traditions. TTM is the standardized form of traditional medicine which was established during the time of the first, second and third kings of the Chakri dynasty and was later codified and standardized by the prominent doctors during the reign of the fifth king. It has been again revamped and re-standardized by the Ministry of Public Health during the last 50 years. Although TTM has some common features with the Lanna tradition (northern tradition) of medicine, it is a separate system.

Cupping can be found in almost every country where traditional medicine is practised. In TLM, it is one of the most popular physical therapies and is used together with bone setting, scraping, bleeding, compresses (cold, hot, dry, wet), liniments, balms, saunas, tok sen (hitting therapy), massage, etc. Traditionally the oldest cupping tools were horns, which were then replaced with clay cups and bamboo cups, and, latterly, with glass cups. In Thailand practitioners use whatever is handy! Sometimes cupping is used in conjunction with bleeding. In northern Thailand the traditional doctors use mantras with the cupping treatment. According to Ajahn Dao (one of my teachers from Thailand), it is quite common for TLM doctors to use mantras with cupping and other Lanna medicine and, in fact, it is an essential part of the tradition.

General Description of the Four Elements

In TLM there are four body elements – Earth, Water, Fire and Wind – that interact with and affect each other. Actually, the term 'element' refers to the qualities and not to the actual substance. For example, when we refer to Water, we are talking about its qualities and not the water itself; regarding any solid substances, we say that they have the qualities of the Earth element. The same applies for the other elements.

Balance and the harmony between the four elements is essential to create a positive effect in the body. A person with a good balance of the four elements will achieve good health, have overall immunity from disease and will be stronger. Conversely, when an imbalance of any body elements occurs – as for example excess or deficiency – this will lead to the development of various symptoms and eventually diseases.

Characteristic Qualities of the Elements in TLM

Earth Element

Experience: Solidity
Function: Resistance and support
Qualities: Hard, stable, heavy
Temperature: Mild
Parts of the body:

- Hair of the head
- Hair of the body
- Nails
- Teeth
- Skin
- Muscles
- Tendons and ligaments, vessels and nerves
- Bones
- Bone marrow
- Kidneys
- Heart
- Liver and pancreas

- Fascia (sometimes the diaphragm or sometimes the pleura)
- Spleen
- Lungs
- Large intestine
- Small intestine
- Stomach and new food
- Digested food and faeces
- Brain and central nervous system.

Water Element

Experience: Aqueousness
Function: Cohesion and fluidity
Qualities: Moist, fluid and soft
Temperature: Cold
Parts of the body:

- Bile
- Mucus and phlegm
- Pus and lymph
- Blood
- Sweat
- Fat
- Tears
- Oil
- Saliva
- Snot (mucus in the nose and throat)
- Synovial fluid
- Urine.

Fire Element

Experience: Heat
Function: Transformation and ripening
Qualities: Bright, reactive and sharp
Temperature: Hot
Parts of the body:

- Fire that causes ageing and decay of the body
- Fire that provides warmth to the body
- Fire that digests
- Fire that causes emotion and fever.

Wind Element

Experience: Movement
Function: Growth and vibration
Qualities: Light, mobile and dry
Temperature: Cool
Parts of the body:

- Wind that moves from the top of the head to the feet / Wind that moves from the top of the head to the abdomen
- Wind that moves from the feet to the head / Wind that moves from the abdomen to the top of the head
- Wind that is within the digestive tract
- Wind within the abdomen but outside of the digestive tract
- Wind that circulates to all parts of the body including the extremities
- Wind that is inhaled and exhaled.

THE WIND ELEMENT EXPLANATION IN TLM

In the TLM system it is understood that the internal environment is affected by the external environment. The Wind element in nature is *movement*, for example the wind rustling the leaves or animating nature. The body's health and harmony depend on the balance and smooth flow of 'internal Wind' within the body. At the same time, internal Wind is the most insubstantial and easily affected and distorted element in the body. The most effective way to keep Wind in balance is through the practice of Reusi Datton (Thai hermit exercise). *When the Wind element flows naturally through the channels in a harmonious way, the body itself will be in balance.*

When the Wind is distorted this will cause different imbalances in the body such as: joint stiffness, pain that moves, bloating from gas, anxiety and problems with mobility. Cold foods, irregular schedule, lack of sleep and over-study can all contribute to a disturbed Wind element in the body. For example, when Wind accumulates at a particular point that can't be dealt in a manner, such as by the skin, it turns into a 'waste product'. This 'waste product' must be purged from the body. Cupping is one of the best ways that this can be done effectively.

Diagnosing Wind in the Body

Wind diagnosis is part of a complex system for diagnosing the pathogenic elements in the body. However, this training can't be learned from a book; a teacher and long practice are required for this kind of training. Therefore, the explanation below will be a limited to a brief introduction.

Diagnosis is performed at the Wind gate points (places where the Wind 'pools') – points that are used for assessing, redirecting, releasing and manipulating the flow of Wind. The points are located in superficial areas around the joints in the extremities, the abdomen, the clavicular fossa and the temples (temporal fossa). These areas are also places where one can easily access the rhythm and flow of Wind in the channels. When palpating these points we are looking for the general characteristics of the invading Wind so, though physically working on a pulse, we are accessing more than this; we are checking the pulse quality – is it hard or soft, fast or slow, deep or superficial, tense or relaxed, smooth or irregular, empty or full?

All channels originate at the navel. We first evaluate this Wind gate and then move bilaterally towards the periphery noticing where the peripheral pulses differ from the navel pulse. By doing so we can evaluate the flow of Wind throughout the channel system and see where it is becoming disrupted or blocked. Primarily the Wind gates are located near the navel, temples, wrists and ankles. Once you have established the location of the Wind disturbance you can work out the treatment protocol.

Causes of Disease

For an explanation of these refer to 'Cupping in Buddhist medicine' (in Part 1 above) as the causes of disease in that tradition are very much the same as in LTM.

Layers of the Body

There are five layers in the body: the skin, tissues, channels, bones and organs. The disease's natural progression is from the outside to the inside. It also *condenses* as it penetrates into the deeper layers of the body. By its suction action, cupping reverses this process. Pathogenic factors such as the Wind element are brought up from the deeper channels to the more superficial channels where they can be expelled from the body. Depending on which layer of the body you are working on, it is important to work on the layers above the blockage when applying the cupping treatment. To make the cupping treatment more effective we can manipulate the channels during a session and move toxins towards the cup. You must pay attention to the direction in which you work the channels and how you are manipulating the flow of the Wind. For example, if the diagnosis indicates toxic Wind, we would work towards the cup and be mindful not to draw the toxins towards the periphery.

How an External Pathogen Enters Through the Layers of the Body

External pathogen enters through the skin → to the tissues → enters the channels → goes the bone → to the hollow organs (those which have contact with outside the body, e.g. lungs, bladder, stomach, intestines) → to the solid organs (those that are solid and considered 'vital', e.g. spleen, liver, heart, etc.).

The defence for the external Wind pathogen is the skin. However, if the body is weak due to an illness or already has a Wind invasion then the skin will not do its job properly (i.e. defending body from the outside attack!). Once the Wind goes through the skin, it penetrates down to the tissue, and once in the tissue it will create pain. If the problem is not treated then the Wind or pathogens will then penetrate to the channels lying just beneath the skin, and from here the Wind and pathogens will circulate throughout the body, and the person will experience more systemic problems. Then once the pathogens reach the level of the bone the problem will become even more serious, difficult to treat and also may cause more permanent damage. The same principle applies when the pathogen is permitted to penetrate to the levels of the organs.

The Sen (Channels) in TLM
(by Ajahn Wit, TLM and TTM Doctor)

In TLM there are different kinds of channels in the body. We can talk about two main kinds: channels of the *physical body* and *the subtle channels*. The difference between these two channels is that the first group of channels is visible, palpable and can be manipulated with medicine, cupping, massage and other therapies including Ruisi Datton (Thai yoga). The subtle channels are not visible and are not physically palpable. But these channels can be manipulated through meditation, visualization, breathing and other methods. These subtle channels are predominantly related to the mind first, and to the physical body later, whereas with the gross channels it is the reverse. When we talk about channels in LTM, we are referring to the gross channels. These are listed under the Earth element: nerves, tendons, ligaments and blood vessels. In Thai yoga, or Ruisi Datton, we work both with these and with the subtle channels, which have their own location and pathways; this is what is meant by the term 'sen'. When we are discussing yoga, meditation and breathing exercises, we are generally working with the subtle channels, which are also called sen. 'Prāṇa' means breath, specifically inhalation; it can also refer to Wind in yoga texts.

Importance of Cupping in TLM

As described above, the pathogens – be they Wind, Damp, Heat, etc. – move through the various layers of the body until they affect the body adversely. The benefit of Thai cupping is that, once those pathogens are drawn to the superficial layer, the body can actually deal with them in a better way and heal itself, or we can employ other therapies such as massage or hot poultices, etc. *Pathogens usually present themselves in the blood, lymph or tissue as Wind.*

Lom Pit / Wind-Poison

'Lom Pit' is the term used to refer to the Wind-Poison (or toxic Wind), which is normally released from the body during cupping. 'Lom Pit' is released both locally where cupping occurs, and also systemically. For this reason a person who has recently been cupped may experience initial cold- or flu-like symptoms. These include general malaise, tiredness, dizziness or feeling cold. In general, these symptoms last only a few hours.

'Lom Pit' also refers to the Wind that accumulates inside the cups. Because of the presence of Wind-Poison, it is important to remove the cups *away from your face!* Also, try not to breathe towards the cup you have just removed. Ventilate the room and burn cleansing herbs or incense.

APPLICATIONS OF THAI CUPPING THERAPY

Cupping is used primarily (in TLM) for:
- common colds
- pain and swelling
- helping scar tissue
- releasing tight fascia
- releasing Heat
- dispersing stagnation
- releasing accumulated waste
- headaches
- regulating Wind in the body.

Types of Cupping

- **Dry cupping:** Refers to cupping that does not promote bleeding.
- **Wet cupping:** Refers to the use of cups in bloodletting.
- **Flash cupping (also known as Empty cupping):** Cups are applied and then rapidly removed, followed by immediate re-application and removal, again and again for about 15 minutes. Flash cupping is a gentle form of cupping.

Tools

- Cups made from horn, clay, bamboo, glass or plastic
- Surgical spirit (alcohol)
- Cotton-wool balls
- Source of fire
- A tray to put cupping tools on
- Massage oil: almond oil, coconut oil, sesame oil, etc.
- A bowl with water to put potentially hot tools on
- Balms, liniments, herbal compresses, etc.

Cupping Treatment Procedure

- Explain to your client what you are about to do and warn him or her of the possible cupping marks. Make sure the person feels comfortable with the use of fire.
- Make sure the room temperature is high enough as people being cupped can become cold.
- Apply oil to the skin, especially if you are working on someone with a lot of body hair.
- Create a vacuum by inserting fire into the cup, quickly removing it and rapidly applying the cup to the skin.
- The strength of the suction can be lowered by gently pressing down with your fingers at the rear of the cup.
- In TLM one to three cups are commonly used in order to allow you to work on surrounding areas.
- The amount of time the cups are left on varies between about 5 minutes and 20 minutes, but usually they are left on for 10 to 15 minutes. There is no set rule, however.
- Different traditions and teachers encourage different degrees of suction. I personally do not like to make the suction very strong.

Cupping Mark Diagnosis

Diagnosis from the coloration of cupping marks is illustrated in Figure 3-4.

A bright red coloration after cupping (Fig. 3-4A) indicates excessive Heat in the area and possible inflammation. Flash cupping is generally used. With inflammation, and especially in acute injuries, bleeding may be indicated. In such a case it is helpful to use cooling balms and liniments to cool the area. Ice is not normally used.

A deep red to magenta cupping mark (Fig. 3-4B) indicates stagnant Heat. Cupping and bleeding are indicated. You can then use a drawing liniment or trauma liniment that is cooling to neutral.

A purple-blue cupping mark (Fig. 3-4C) indicates stagnation with the absence of Heat. Wind is stuck in an area and it is unable to move. Cupping is indicated. Heating therapy can be used to disperse the area. With the presence of stagnation, you may want to cup more often and bleeding may be indicated.

A dark blue to purple-black cupping mark (Fig. 3-4D) indicates chronic build-up of 'Wind-Poison'. The blood in the area is toxic and needs to be drained.

A dark coloration receding after the cup is removed (Fig. 3-4E) means that the toxins are sinking back into the body and need to be drawn out with more cupping and drawing liniments, balms or poultices.

A pale whitish cupping mark (Fig. 3-4F) indicates the area is lacking in circulation because of a blockage somewhere around the area. Cupping is contraindicated in this condition. Stop cupping immediately and apply external warmth. Use hot compresses or a heating balm.

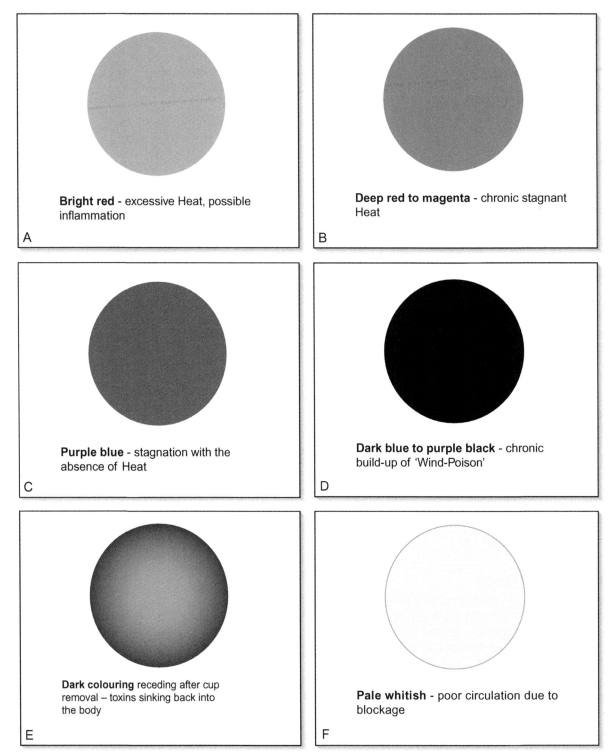

A **Bright red** - excessive Heat, possible inflammation

B **Deep red to magenta** - chronic stagnant Heat

C **Purple blue** - stagnation with the absence of Heat

D **Dark blue to purple black** - chronic build-up of 'Wind-Poison'

E **Dark colouring** receding after cup removal – toxins sinking back into the body

F **Pale whitish** - poor circulation due to blockage

FIGURE 3-4 (A–F) Diagnosis through cupping marks (See Plates 41A–F in the colour plate section).

ACKNOWLEDGEMENTS

If you would like to study and know more about this tradition, I am happy to help and, if necessary, suggest the right teacher for you. I am forever grateful to Ajahn Wit for his teachings and guidance on cupping in traditional Lanna medicine. And to all my other teachers: Ajahn Chandor, Doctor Ang Lai Hiang, Ajahn Pichest, Thai Hill Tribe Cupping Practitioners from the market, Ajahn La, Ajahn Dao, Mama Lek Chaiya, Master Jack Chaiya, Ajahn Sinchai and last but not least to my first Thai massage teacher Dimpa.

BENEFITS OF CUPPING THERAPY

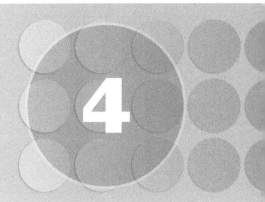

4

CHAPTER CONTENTS

SKIN, 47
LYMPHATIC SYSTEM, 48
CUPPING THERAPY AND LYMPHATIC DRAINAGE, 56
BLOOD, 56
QI, 58
WEI QI, 58

STAGNATION, 59
BLOODLETTING, 60
GUA SHA, 60
CUPPING, 61
EFFECTS OF CUPPING THERAPY, 63
REFERENCES, 64

Before listing the benefits of cupping therapy, let us take a closer look at the skin and its relation to the internal organs, the lymphatic and the immune system, and at terminology as seen in traditional Chinese medicine (TCM), such as Blood, Qi and Wei Qi phenomena, stagnation, bloodletting, Gua Sha and cupping. I am a great believer that cupping therapy has the most profound effect on the movement as well as the substance of the Blood, quality of Qi, the Wind element, and all the bodily functions that comes under their influence. Qi and Blood circulate throughout the entire body (internally as well as externally), on the skin, through the channels and collaterals and reach the organs.

SKIN

Any topical stimulus destined to influence and manipulate internal or external organs must start at skin level. The skin is our largest organ, containing fluid, blood, blood vessels, connective tissue, muscle and rich nerve supplies. Our body's first direct contact with the outside world is through the skin. It is also true to say that the skin is the mirror of our health: in good health the skin is shiny, tight and has a smooth texture. It responds to changes in temperature and is generally warm when touched. When the body is unhealthy, however, a dull, rather lifeless skin appearance is evident, with little natural colour and often cold to the touch.

As well as protecting the body from external pathogens, the skin has a major role in a number of body functions. It is the main organ of sensation, through many millions of nerve endings contained in its structure. A rich network of blood vessels and glands provides an effective means of temperature control. There are two main layers of the skin proper: the outer epidermis and the inner dermis. The fatty subcutaneous region lies beneath these two. The epidermis is the cellular layer of the skin, varying in thickness from 0.1 mm in the eyelid to over 1 mm on the palms of the hands and soles of the feet. It has no nerves, connective tissue or blood vessels (Fig. 4-1).

The main 14 channels with a direct link to the internal organs (Zang-Fu) also lie within the skin. In stimulating a particular point, with acupuncture, massage, Gua Sha or cupping, the objective remains the same: through manipulation of the skin to influence and change a particular organ's Blood and Qi. If we look at this through the perspective of Western medicine, it is the blood vessels, veins, arteries, the nervous system and connective tissue, and through this network, each cell in a particular area, that are

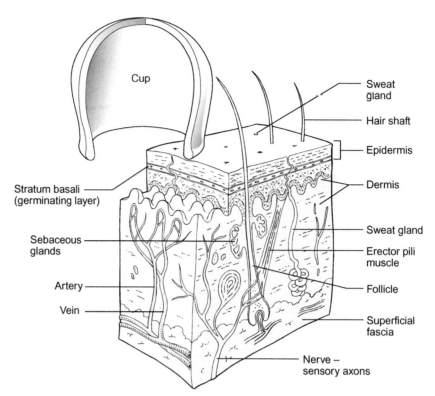

FIGURE 4-1 Section of skin with cupping application.

responsible for the above. However, from the TCM point of view it is the responsibility of the channels, collaterals, Blood and Qi. According to TCM, the skin is influenced by and under the direct control of the Lungs. When the Lung's Qi is in abundance the skin is nourished, glows and performs well, and hair and nails all receive nourishment and look healthy. Lungs spread the Qi and fluids all over the body through the skin. Therefore, skin moisture is also dependent on healthy lungs. Each Zang-Fu organ is represented by a channel on the skin; therefore, a connection, or an open door, mediates with external pathogens via the skin (Figs 4-2–4-15).

LYMPHATIC SYSTEM

The lymphatic system is made up of lymphatic vessels (similar to blood vessels) and lymph nodes (glands) that extend throughout the body. It helps maintain the balance of fluid in the body by draining excess fluid from the tissues of the body and returning it to the blood system.

Closely related to the cardiovascular system, the lymphatic system has several major functions. It is important in the body's defence mechanism, filtering out bacteria and also (along with the spleen) producing disease-fighting lymphocytes (white blood cells), generating antibodies that are so essential to the body's immune system. The fluid that circulates in the system is called lymph. In addition to lymph, the system includes lymphatic capillaries and large vessels, lymph nodes (glands), the spleen, the tonsils and the thymus. Besides forming lymphocytes and antibodies, the lymphatic system is also responsible for the collection of fatty globules from the intestine and their transmission through the mesenteric glands and the thoracic duct into the bloodstream.

The lymphatic system also prevents infection entering the bloodstream. It also preserves the fluid balance throughout the body. After an injury, the affected tissue generally swells. It is the lymphatic system that removes most of the excess fluid, and then returns it for circulation. All forms of massage or tactile therapy that involve stimulation of the skin surface will result in improvement of blood and lymph circulation. One advantage that blood circulation has over lymph circulation is that blood is pumped around the body by means of the heart. In contrast, the circulation of lymph relies on breathing, movement (walking or exercising) or external pressure, which is usually administered by various

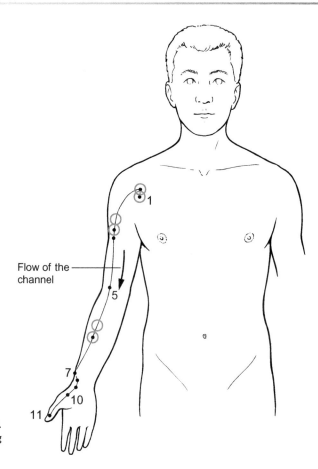

FIGURE 4-2 Course of the Lung (LU) channel. Conditions of the chest, nasal and fluid. Moving cupping or Gua Sha on the channel can be employed.

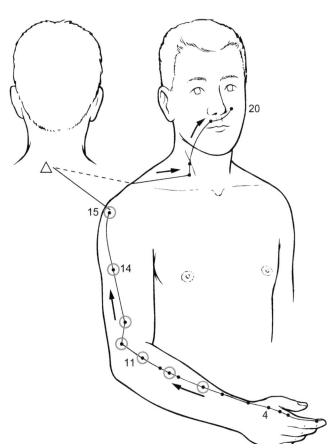

FIGURE 4-3 Course of the Large Intestine (LI) channel. Conditions of the head, nose, throat, intestines, febrile diseases and face (facial paralysis). Fixed cupping therapy on the facial points and moving cupping or Gua Sha to the rest of the channel can be applied.

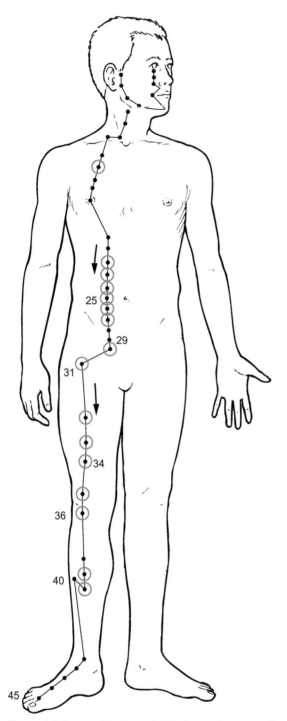

FIGURE 4-4 Course of the Stomach (ST) channel. Conditions of the head, face, throat, digestion, leg and Qi. Cupping therapy on the facial and abdominal points can be employed.

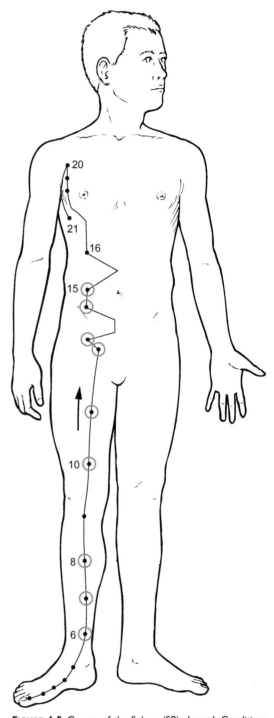

FIGURE 4-5 Course of the Spleen (SP) channel. Conditions of the stomach, spleen, intestines, lower extremities, Qi and urogenital. Cupping therapy on the abdominal points can be employed.

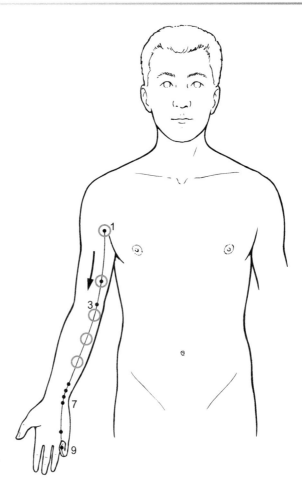

FIGURE 4-6 Course of the Heart (HT) channel. Conditions of the chest, heart, emotions and sleep.

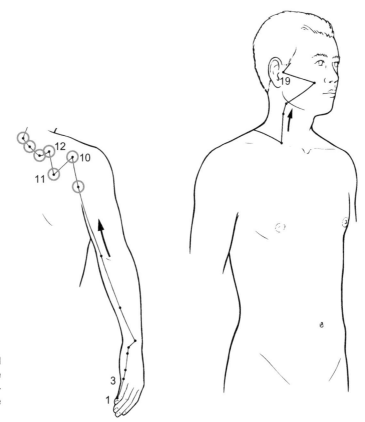

FIGURE 4-7 Course of the Small Intestine (SI) channel. Conditions of the head, neck, shoulders, eyes and emotional nature. Cupping therapy on the facial and shoulder points is applicable.

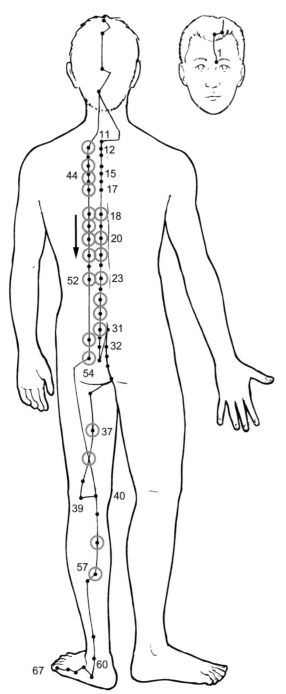

FIGURE 4-8 Course of the Bladder (BL) channel. All Back-Shu points are located on this channel; consequently, this is the most-used channel in cupping therapy. All 10 methods can safely be employed on this channel.

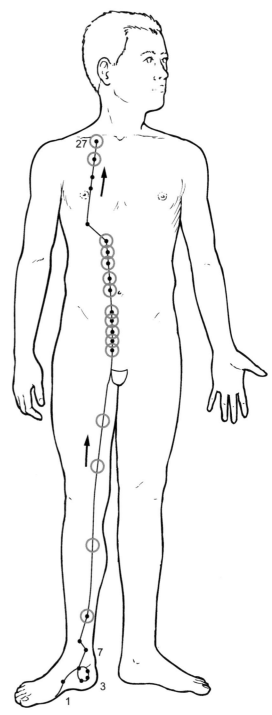

FIGURE 4-9 Course of the Kidney (K) channel. Conditions of abdominal, urogenital, Qi and emotional origin. Cupping therapy on the points on the trunk and leg can be employed.

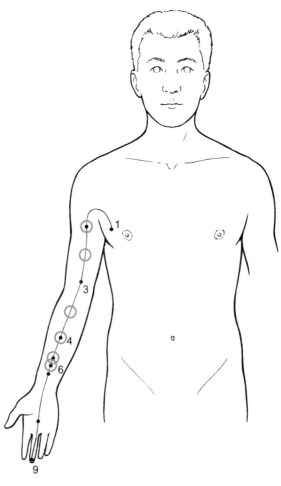

FIGURE 4-10 Course of the Pericardium (P) channel. Conditions of the chest, heart, nausea and emotional complaints.

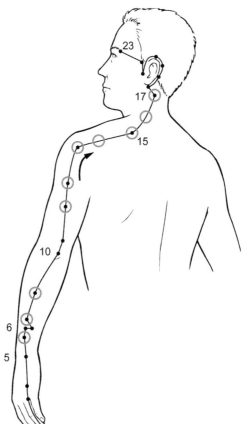

FIGURE 4-11 Course of the San Jiao (Triple Warmer – SJ or TW) channel. Conditions of the chest, ear, eye, throat and shoulders. Cupping therapy to the upper arm and shoulder points can be employed

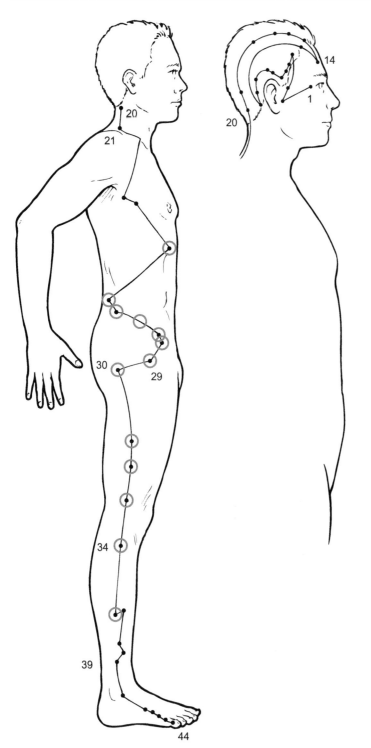

FIGURE 4-12 Course of the Gall Bladder (GB) channel. Conditions of the head, i.e. migraine, eye, chest, muscular complaints and febrile diseases. Cupping therapy to the trunk and moving cupping to the leg points can be employed.

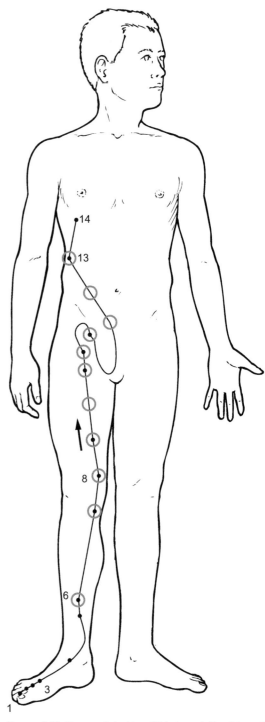

FIGURE 4-13 Course of the Liver (Liv) channel. Conditions of mental, emotional, digestive and urogenital systems. Cupping therapy on the abdominal and leg points can be employed.

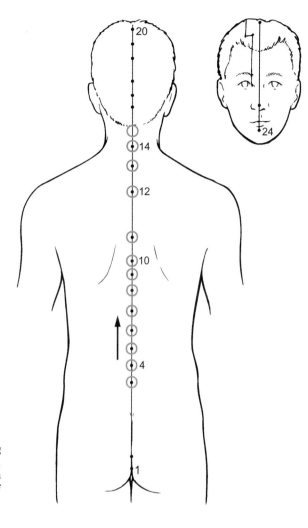

FIGURE 4-14 Course of the Du Mai (Governing Vessel – DU or GV) channel. Conditions of the head, neck, febrile diseases and Qi. All 10 cupping methods can safely be applied to this channel, on the trunk of the body.

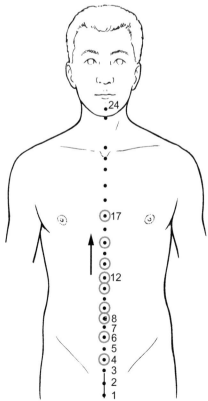

FIGURE 4-15 Course of the Ren Mai (Conception Vessel – Ren or CV) channel. Conditions of abdomen, digestive, urogenital and Qi. Limited cupping methods can be applied on this channel.

types of compression garments or bandages, and gravity. Since the origin of the lymph is the blood plasma, the two fluids are very much interconnected and inseparable physiologically.

As the lymph circulates between the cells, it collects waste matter including dead blood cells, toxic material and, if present, some cancer cells. While blood is responsible for collecting and distributing oxygen, nutrients and hormones nourishing the entire body, the lymphatic system is responsible for collecting and removing waste products in tissues, acting as a systematic garbage collection service! When this waste is not collected adequately or effectively, it congregates as a localized congestion. Waste-laden lymph is filtered by lymph nodes that are located throughout the body, some superficially under the skin and others situated deeper in tissue in the abdomen and neck, under the arms and the intercostal spaces both to the front and back of the rib cage. The function of these lymph nodes is to remove some fluid and toxic matter as well as killing many pathogens. They are also sometimes responsible for trapping cancerous cells, slowing down the spread of the disease.

During cupping therapy, in particular when 'Moving cupping' is employed, both blood and lymph circulatory systems are simultaneously stimulated to work more efficiently. This results in a more efficient collection and transportation mechanism for toxic substances, depositing them into the lymphatic system to be destroyed, and allowing the circulation of fresh lymph in order to nourish the tissues and generate a booster to the immune system (Fig. 4-16).

CUPPING THERAPY AND LYMPHATIC DRAINAGE

As mentioned above, during a normal course of cupping therapy blood and lymph are activated simultaneously. In a healthy person this improved circulation of the cardiovascular system is a beneficial outcome and one that the practitioner and the patient both desire. However, this might not be the case with patients suffering from lymphoedema (swelling caused by obstruction of the lymph vessels or abnormalities in the development of lymph vessels) or lymphomas (cancers that occur from within the lymphatic system).

Definition and Signs of Lymphoedema

Lymphoedema is a swelling caused by a build-up of lymph fluid in the tissues due to a compromised lymphatic system. This condition is considered not to be a serious health problem and it is often neglected. Lymphoedema is caused by injury to the lymphatic vessels. It is most frequently seen after surgery or radiation therapy, which can cause unintended damage to the lymphatic drainage system. It is especially common after surgery and radiation therapy are used in combination to treat breast cancer. Lymphoedema can also be associated with accidents or any other sort of disease or problem that can inhibit the lymph from proper function. Symptoms include severe fatigue, a heavy swollen limb or localized fluid accumulation in other areas, deformity, and decolourization of the skin overlying the lymphoedema.

Signs and Symptoms of Lymphoma

Lymphoma is a type of cancer that occurs when there is a fault in the way a lymphocyte is produced, resulting in an abnormal cell. Like normal lymphocytes, the cancerous lymphocytes can grow in many parts of the body, including the lymph nodes, spleen, bone marrow, blood or other organs. There are two main types of cancer of the lymphatic system: Hodgkin's disease and non-Hodgkin's lymphoma. A painless swelling in the neck, groin or axilla (armpit) may have been a reason for a visit to the practitioner. Other symptoms may accompany the swelling, such as fevers, night sweats, tiredness, weight loss, itching and, sometimes, pain after consuming alcohol. A lymphoma can occur in any part of the lymphatic system or outside it. Metastasis (spread of the cancer) can be within the lymphatic system or outside it.

Cupping therapy is categorically contraindicated and should be avoided on limbs affected by cancer or on limbs at risk of lymphoedema.

Beverley de Valois, personal communication, 2013

BLOOD

A kind of material transformed from the essence of food produced through functional activity of Qi, which circulates through the blood vessels and nourishes the body tissue.

Wang Bao Xiang, Dong Xue Mei, 1992

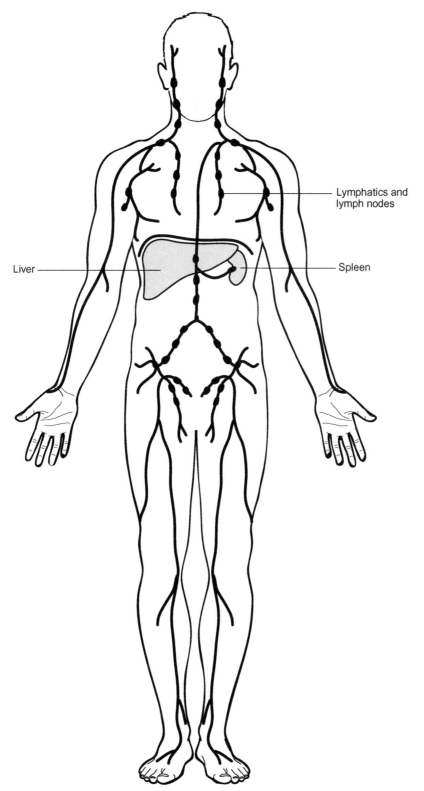

FIGURE 4-16 The lymphatic system.

Whenever Blood is mentioned throughout this book, it is within the context of TCM teaching (i.e. that the Blood is derived from Food and Qi and produced by the Spleen).

Like the skin, Blood has a different role to play in TCM from that of Western medicine. One of the most important characteristics of the Blood in TCM is that it contains Qi (life force). Qi is the locomotive of Blood. 'Blood is inseparable from Qi itself, Qi infuses life into Blood; without Qi, Blood would be an inert fluid' (Maciocia, 1989). Where Qi moves, Blood also moves, and vice versa: where Blood moves, Qi follows. When compared, Blood is Yin where Qi is Yang. Blood circulates in blood vessels as well as in the channels and collaterals. The Liver, Heart and Spleen have a special relationship with Blood. The Liver stores the Blood and is also responsible for the smooth flow of Qi within the organs. The Heart governs and harmonizes the smooth flow of Blood and blood vessels. The Spleen's responsibility is to rejuvenate Blood as well as control and keep the Blood within the vessels.

Blood Stagnation/Stasis

The TCM patterns 'Blood stagnation', 'blood stasis' and 'Blood congealing' all describe the same disorder. For some reason, Blood is obstructed and is not *moving freely* within the organs or blood vessels, causing discomfort. The most distinct symptom of Blood stasis is pain with a fixed, sharp or stabbing character. This type of pain can be felt deep in the internal organs or quite superficially at the muscular and skin level. *Light, Medium, Strong, Moving and Bleeding cupping methods are employed during the treatment of Blood stasis/stagnation syndromes.* During Bleeding cupping, however, *Blood stasis* is achieved by removing some blood from the stagnated location, thus encouraging a fast supply of fresh blood to the area. All other cupping methods have a similar action but tend to be milder.

QI

Many people frequently ask the question: 'what is the true meaning of Qi?' My understanding of Qi is the life force itself. It is the invisible force behind all happenings – like air and wind, immaterial yet with substance. When I travel in a car I often put my hand out of the window and feel the force of the wind, trying to hold it in my palm. It is so real, yet so immaterial and elusive.

'The Qi of life', 'vital force' and 'life force' all are Western attempts to describe the meaning of Qi, but there is no Western equivalent. Often we hear comments such as, 'last week I was very ill and lethargic, my Qi level was so low that all I did was stay in bed. Today I feel better and more upbeat and much brighter too.' In other words, we all experience the existence of Qi continuously.

Movement and heat signify Qi. Movement of any kind requires Qi, and often this is manifested as heat. Lack of Qi, on the other hand, is signified by cold and sluggishness. In the clinical situation too, when a patient complains of feeling cold, tiredness often accompanies their symptom. It is an old Turkish custom that, when a chair is vacated it must be allowed to cool down before someone else takes it. There is a genuine concern and fear of catching another person's unknown or hidden illness through their body warmth left on the chair. When treating a disease that is in the Qi Level, according to the 'Four Levels of Differentiation of Syndromes', the external pathogen is still fighting at the skin level and the body's overall resistance is still good. Some of the clinical manifestations are a high fever, a cough with thin yellow phlegm, wheezing and thirst. Cupping treatment at this level is very effective. There are two major conditions associated with Qi phenomena: Qi deficiency and Qi stagnation. Within these two main categories there are subcategories (for more information, see Kaptchuk [1983], p. 38).

Qi deficiency symptoms include unexplained tiredness, breathlessness, speaking with a very low voice ('like an ant'), poor appetite and an empty pulse. The clinical manifestations of Qi stagnation are moving pain (wandering pain), feeling of distension (breast or stomach) emotional conditions such as depression, mood disorders or irritability, and a wiry or tight pulse.

WEI QI

Wei Qi is the protective/defensive Qi that travels just under the skin within the membrane (thin layer of tissue which lines or covers an organ). It forms the outermost defensive wall against all external pathogens, such as Wind, Cold, Damp and Heat. Wei Qi also regulates the opening and closing of the pores of the skin, and is therefore in control of perspiration. It warms and nourishes the skin, its source is Blood and Qi, and it is governed by the Lungs.

Wei Qi is one type of Yang-Qi, the result of the digestion and absorption of food by the Spleen and Stomach, having the functions of protecting the integument (skin, outer layer) and musculature against external pathogen, adjusting sweat secretion and nourishing the skin portion.

Failure of Wei Qi to protect the body against diseases: a morbid state marked by spontaneous sweating and aversion to wind, caused by deficiency of the superficial Qi, lowering the ability of the body to resist diseases, leading to the invasion of exopathic factors.

Wang Bao Xiang, Dong Xue Mei, 1992

Clinical manifestations at this level include fever with little or no sweating, occipital headache, stiff neck, thirst, sore throat, cough and a feeling of chill. Treating conditions at this level with cupping therapy is highly effective.

STAGNATION

In TCM the term 'stagnation' usually refers to congestion or accumulation through lack of movement – movement of any kind (i.e. Food, Body Fluids, Qi or Blood).

Stagnation of Food (Food Accumulation)

This pattern is often seen in children, where the parents are eager to feed the child with rich foods, sometimes with force.

High sugar intake, cold drinks and foods or irregular feeding habits can also cause accumulation problems. In adults, food accumulation occurs with the consumption of sugary, rich and fatty foods, often eating before feeling hungry, and lack of exercise, in particular walking. Food stagnation syndrome is also prevalent in today's young generation, where eating out late, ordering fast food, high-sugar drinks, or a takeaway meal is considered to be 'fashionable' instead of time-consuming home cooking! This impairs the Spleen's function of transformation and transportation. Clinical manifestations of Food stagnation are restlessness, vomiting and the production of phlegm, diarrhoea, constipation, a hardened stomach and painful abdomen.

As far as Western medicine is concerned, the spleen is the largest single organ of the lymphatic system in the body. It is responsible for manufacturing cells of the immune system and for filtering from the bloodstream the old and damaged cells, as well as foreign matter, such as bacteria, which circulate through its rich network of blood vessels. For this reason when damage to the Spleen's Qi transpires through poor eating habits, the risk of compromising the immune system is a very real one. *Empty (Flash), Light, Medium and Light–Moving cupping methods can be applied during the treatment of Food stagnation complaints.*

Stagnation of Body Fluids

The Stomach is the origin of Body Fluids. The Lung is responsible for regulating water circulation throughout the body (between three [San] Jiao). The Lungs support the skin, which in its turn nourishes the Kidney. The lungs also excrete about 500 mL of water, as vapour in the expired air, under average conditions in a day. Under similar conditions the skin loses about 1000 mL as perspiration.

Body Fluids are the necessary Yin substance in the Stomach that helps it carry out the proper digestion process. When this process is impaired by Cold and Heat pathogens, or too many raw foods, this in turn damages the Spleen's functions. Clinical manifestations of Fluid stagnation are very similar to those of Food stagnation, with the exception of fluids accumulating in the extremities (i.e. the hands and feet). Fluid build-up is also likely when the lymphatic system is overloaded or damaged (by operation, radiation or accident) and in elderly people who might suffer from Heart- or Kidney-Qi deficiency. *Empty (Flash), Light and Light-moving cupping methods are particularly effective methods when dealing with Fluid stagnation conditions.*

Qi Stagnation

This is the failure of Qi to flow smoothly throughout the body. The main clinical manifestations are a feeling of distension, distending pain that moves from place to place, abdominal masses that appear and disappear, mental depression, irritability, a gloomy feeling, mood swings, frequent sighing, a wiry or tight pulse and a slightly purple tongue. This condition is very apparent during the menstrual cycle, where the liver Qi is often impaired. Mental depression and associated conditions also come under Qi stagnation syndrome (see Chapter 14). One way of dealing with Qi stagnation is to administer 'channel/meridian cupping' as described in the channel illustrations. *Empty, Light, Light-moving and Medium cupping methods can all be employed when treating the Qi stagnation syndromes.*

Stagnation of Blood and Blood Stasis

See the section on Blood, above.

BLOODLETTING

For the history and practice of bloodletting, see Chapters 1 and 9.

GUA SHA

Professor Wong Lun of the School of Traditional Chinese Medicine in Melbourne, Australia, who was my first Chinese medicine teacher, was a great believer in and practitioner of both cupping and Gua Sha. Like cupping, very few practitioners use Gua Sha, and this includes the Chinese doctors in China. The only comprehensive study to date is the work of Arya Nielsen (1995). Gua Sha is a technique very similar to cupping, inasmuch as it creates a deliberate hyperthermia in order to bring the Heat and Wind pathogens to the surface. Nielsen explains that 'Gua means to scrape or scratch', and Sha is 'cholera, heat, skin rash'. 'The technique of Gua Sha intentionally brings the Sha rash to the surface. By expressing the rash that marks the crisis of the Sha syndrome, Sha-evil is eliminated and the Sha syndrome resolved.'

Gua Sha is used where pain, Heat and stagnation are present. The treatment itself is very simple and pain free in practised hands. However, in untrained hands it can be rather uncomfortable and sometimes painful, especially when used on the bony parts of the body and on rather thinly built patients.

Traditionally, a porcelain Chinese soupspoon is used to scrape the skin (Fig. 4-17). Before scraping the desired area, oil or talcum powder must be applied to facilitate smooth rubbing. Long, gentle strokes are applied until bruising appears on the skin. The colour of the rash and the time it takes to appear guide the practitioner. One of my favourite conditions to treat with Gua Sha is a muscular 'Bi',

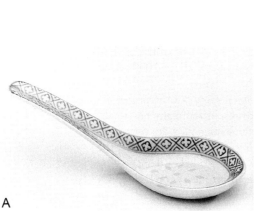

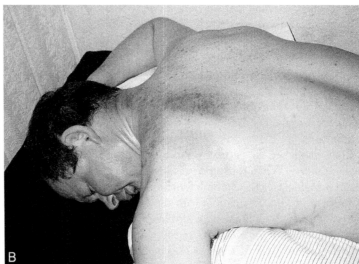

A   B

FIGURE 4-17 (A) Gua Sha. The traditional porcelain soupspoon used during Gua Sha. (B) Following the Gua Sha treatment, a mark (Sha) appears.

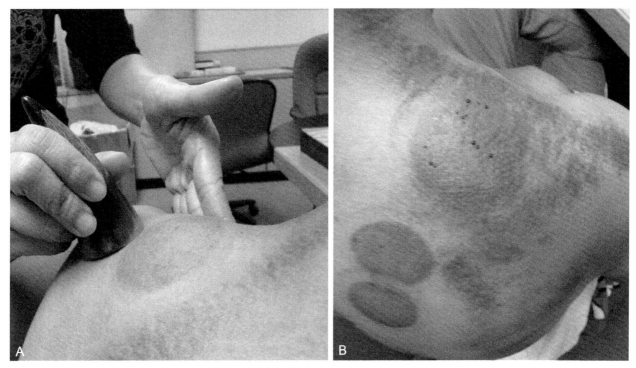

FIGURE 4-18 (A, B) Gua Sha over cupping points.

and 'plum-stone throat' syndromes. For longstanding muscular pains that also bring about stagnation of Qi and Blood, Gua Sha is extremely effective in releasing the stagnation and restoring the flow of Blood and Qi to the area. For the treatment of 'plum-stone throat' syndrome, which appears in extreme emotional conditions, the sternum is treated by Gua Sha from the top to the end of the xiphoid process, using gentle, even strokes as this area is very bony and rubbing can be painful. As a diagnostic tool in people with long-term emotional problems (i.e. Liver-Qi stagnation), palpating this area can also be painful. To Gua Sha this region releases the chest stagnation and opens the Heart. For muscular pain in the arms, legs and neck, where cupping can be difficult, Gua Sha is very effective, especially to the upper neck, where cupping is almost impossible. On my recent visit to Taiwan (February, 2012), I witnessed many practitioners applying Gua Sha following cupping therapy, in particular to the areas where cupping has left a dark or purple cupping mark. This action helps the local stagnation to disperse much quickly (Fig. 4-18).

CUPPING

The following paragraph reflects my own theory on the mechanism of cupping therapy, in which I passionately believe.

Cupping application on its own is a unique expression of a considerable energy exchange between the cells of the physical layers of the body, which incidentally triggers and kick-starts the healing process. The moment a cup is placed upon the skin this amazing energy exchange begins to unfold! The negative power inside the cup forces almost every molecule, cell, and tissue into a *movement*, i.e. towards the source of the power, which is the suction cup on top of the skin. When the pressure is released from the cup at the end of a treatment, the skin and each physical parts and particles directly under the cup returns to their original state. As a direct result of this forced activity, Qi (life force/energy) is created. With this newly found Qi, Heat is also generated. Heat in turn accelerates the metabolic rate, hence triggering the chain of activity and communication between the cells, tissues, channels and finally the organs! (See Fig. 4-1.)

Cupping regulates the flow of Qi and Blood. It helps to draw out and eliminate pathogenic factors such as Wind, Cold, Damp and Heat. Cupping also moves Qi and Blood and opens the pores of the skin, thus precipitating the removal of pathogens through the skin itself. In my opinion, *nothing moves Qi and Blood faster than cupping*. From the very start of its application one can observe the Blood moving in the direction of the cup. Where a patient's Qi is deficient this movement will be slow; if the Qi is abundant it will be much quicker. One can actually observe this process if glass cups are used.

As discussed earlier, cupping is particularly effective when the external pathogen still resides in the superficial energetic area of the body, the defensive/protective level (Wei Qi). Whatever the vessel used, the objective of the treatment remains the same: to remove the external pathogens from the deeper layers of the body and restore the circulation of Qi, Blood and the Body Fluids, thus bringing health to the sick.

Below is a rare Japanese account on the subject of cupping therapy, taken from a Japanese cupping-set manual (no author is mentioned).

The effect of this therapy can be classified into two categories: the general (purification of blood, improvement of circulatory functions of blood and lymph, regulation and betterment of automatic nervous system, etc.) and the local (removal of pain, relaxation of stiff muscles, etc.). The former effects, that is, effects upon the bodily tissues and organs, are as follows:

1. EFFECTS UPON THE SKIN

According to one experiment on a 35-year-old male subject, fine hair on his back grew to thick hair of 1 to 1.5 cm long after about 140 applications of treatment by this method. This is because the direct physical stimuli on hair roots and the expansion of blood vessels of the skin, by means of the pull of low pressure, cause an increase in blood circulation, a rise of skin temperature, the promotion of metabolism within skin tissue, better functioning of sweat and sebaceous glands and of cutaneous respiration and sufficient supply of nutrition to the tissues. The essential point of 'cupping therapy' is not only to withdraw stagnant old blood within the skin but also to remove poisonous substances from the surface of the skin. This is why, when a doctor continues this therapy on a patient with his bare hands, they become yellowy. It accelerates secretion of salts and sebaceous matter and the excretion of water. Another important point is that it strengthens the renewing power of the skin and its resistance to various harmful conditions.

2. EFFECTS UPON MUSCLES

The pull of low-pressure 'cupping therapy', the functioning of blood vessels within the muscles is activated in response to the stimulation of the subcutaneous capillary vessels. Thus the expansion of the blood vessels in the muscles facilitates the flow of blood and has a remarkable effect on a stiff shoulder, for example, removing congested blood. Moreover, this facilitates the flow of lymph. After the 'cupping therapy', the skin will be all aglow as a result of the rise in skin temperature and muscles by the increase of the blood flow.

3. EFFECTS UPON JOINTS

Chronic joint rheumatism is one of the conditions for which 'cupping therapy' is effective. In this case the treatment is concentrated on the area of the joints concerned. When the condition is mild, an almost complete cure is possible, and this results from the better flow of blood within the joint, the activity and secretion of synovial fluids. In case of muscular spasms around the joints, they can be removed.

4. EFFECTS UPON THE DIGESTIVE ORGANS

Most patients feel hungry after the cupping therapy on the stomach region. As the digestive organs, especially spleen and stomach, looked upon as the 'engine' of the human body are regarded as the most important; and the treatment of the middle Jiao is considered equally important. In other words, as the natural healing power of the body derives its energies mainly from the digestive organs, a great emphasis is laid on the treatment of the stomach, spleen and intestines. The pulling power of low pressure upon the belly stimulates the inside of the organs, their peristaltic movement and secretion of digestive fluids, and strengthens thereby the power of digestion and absorption of nourishment as well as the power of secretion. Therefore, this therapy has remarkable effects upon chronic gastroenteritis disorders and the constipation as a whole. These organs are affected favourably even during the treatment of the back by way of the stimulation of the spinal nerves and the automatic nerves. Besides these the therapy strengthens the muscles of the respiratory organs.

EFFECTS OF CUPPING THERAPY

Purification of Blood

Among the general effects, the most important is the effect upon the circulatory system. Professor Kentaro Takagi of Nagoya University says that the skin-stimulating therapies are significant in that they awaken the greatest responses in the circulatory system. His remarks were not necessarily directed towards cupping therapy, but I think it has much in common with the skin-stimulating therapies he mentioned. Owing to the pull of low pressure, the flow of blood in the arteries and veins increases, although in the case of the latter, localized spots of congested blood appear and then disappear. It is possible to ease the interruption of blood circulation and congestion and to stop the inflammatory extravasation (escaping of body fluids such as blood) from the tissues. Therefore, facilitation of the flow of blood is the most important characteristic of this therapy. It is very beneficial for hardened arteries, stiff shoulders, etc.

Dr Katase of Osaka University suggests that this therapy may influence the composition of blood: it may help to increases red and white blood cells and changes acid blood into alkaline or neutral. This leads to the purification of blood.

Effects on the Nervous System

Cupping therapy stimulates the sensory nerves of the skin. As demonstrated in a clinical experiment conducted at Kobe University, the inhibitory effects on hypersensitive pain are not limited to the area of direct treatment, but include the areas controlled by the relevant nerves. Treatment on the back is mainly directed to the central line (spinal nerves and parasympathetic nerves) and the sympathetic nerves beside it. The stimulation of these has, it can be said, a good influence not only on the automatic nervous system itself but also on various organs under its control.

Cupping therapy is, like massage, effective against the so-called syndrome of general malaise, such as chronic headaches, dizziness, languor (mental or physical weariness), stiff shoulders, fatigue, etc. These are said to derive from anxiety, worry and bodily pain. It is also effective against endogenous chronic diseases such as high blood pressure, neuralgia and rheumatism. During treatment with this therapy on the back or the loins, for example, some middle-aged or elderly patients fall asleep, snoring loudly. This clearly shows one of the effects upon the nervous system. The mechanism of its effectiveness will be clarified some day. Thus the general and localized effects of this therapy strengthen the healing power against diseases and, together with a healthy diet and psychotherapy, cure or prevent disease completely. *All cupping methods have some degree of influence on the nervous system.*

In October 1995, the World Federation of Acupuncture Societies held a 4-day symposium in Istanbul, Turkey. The theme of the gathering was acupuncture and Qi, and I presented a paper on cupping and Qi. Over 200 acupuncturists from around the world attended the seminar, of which only a handful were using cupping in their practice. Most lacked the basic knowledge and skills necessary for cupping and were unaware of the benefits this technique can offer their patients.

Cupping therapy, following a few thousand years of use, development and perfection, has been increasingly accepted by variety of cultures and people. Its application is extensive, its efficacy is good, its cost is low, and its easy application and safety without adverse side-effects resulted in many practitioners introducing cupping therapy into their practices.

Cupping therapy is suitable for the treatment of pains, Bi syndromes, inflammatory conditions, diseases of the digestive, circulatory and respiratory systems, some skin conditions such as boils and eczema, wind-stroke (facial paralysis), weakness of the muscles, sports injuries, high blood pressure, the common cold, emotional conditions and cosmetic purposes such as treating cellulite and during weight-loss programmes.

Wind Element

My personal opinion is that cupping is the most powerful complementary medicine tool to fight against the Wind pathogen. Given all the 'external pathogenic factors', the Wind element is by far the most affected and influenced as a result of cupping application. In almost all traditional medicine practices from around the world, the Wind element is seen as the most perilous external pathogen of all. Wind pathogen can cause external as well as internal diseases, therefore it is always recommended to avoid situations or exposure to the Wind element. In TCM too, when we look at the disease pathogenesis,

Wind pathogen is considered as a major causative factor. As well as external Wind attacks such as Wind-Cold, Wind-Heat or Wind-Damp, which are considered as the 'root' of many diseases, cupping therapy is shown to be quite an effective treatment tool. The 'internal Wind patterns' too respond well to cupping therapy. These patterns are usually the result of chronic deficiencies, such as Blood or Yin deficiency, or extremely hot weather conditions. In TCM, for instance, 'trembling or shakes' (muscular as well as internal tremors) are considered to be a sign of 'Wind-attack' pattern.

Cupping: the Multi-function Therapy

Finally, **cupping therapy has a multi-function action**. For instance, it can treat pain, improve the metabolism, improve blood microcirculation, activate the lymphatic system and the toxin elimination process, tone up the skin, and remove pathogenic factors such as Wind, Heat or Cold, all at the same time! To reiterate my earlier statement:

Nothing moves Qi and Blood faster than cupping!

Diseases and treatments will be discussed in detail later in this book.

REFERENCES

Kaptchuk, Ted.J., 1983. The Web that has no Weawer. Rider and Company, London, UK.
Maciocia, G., 1989. The Foundations of Chinese Medicine. Churchill Livingstone, Edinburgh, UK.
Nielsen, A., 1995. Gua Sha, a Traditional Technique for Modern Practice. Churchill Livingstone, Edinburgh, UK.
Wang Bao Xiang, Dong Xue Mei, 1992. Chinese–English Bilingual Glossary of Traditional Chinese Medicine. Jian, Shandong Province, China.

PREPARING THE PATIENT FOR CUPPING TREATMENT

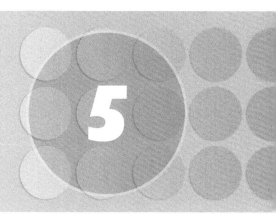

5

CHAPTER CONTENTS

CUPPING ON THE HEAD AND NECK, 68

TREATING WHILE THE PATIENT IS STANDING, 69

TREATING THE JOINTS, 69

CUPPING THE FACIAL POINTS, 70

CUPPING UNDER THE FEET, 70

CUPPING THERAPY TO THE ELDERLY PATIENT, 70

CUPPING ON THE ABDOMINAL POINTS, 71

Once the practitioner decides to perform therapy they should then proceed to prepare the patient for treatment. When I use the term 'prepare' I really mean just that. Do not suddenly appear in the cubicle with a set of cups in one hand and a fire in the other ready for cupping! One should perhaps explain the reason for this therapy and the benefits of cupping treatment, while enlisting the patient's consent (and that of the parent if the patient is a child) without forcing the issue of this particular treatment. Each individual is different: old, young, men, women or children, and we all have different levels of pain tolerance. What may be tolerable and acceptable for one person could be quite painful and unacceptable for another. Enquire about the person's pain threshold by asking and by palpating the area to be cupped. If necessary, gently massage the area to be cupped as this will help to relax the patient and also warm the cupping location. An alternative method of massaging and warming the skin is the palm/hand cupping method. With this technique the practitioner uses both his/hers palms to make a cup, then proceeds to gently palpating the skin, moving constantly over the treatment area (Fig. 5-1).

As cupping is performed on naked and exposed skin, the treatment room should be comfortably warm. *During the cupping treatment sessions all air conditioning systems should be turned off as cold air/wind is seriously contraindicated. Also keep a glass of drinking water close by as in some patients cupping may cause dehydration during the treatment.* Make absolutely sure that your patient is relaxed and not suffering from any degree of anxiety. Choose the best position to suit your patient and not you. For many people it might be a frightening experience to hold fire so close to their flesh. If necessary, show the cups to the patient and let them hold them. Apply a single cup to your own forearm and let the patient touch the cup. This will reassure and go a long way towards relaxing the person. Most people will tell you that they have indeed heard of cupping, or seen it on a television programme, but have not experienced it themselves. Explain that introducing fire into the cup will create a vacuum, and when the cup is turned on the skin it will pull the skin into the cup, and that this pulling action is the desired outcome.

Most cupping techniques have a mild and tolerable pulling action on the skin. Some, however, produce a stronger negative force and can be slightly painful – for example, strong and moving techniques. Good suction is noticeably more difficult to obtain and sustain for a longer period of time on dry and hairy skin than on oily and smooth skin. Some skins are so dry that they look and feel like tree bark: very porous and rough to touch. Fine hair covering the skin will present no problem during cupping, but a long, bushy growth, especially on a male back, may present a problem when trying to maintain good suction. Both situations require a little patience. Dry and hairy skin surfaces will prevent the cup

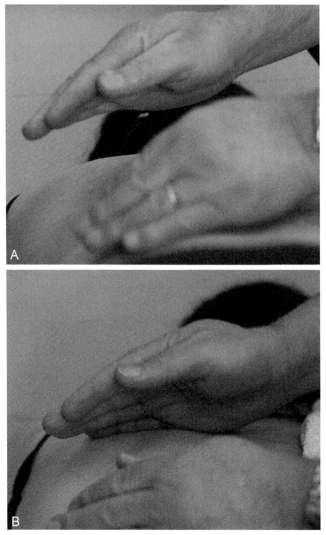

FIGURE 5-1 (A) Palm and (B) Hand cupping technique.

making perfect contact with the flesh: the suction created is usually strong enough to draw some air into the cup, and as a result the pulling action will cease in a much shorter time and the cup will come off in less than 5 minutes or so. In order to achieve a better contact between cup and flesh, and obtain good suction, apply massage oil liberally to the area to be cupped; this usually works satisfactorily. It is equally important that you ask the patient to sit or lie still during the treatment, as sudden movements are definitely not recommended.

When treating children less than 16 years of age, always invite the parents into the cubicle with you. Here again, show the cups to the child but perhaps not the fire, as they may be a little apprehensive about the whole procedure. Maybe the pistol handle or the silicon cups will be more appropriate to use, which do not require the use of fire! When parents are present then children are quite relaxed and cooperative during the treatment.

The location to be treated is important in deciding the position of the patient (Fig. 5-2). If the cupping is to be performed on the back, the most comfortable position will be prone on the couch or the floor; if on the area of the stomach, a supine position is preferred. For the face, knees, neck and shoulders, a sitting position in a chair may be chosen. For the elderly, severe asthmatics or patients who have recently suffered from any heart condition, an upright sitting position should always be preferred.

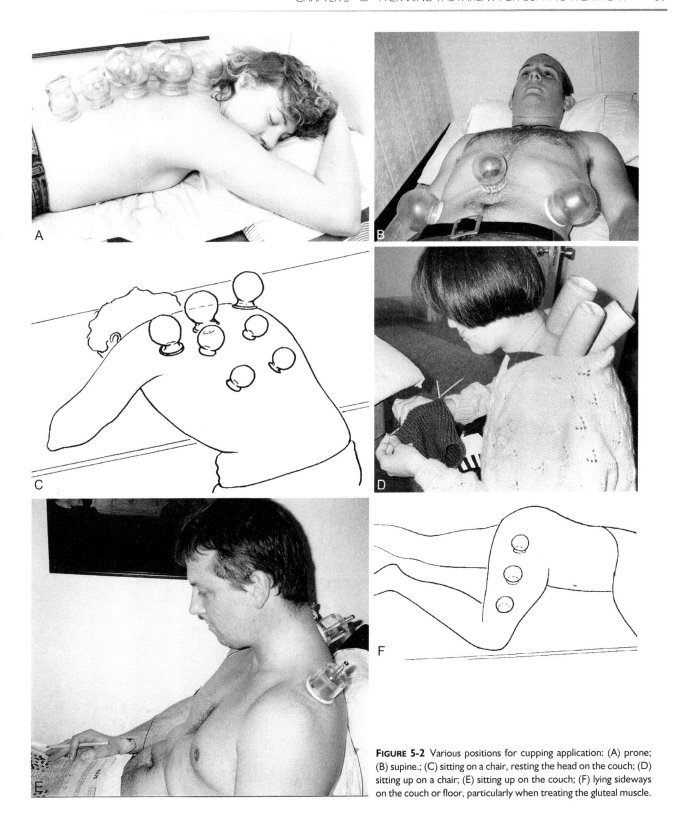

FIGURE 5-2 Various positions for cupping application: (A) prone; (B) supine.; (C) sitting on a chair, resting the head on the couch; (D) sitting up on a chair; (E) sitting up on the couch; (F) lying sideways on the couch or floor, particularly when treating the gluteal muscle.

CUPPING ON THE HEAD AND NECK

When treating the points on the head and the neck, it is best to have the patient in a sitting up position on a chair while resting the hands on the couch in front (Fig. 5-3). Sometimes it might be necessary to shave the head. Applying non-flammable gel on the head might also help to obtain a good suction.

Applications

Headache, migraine, eye conditions, ear complaints, nasal condition, neck pains, neck spasms, post stroke, paralysis, Bell's palsy, torticollis (wry neck), whiplash injury, toothache, throat complaints such as dry mouth, tonsillitis and laryngitis and during the facial rejuvenation programme.

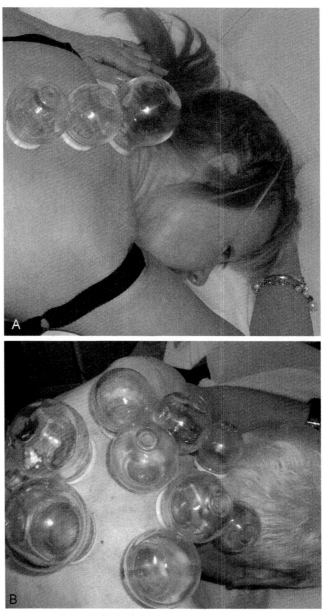

FIGURE 5-3 (A, B) Cupping of the head and neck.

TREATING WHILE THE PATIENT IS STANDING

Sometimes it might be necessary to treat the patient while standing up. This position is mostly used when treating leg, sciatica and back pains (Fig. 5-4).

Application

Sciatica.

TREATING THE JOINTS

When the area to be treated is around a joint, such as the elbow or the ankle joint, small-sized cups are more appropriate (Fig. 5-5).

Application

Swollen joints, oedema, all Bi syndromes, arthritis, rheumatic pains and paralysis conditions.

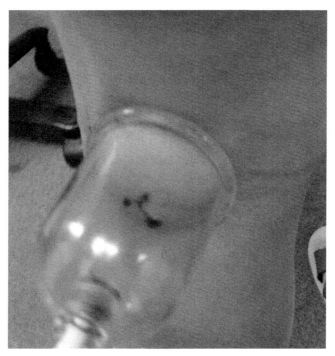

FIGURE 5-4 Cupping while standing.

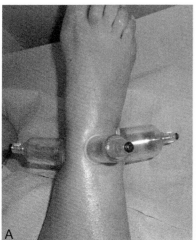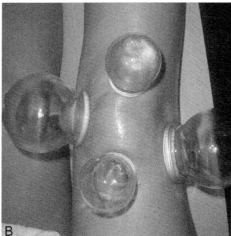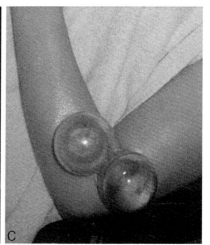

FIGURE 5-5 (A–C) Treating the joints.

CUPPING THE FACIAL POINTS

During the facial cupping procedures, extra care is necessary as the facial skin is quite sensitive and could easily cause cupping marks on the skin to appear. In order to avoid cupping marks to the facial skin, always choose the Light cupping technique and do not keep the cup in a one position for more than 2 minutes at a time. As far as the equipment is concerned, non-fire cupping sets such as the pistol handle or the rubber and the silicon cups are more manageable while working on the facial points (Fig. 5-6).

Application

Facial paralysis, Bell's palsy, stroke, toothache, nasal congestion, eye conditions and facial rejuvenation programme.

CUPPING UNDER THE FEET

Treating under the feet with cupping is similar to reflexology stimulation but the pressure to the sole of the foot is the opposite direction: it is an outward negative pressure. With this cupping method the finger pressure to the sole of the foot is replaced by a negative cupping suction to the sole. *Cupping to the feet or under the feet in diabetic patients is contraindicated* (Fig. 5-7).

CUPPING THERAPY TO THE ELDERLY PATIENT

Extreme care is needed when cupping elderly patients. As we get older our skin looses the fatty layer and becomes thinner. This can cause cupping marks and blisters to form much quicker than normal. Another common cause for the frail skin on the elderly is dehydration; somehow the elderly fail to drink enough liquid, which results in dehydrated skin. During cupping sessions on the elderly always use Light to Medium cupping methods in preference. All the strong techniques including Moving cupping are contraindicated in elderly patients (Fig. 5-8).

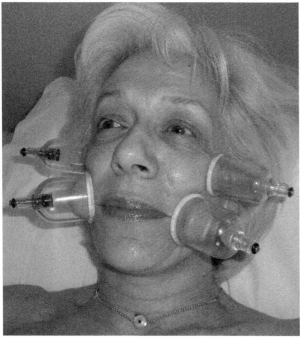

FIGURE 5-6 Cupping the face.

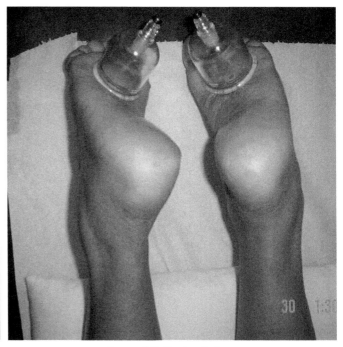

FIGURE 5-7 Cupping the feet.

CUPPING ON THE ABDOMINAL POINTS

Cupping therapy to the abdominal points will always result in more flesh being sucked into the cup! This is quite acceptable and normal since the flesh around the abdomen is soft, loose and has no attachment to the bone structure. We can see this more clearly when cupping below and around the umbilicus points. Suction of more skin into the cup could be deceiving and can be mistaken for a Strong cupping method. Confer with your patient and make sure that the pressure inside the cup is not excessive (Fig. 5-9).

Application

Gynaecological complaints, infertility, abdominal pain, abdominal spasm, indigestion, flatulence, constipation, diarrhoea, liver-related conditions and during a weight-loss programme.

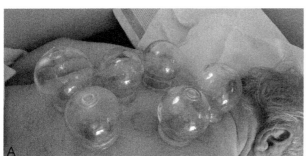
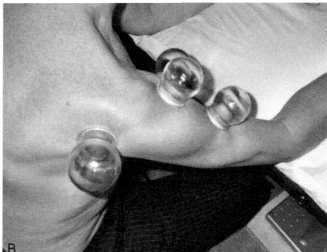

FIGURE 5-8 (A, B) Cupping the elderly patient.

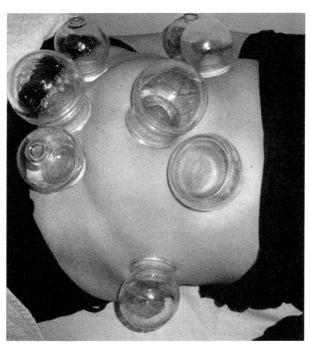

FIGURE 5-9 Cupping on the abdominal points.

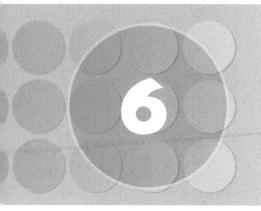

6

COMPLEMENTARY AND ALTERNATIVE MEDICINE (CAM) THERAPIES THAT CAN SAFELY INTRODUCE CUPPING TO THEIR TREATMENT PROTOCOL

CHAPTER CONTENTS

AROMATHERAPY, 72

MASSAGE, 72

CHIROPRACTIC, 74

OSTEOPATHY, 74

KINESIOLOGY, 75

ALEXANDER TECHNIQUE, 75

SHIATSU, 75

REFLEXOLOGY, 76

POLARITY, 76

PHYSIOTHERAPY, 76

FOUR-ZONE CUPPING THERAPY, 77

MERIDIAN/CHANNEL CUPPING, 78

Generally speaking, most hands-on complementary and alternative medicine (CAM) therapeutic practitioners can safely incorporate cupping therapy to their practice. The ultimate aim of all hands-on techniques is to stimulate the body's natural healing powers by balancing the physical, mental and emotional energies and restoring health to the individual. Therapies such as aromatherapy, massage, chiropractic, osteopathy, kinesiology, Alexander technique, shiatsu, reflexology, polarity and physiotherapy can all incorporate cupping therapy into their skills. For the non-Chinese-medicine-trained practitioners I have devised the 'four-zone cupping therapy map' (Fig. 6-1).

AROMATHERAPY

This is a massage technique that matches suitable essential oils to the condition of the patient. Essential oils have been used therapeutically throughout history, therapists recognizing the therapeutic values of flowers and plants and using them regularly for treatment purposes. They have been particularly successful in the treatment of aching muscles and joints, and of stress-related conditions. It is recommended that the therapist should apply cupping therapy *before* the aromatherapy session begins. This way you move and stimulate the Qi and Blood first and finish off the treatment with the soothing action of aromatherapy.

MASSAGE

Whenever we feel pain in any part of our body, our hand automatically goes to that part and we begin to rub, squeeze or simply massage the painful spot. This usually brings some instant relief. Massage must be the oldest and the most effective form of cure, used either therapeutically or as a preventive. Rubbing the skin increases the blood circulation and metabolism in the affected area. This action will not only directly benefit the immediate skin and muscles, but also the lymphatic system, nerves, blood vessels, cells and organs beneath the skin. A good body-worker is able to feel the tension on the skin and identify the stress zones. Once identified, different massage methods can be applied to eliminate these stress zones. Cupping directly on or next to stress zones can bring relief to sufferers.

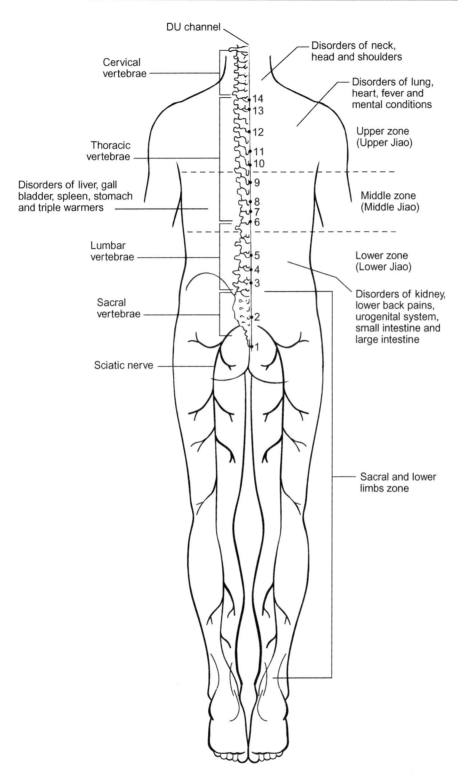

FIGURE 6-1 Four-zone cupping therapy map. All non-Chinese medicine-trained practitioners can refer to the map.

As a rule, treatment should begin with massage and, when the stress zones are identified, cupping should be applied for the desired time, again followed by massage and rest. Provided the practitioner keeps in mind the patient's energy level, various forms of cupping can be employed during massage therapy. Light, Medium, Strong, Moving, Light-moving and Empty methods can all be safely employed.

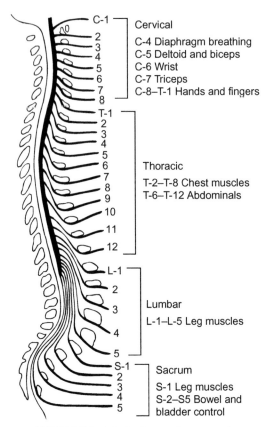

FIGURE 6-2 Vertebral column and nerve supply.

CHIROPRACTIC

Chiropractic was developed by Daniel David Palmer in the USA in 1895. This system of treatment sees the root of the disease in the displacement of the vertebrae, which causes blockages in the energy to a particular organ (Fig. 6-2). By manipulating and adjusting the spine manually, the blockage and the pressure are relieved; this is known as 'subluxation'. Chiropractors also advise the patient on nutrition and exercise.

Cupping during chiropractic manipulation reduces the local pressure on the vertebrae and improves the flow of the Qi and encourages the blood circulation to the muscle and tendons of the spine. Cupping is used next to the subluxation and not directly over it. Also direct cupping application to the inflamed disc should be avoided.

OSTEOPATHY

The principle of osteopathy is that disease is primarily the result of derangement of the spinal column, which consists of 24 movable vertebrae. These enclose and protect the spinal cord. When vertebrae are displaced they press on a nerve and, as a result, muscular or organ dysfunction occurs. If we think of the nervous system as an electric wiring configuration carrying uninterrupted power (energy) from site A to site B, all the expected bodily functions will occur continuously and without interruption. However, when there is a 'short' (blockage) anywhere in the system, the power (Qi/energy) will not reach the desired point and dysfunction will follow. An osteopath is trained to locate this blockage and unlock it using manipulation techniques, which may sometimes be followed by drugs or surgery. The more traditional osteopaths prefer to use manipulation as the only method. The objective is to restore the Qi/energy flow to the organs uninterrupted.

Cupping can be applied to the local and distal points on the lesion during manipulation or at the end of the session. Light, Medium, Strong and Empty cupping methods can all be employed. Avoid direct cupping therapy on the inflamed disc.

KINESIOLOGY

Developed by Dr George Goodheart, a chiropractic practitioner, in the early 1960s, this is a system that uses muscle reflexes and their effects on corresponding organs. Weak and strong muscles are identified through a series of muscle tests. Herbal remedies, together with nutritional therapy, may also be prescribed. Shiatsu/acupressure and massage are applied to the weak muscles in order to strengthen them and the associated organs. Although this is by no means a form of relaxation massage, the patient feels light, alert and full of energy following the treatment.

Cupping can also be applied to strengthen the weak muscles and associated organs through its ability to influence the flow of Qi and Blood. Light, Medium, Strong, Moving, Light-moving and Empty cupping methods can be employed to the local muscles. Cupping should be used at the end of a kinesiology session, followed by a massage.

ALEXANDER TECHNIQUE

This is a system of posture-correction techniques and body awareness methods and movements that help us to understand how best we can use our bodies when talking, walking, reading, singing and even during relaxation. F. Matthias Alexander, an Australian, came to the conclusion that faulty posture was responsible for a great many medical symptoms. When people habitually misuse their bodies by adopting poor postures, this will have an adverse effect on the muscular or nervous system.

Cupping therapy can assist in maintaining a strong and healthy spinal column. Apply symmetrically up to seven cups, on each side of the Bladder meridian (1.5 cun lateral on both sides of the spine), starting from BL-11 Dashu (location 1.5 cun lateral to the lower border of the spinous process of the first thoracic vertebra) and ending at BL-25 Dachangshu (location 1.5 cun lateral to the lower border of the spinous process of the fourth lumbar vertebra). The entire spinal cord is stimulated by the pulling action of cupping and the blood flow to the spinal cord will be increased, resulting in a greater energy flow and wellbeing. Light, Medium, Strong, Moving and Empty cupping methods can all be applied (Fig. 6-3).

SHIATSU

The principle of shiatsu, or acupressure as some practitioners call it, is the same as that of acupuncture. The 14 main meridians are used as energy pathways and the classic acupuncture points are used as point of treatment. Diagnosis is performed in exactly the same way as in acupuncture: pulse, tongue, palpation, listening and observing. However, instead of using needles for the treatment as in acupuncture, finger pressure is used in shiatsu treatment (Japanese 'shi', finger, and 'atsu', pressure). This form of treatment was introduced in Japan as a healing technique, although the theory and application both stem from the same principle as acupuncture.

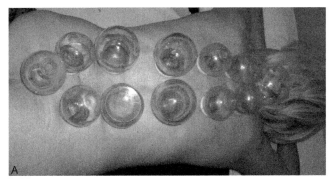 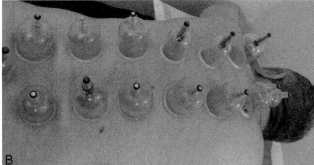

FIGURE 6-3 (A, B) Cupping during Alexander technique.

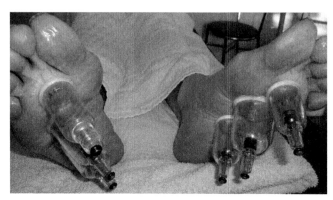

FIGURE 6-4 Cupping under the feet.

Cupping is extensively used during shiatsu sessions, and the treatment principle should be the same as in acupuncture. The same meridians and acupuncture/acupressure points are selected during the treatment. Cupping is performed in the middle of a shiatsu session and terminated by a light massage. Light, Medium, Strong, Moving, Moxa, Empty, Herbal and Water cupping methods can be employed during shiatsu sessions.

REFLEXOLOGY

Reflexology is another form of energy balancing therapy, focusing on the relationship between granulated points found on the soles of the feet and reflexes on the body. The reflexology practitioner, by means of a gentle touch or rub, is seeking points that are sensitive and granular. These are treated as uric acid crystallizations in the feet and are used in diagnosis and treatment. When massaging or rubbing the granules, therapeutic benefits can be expected on the corresponding organs of the body. Reflexology is based on the principle that there is a connection between the nerve endings in the feet and the organs of the body. Cupping is applied directly under the feet. Light, Medium, Strong, Moving and Empty cupping methods can all be used during a reflexology session (Fig. 6-4).

POLARITY

Developed by Dr Randolph Stone, this system of energetic healing consists of analysing the magnetic field and its patterns of movement in the body. Massage, manipulation, mental exercises and nutritional advice are all used to eliminate energy blockages and restore harmony and wellbeing. Pressure is systematically applied on two points at the same time using both hands. For the polarity therapist, the universe and everything connected with it has two opposing sides (poles) to it, very much like Yin and Yang: day and night, male and female, inhaling and exhaling, negative and positive electrical energies.

During cupping therapy, an equal number of cups should be applied bilaterally, and the four-zone cupping therapy map should be used. Light, Medium and Strong cupping methods can all be employed.

PHYSIOTHERAPY

This manipulative therapy is the most accepted and utilized by the medical profession all over the world, especially in the Western hemisphere. The aim is to retrain and restore the bodily functions lost as a result of operations, trauma, strokes, disease, etc., by applying mild pressure, heat, water and/or manipulation or strengthening techniques to the moving parts of the body. During physiotherapy the use of equipment is common, but nothing can substitute for the touch of the physiotherapist (the healer).

Cupping can be a great help in restoring the blood flow and improving the lymphatic circulation to the immobile or dormant parts of the body, and is especially beneficial when treating stroke patients or any other muscle-wasting disorder (Fig. 6-5). Four-zone cupping therapy can be integrated with the physiotherapy.

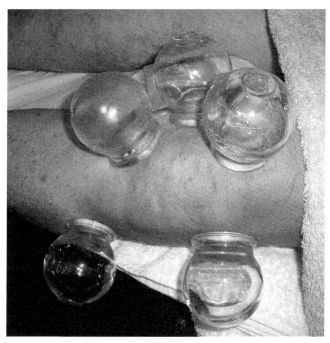

FIGURE 6-5 Treating a knee injury.

NB: Cups should not be applied to any part of the body affected by bone fractures of any kind. Light, Medium, Strong, Moving, Light-moving and Empty cupping methods can all be employed alongside the physiotherapy.

FOUR-ZONE CUPPING THERAPY

For non-Chinese medicine-trained practitioners I have formulated the four-zone cupping therapy map (see Fig. 6-1).

Zone 1: The Upper Zone

- *Front aspect:* This zone includes the upper chest under the clavicles; it is mostly used to treat respiratory conditions such as asthma, emphysema, the common cold and emotional complaints.
- *Back aspect:* The cervical spine from C4 to C8 and continuing through the first thoracic vertebra (T1) to the sixth thoracic vertebra (T6).

Disorders of neck and shoulders, occipital headache, stress-related tension, deltoid and biceps pains and weaknesses, wrist pains and weaknesses, triceps and hand and finger problems, disorders of the lungs such as cough, asthma and other breathing problems, colds, chills and fever, dizziness and high blood pressure can all be treated by cupping therapy to the upper zone.

Zone 2: The Middle Zone

- *Front aspect:* This zone is the stomach and the lower abdomen area. It is used for most gastrointestinal complaints as well as menstrual problems in women.
- *Back aspect:* This zone begins from the sixth thoracic vertebra (T6) to the 11th thoracic vertebra (T11).

Disorders of the liver, gall bladder, spleen and stomach, poor appetite, belching, hiccup, the triple burner, chest and abdominal muscles, emotional conditions such as nervous dispositions, anger and frustration, and blood disorders such as anaemia can all be treated at this zone.

Zone 3: The Lower Zone

- This zone starts from the 11th thoracic vertebra (T11) and terminates at the fourth lumbar vertebra (L4).

Disorders of kidneys, lower back problems, bladder and other urogenital conditions, small and large intestine complaints, sexual disorders, menstrual disorders (including painful menstruation) and infertility problems (men and women) can all be treated at this zone.

Zone 4: The Sacral and Lower Limbs Zone

⊙ This zone starts from the fourth lumbar vertebra (L4) and includes the sacrum, hips, thighs (hamstrings) and the calf muscles (gastrocnemius).

Conditions such as lumbago pains, sciatica pains, numbness and weakness of the lower extremities, paralysis and other muscular weaknesses to the lower part of the body, infertility in men and women, menstrual problems and genitalia pains can all be treated at this zone.

MERIDIAN/CHANNEL CUPPING

It is also possible to apply cups directly over the traditional energy pathways (the meridians/channels). This form of cupping is predominantly administered when dealing with meridian-related Qi problems such as *blockages* or *stagnations*. Between 8 and 12 cups can be administered on the same meridian without any adverse effect to the patient. Smaller cups (number 1, 2 or 3) should be used over the bony parts (over the limbs) and larger cups (number 3, 4 or 5) on the more fleshy parts of meridians (see the meridian charts and the associated therapeutic characteristics in Figs 4-2–4-15; 'O' circle markings on the channels indicate the possible cupping locations).

THE CUPPING PROCEDURE

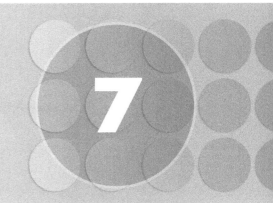

CHAPTER CONTENTS

SAFETY MATTERS, 79
HOW TO INTRODUCE FIRE SAFELY INTO THE CUP, 79
SYMMETRIC APPLICATION, 83

DECISION TIME, 84
OBTAINING THE PATIENT'S CONSENT, 86

SAFETY MATTERS

I remember a tragic story that my mother told me as a child to discourage us from playing with fire and cups. A woman in the village decided to use cups on her husband after he caught a cold. A traditional Cypriot remedy after cupping treatment is a homemade alcoholic drink called Zivania, which is rubbed over the body to produce warmth and promote perspiration. Unfortunately, in this case the woman decided to rub on the alcohol before she put the cups on! She then proceeded to light the cotton wool and apply the cups. To her horror she set fire to her husband, who stood no chance of surviving. He ran out of the house, but collapsed and died in the garden. This story also illustrates how such a simple and unsophisticated treatment as cupping can have undesirable consequences if not used correctly. Because the treatment involves handling oil, alcohol and fire at the same time – a potentially hazardous cocktail – it is not difficult to imagine the implications of careless practice. For the uninitiated I would strongly advise beginning with silicon, rubber or pistol-handled cupping or other non-flame cupping equipment.

There are different ways to create a negative pressure inside the cup: expelling the air by ignition (some form of flame) or by using manual or mechanical air extraction pumps.

HOW TO INTRODUCE FIRE SAFELY INTO THE CUP

Suction, or a negative pressure, is achieved by briefly launching fire into the cup. There are several safe and proper ways to perform this simple but rather risky process.

The Cotton Ball Method

Hold a ball of cotton wool soaked in 95% alcohol with a pair of long forceps (locking forceps are preferred) and set fire to it (Fig. 7-1A). Any excess alcohol must be squeezed out of the cotton wool before setting it alight (poor handling skills and dropping saturated cotton wool on the patient is the most commonly seen accident during cupping treatment).

Cupping Torch Method

This is relatively a new flame device, which has been introduced to the TCM clinics in the last 10 years. It is a flame holder that has a long metal holding arm, and a head that is made from an absorbent material. Prior to setting light to the torch, the practitioner presses on the alcohol dispenser, which brings the alcohol to the surface ready for soaking the torch. Once soaked in alcohol it is lit for use. (See Fig. 7-1B.)

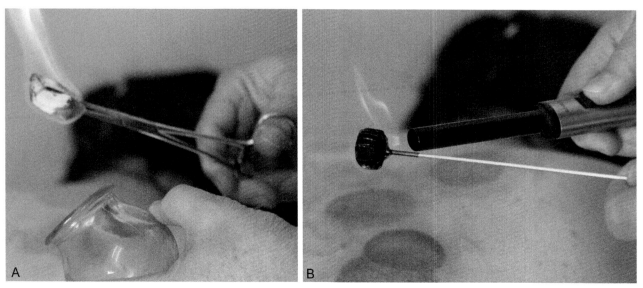

FIGURE 7-1 Choice of methods for introducing fire into the cup. (A) Holding cotton wool with locking forceps. (B) Cupping with wax torch flame.

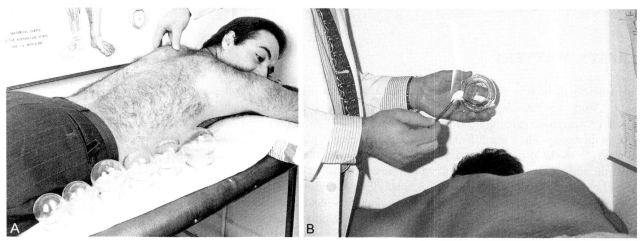

FIGURE 7-2 (A, B) Standing close to the patient during the cupping application.

The practitioner places the cups next to the patient beforehand. Holding a cup in one hand and the fire in the other, the practitioner approaches as close as possible to the site to be cupped. Holding the mouth of the cup towards the patient, the practitioner quickly and briefly introduces the fire into the cup, simultaneously turning and placing the cup on the desired point on the flesh (Fig. 7-2). There is no need to press the cup against the flesh; the suction inside is more than sufficient to hold the cup on the skin. To obtain good suction, a well-lit cotton wool ball is needed. Remember, *the bigger the fire, the greater is the suction*. Even the smaller cups need a large flame inside the cup in order to achieve good suction.

The Wick Method

(*Not suitable for children under 16 years old.*) Pure cotton or linen fabric is wrapped and secured around a coin and the excess material cut 2–2.5 cm above the coin. The ends of the wick are dipped in oil (any natural oil will do). *Do not use alcohol to wet the wick as the alcohol will run down the coin and cause fire when the wick is lit.* Light the tips of the wick and wait for a few seconds before the wick is fully alight (as the wick burns the coin remains cold). Gently lower the cup over the burning wick without delay (any delay at this junction will heat up the coin!). Do not use pressure or press the cup over the wick. Gentle lowering of the cup will be sufficient to obtain a very firm and strong suction. The strength of the suction can be adjusted simply by thumb pressure on the edge of the cup, letting a small amount of air into the cup to reduce its pulling power. This reducing technique is often used, especially when the desired cupping method is light or medium strength (Fig. 7-3).

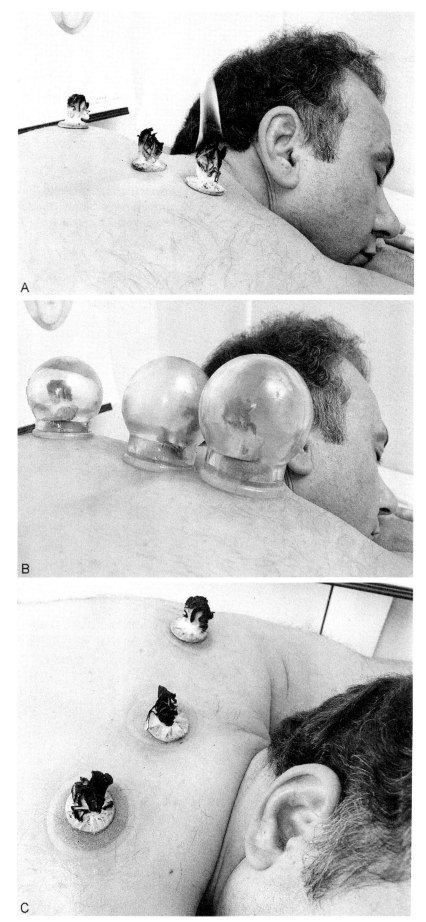

FIGURE 7-3 (A,B) Cupping using wicks. (C) Cupping using wicks. The wick is prepared using a coin wrapped in pure cotton fabric and dipped in oil. The wick is lit and a cup placed over the fire. This method is used when a particularly strong suction is desired. It is also a very slow method of cupping.

The Alcohol Rub Method

Cotton wool is held and locked with forceps and soaked in alcohol. Light the cotton ball and rub the flame inside to the bottom of the cup. Following the rubbing action simultaneously turn the cup on the desired location. Again, before lighting the cotton wool remember to squeeze out the excess alcohol. Otherwise there is a real risk of fire with alcohol running down the edges of the cup and to the skin causing burns (Fig. 7-4).

The Lighter Flame Method

An ordinary gas cooker flamethrower is used to briefly introduce fire into the cup. Although this may seem as a 'much safer' option for cupping, due to the poor quality volume of the flame the suction strength is somewhat weak. This method is preferred by some practitioners as no alcohol is involved (Fig. 7-5).

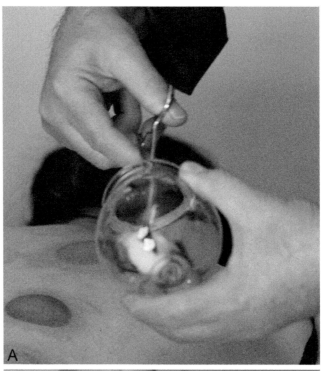

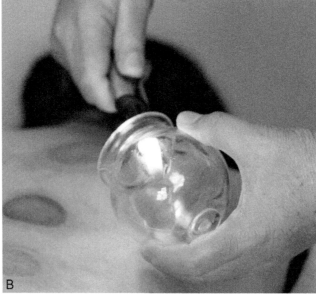

FIGURE 7-4 (A, B) Alcohol rub method.

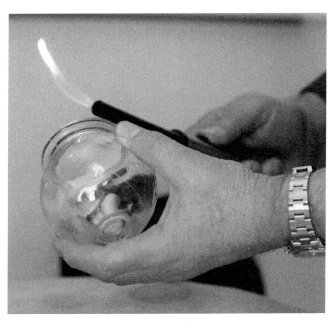

FIGURE 7-5 Lighter flame method.

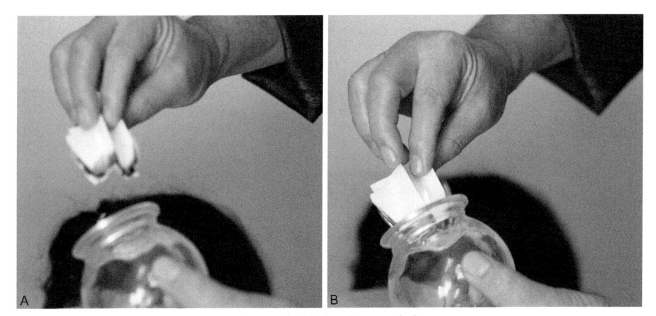

FIGURE 7-6 (A, B) Paper burning method.

The Paper Burning Method

A piece of paper is cut to the size of the cup and folded several times (this stops the paper falling back on the skin when lit). Once the paper is lit, it is then thrown into the cup (flame facing the bottom of the cup) and simultaneously turned on the skin. This method usually manages to attain Light to Medium cupping strength (Fig. 7-6).

SYMMETRIC APPLICATION

During the cupping application, since the aim is to manipulate the channels, Qi, Blood or Wind elements, it is imperative to apply cups symmetrically. Unless the treatment location has a limited cupping space, that will not allow symmetric application to take place. This rule is particularly justifiable when cupping on the face, abdominal points and the bladder channel at the back of the body. From the patient's perspective too, when the cupping sensation on the skin feels more equally distributed it makes the treatment more pleasurable. Symmetrical method allows equal channel manipulation to both sides of the body.

DECISION TIME

This is the crucial time when the practitioner has to decide which type of cupping procedure to follow. The first question comes to mind is: which cupping method do I employ – the fire cupping (Hot method), or the non-fire manual suction cupping (Cold method)? The second question is: will it be a Dry cupping method (without bleeding), or Wet cupping method (with bleeding)?

I am often asked which type of cupping is more beneficial: the fire cupping, or the manual suction (cold) cupping version? The answer to both of these questions lies with the patient's Qi condition! Throughout this book I have advocated the importance of the patient's Qi state when they present themselves at the clinic. This will help in determining the most appropriate cupping method to suit the individual. Therefore, the most *fundamental* question to be asked by the practitioner is: what *pattern* is the patient presenting – a *Heat pattern* or a *Cold pattern?* The treatment modality will be easier to decide when the differentiation is established. Cold cupping therefore will be more appropriate on patients with Heat pattern and the fire cupping (Hot cupping) will be more suited to the patients with a Cold pattern. When treating the children, however, I prefer the manual pump type cups (rubber and silicon cups can also be warmed up in hot water before the application). To begin with, I first put cups on the parent's arms and then encourage the children to apply the cups on their own arm! This helps to gain their trust and build up confidence. Each treatment, therefore, is 'tailor made' to suit each individual patient's need, there is no 'one fits all' formulae during cupping therapy! Look in Chapter 9 'Twelve methods of cupping therapy' where Cold cupping is presented as a 'draining method' and the Hot cupping is presented as a 'tonifying method'.

To Bleed Or Not To Bleed?

This is the other most frequently asked question by the practitioners: '*shall I bleed or not bleed?*' Or, 'which is the most effective method; the Dry or the Wet type?'

Once again, the answer similarly lies within the patient's pattern differentiation. In general, the Wet (Bleeding) cupping is considered a 'draining' method, which makes it *only suitable* for patients presenting with 'full (excess Shi) conditions'.

Dry cupping on the other has a wider range of application and is further divided into 10 different cupping methods, of which some are 'draining' and some 'tonifying'. Dry method gives the practitioner more overall control in the treatment and management of the disease. I therefore neither advocate nor approve a blanket 'bleeding is best' approach. Most Middle-Eastern-trained practitioners, however, prefer only Bleeding cupping (Hejama) for all types of conditions and for everyone including the children! Once more, I would like express my deep trepidation regarding this approach. First and foremost, the Bleeding cupping method is considered to be an 'extremely draining' method, which may not be the best method for patients presenting with 'deficiency patterns', in particular when treating the old and frail or children. This method is described in detail in Chapter 9.

General Safety Procedures

As mentioned earlier, the practitioner must make sure that the room or the treatment cubicle used is comfortably warm, that the patient is well informed and relaxed, and that there are no inflammable materials or coverings. It is also important to ask the patient to remove clothing from the part of the body to be cupped. If the upper body is to be cupped, the patient must tie back their hair (and, if necessary, hold it with one hand). This eliminates the risk of hair and clothing catching fire.

Choose the position most suitable for the patient's ailment and mobility limitations. Do not ask the patient to lie down or to sit up if this will cause discomfort. Seek their views on the most comfortable position, especially when treating the pregnant or the elderly. Once the patient is ready, moisturize the area to be cupped with massage oil (any commercial massage oil or olive oil will do), prepare the cups close to the patient and, if possible, place them next to the area to be treated. This will save time and effort during the treatment and at the same time eliminate the risk of dropping a flame onto the patient or the floor. Prepare small cotton wool balls, having soaked them in an airtight jar of alcohol beforehand so that they are ready for igniting. When both the practitioner and patient are ready, apply the cups quickly, covering the patient with a blanket for warmth. To remove the cups when the desired cupping time is over, gently press the edge of the cup with an index finger and let in some air (Fig. 7-7). This will release the cup without effort or discomfort to the patient. When removing the cups, special care is needed to make sure that the cup is held *away* from the practitioner's face, to prevent any possible inhalation of vapour from inside the cup (Fig. 7-8). The vapour and odour inside the cup represent the internal pathogenic factor unique to that individual patient (pathogenic Wind). Therefore, every effort should be made to avoid inhaling the discarded energy.

Used cups should be immersed in water containing 2% sodium hypochlorite solution immediately after removal, and washed with soapy water before being stored. This will reduce any risk of cross-infection. Sometimes small amounts of blood may be drawn into the cup during treatment. This is more likely when cupping has followed the removal of acupuncture needles, or when applied directly over skin pustules or acne. In such cases where blood is drawn into the cup the practitioner should wear surgical rubber gloves when removing the cups. A clean paper towel should be held over the mouth of the cup to prevent spillage during removal. Usually any blood drawn into the cup will coagulate within

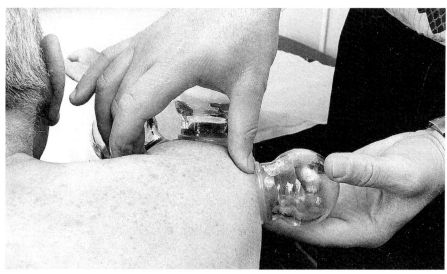

FIGURE 7-7 Cup removal, showing a finger pressing technique to let air into the cup. Remove the cup away from the practitioner's face.

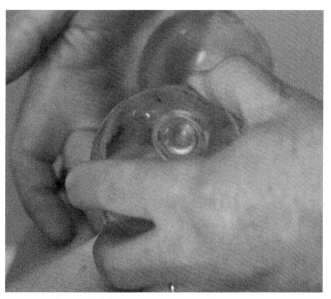

FIGURE 7-8 Removing the cup *away* from your face.

a short period of time and therefore not spill. I would recommend the commercially available antibacterial skin-cleansing agent containing 20% chlorhexidine gluconate (Hibisol) solution, to wash and sterilize the hands after each treatment.

OBTAINING THE PATIENT'S CONSENT

It is good practice to ask the patient to sign a 'patient consent form' (particularly when the patient is under 18 years old and before the cosmetic cupping) before the treatment begins and after explaining the benefits and the side effects of cupping therapy, such as the possibility of a small amount of bleeding from the cupping site and that the cupping marks may last for up to 15 days. It makes good sense to obtain written consent from your patient or the parent. Table 7-1 shows a sample consent form used in my clinics.

TABLE 7-1   Sample Patient Consent Form

[Your name and address]

Cupping Therapy Patient Consent Form

I, (print patient's full name) ……………………….. confirm that the cupping therapy practitioner (your name) ……………………… has fully explained to me the benefits, side effects and contraindications of cupping therapy, and that I understand that slight bleeding may occur from the cupping site and some degree of skin marking or bruising, lasting for between 10 and 20 days, may result.

Signed: …………………………..

Date: ……………………………..

WHAT TO EXPECT DURING AND AFTER CUPPING THERAPY

8

CHAPTER CONTENTS

INTRODUCTION, 87
IS THE CUPPING MARKING A BRUISE OR
AN ECCHYMOSIS?, 89

DIAGNOSIS THROUGH CUPPING
MARKS, 90
REFERENCES, 90

INTRODUCTION

The primary object of cupping therapy is to move Blood and Qi, remove Wind and Cold pathogens as well as Heat pathogens and eliminate stagnation of any kind from the body (and not to 'remove the evil spirit' as was claimed by one untrained therapist, leading to a police investigation in England in July 2005). To achieve this, different cupping techniques can be employed (there are 12 different cupping methods). Almost without exception, in every case where cupping is performed for the first time there will be slight reddening or a ring mark caused by the edge of the cup at the site of the treatment (Fig. 8-1). The extent of the cupping mark depends very much on the length of treatment time and the strength of the suction achieved. To reduce the risk of severe marking, always start with empty, light or medium strength suction, increasing the strength and duration on subsequent visits. The patient should experience a warm, pulling or stretching sensation on the skin, but not pain. If the patient complains of pain at any time during treatment, remove the cups immediately and reapply using reduced technique. The skin of some patients is very sensitive and their pain threshold extremely low, especially children under 16 years old, the elderly, North Americans, Scandinavians and northern Europeans including the UK patients. On several occasions I have come across some unsightly cupping marks that were caused by over-eager or untrained cupping practitioners (Fig. 8-2).

Normally the ring or cupping mark will fade away within 10 days. In some cases a blister may appear on the skin inside the cup. This is an indication of both excessive duration and strength of suction. When this happens, remove the cup without delay and pierce the blister with a sharp sterilized instrument, such as an acupuncture needle, to release the fluid. Do not reapply cups at the site of the blister until it has completely healed. Elderly and very young patients are particularly susceptible to severe marking and blistering. This is another reason for monitoring the patient during treatment. If the blister is not noticed at an early stage, it may result in an unnecessary large, open wound.

During the holiday season, cupping treatment should be terminated a week before the patient goes away (unless the patient does not mind showing off the marks) or the marks may draw attention from onlookers at the beach or the pool. The cupping marks usually appear worst of all after the first application, because of stagnation of Blood and Qi; follow-up treatments to the same point will result in much less marking, as the circulation improves and the stagnation is removed. The fine capillaries under the skin fill and empty freely and, as a result of improved metabolism following treatment, a sense of warmth and wellbeing pervades the patient's body, sometimes accompanied by a feeling of lightheadedness and a slight thirst.

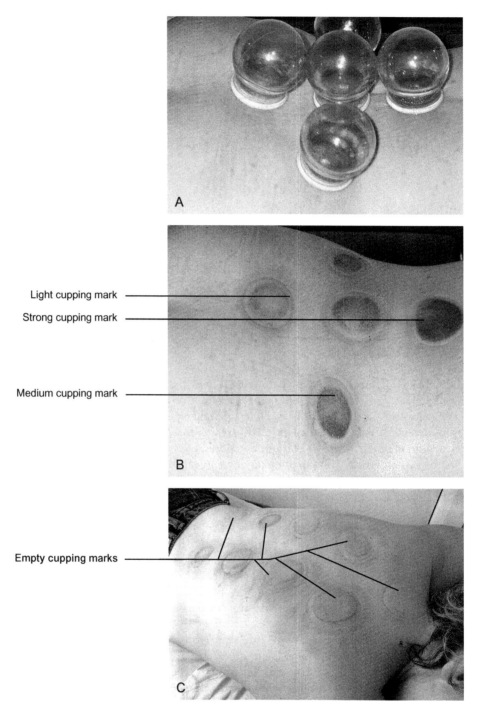

Light cupping mark

Strong cupping mark

Medium cupping mark

Empty cupping marks

FIGURE 8-1 (A–C) Cupping marks following cupping treatment. Cupping marks should not appear after Empty, Light or Water cupping methods.

When the cupping session is over there is a short period of tenderness at the points where the cups have been applied. Using massage oil, the area can be massaged gently and, time permitting, the patient can be covered with a blanket for a few minutes' rest before leaving the clinic. Blood pressure may vary by a few points owing to the unfamiliar suction and its effects on the circulation. As patients with low blood pressure are particularly susceptible to these fluctuations, care must be taken not to send patients away too soon following treatment. Patients coming for cupping therapy should also be advised to eat a light meal at least 2 hours before the treatment commences. Do not administer cupping therapy when the stomach is full or when it is completely empty, and particularly when the patient is fasting. In both situations the Qi is either 'stagnant' or 'empty', in which case it may contribute to the patient feeling unwell.

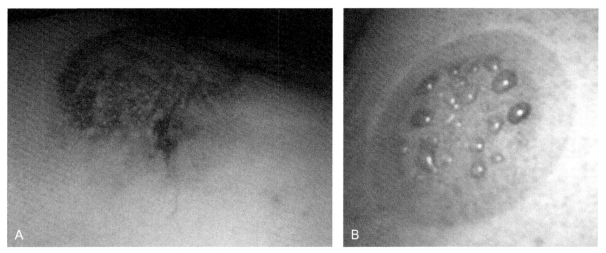

FIGURE 8-2 (A, B) Cupping marks that were caused by an untrained practitioner.

During the cupping days or weeks ask the patient to refrain from eating rich and greasy foods. Light, warm meals in winter and salads in the summer are preferred. The fluid intake should also be increased at least 20% during this period, which will help with the metabolism and the detoxification process. A warm feeling throughout the body, some perspiration and a sense of relaxation normally follow the treatment owing to improved circulation and muscle relaxation. Should the patient feel cold, shivery or extremely tired after the treatment, a warm drink and up to 30 minutes of rest are highly recommended before the patient leaves the clinic.

Like many other therapies, cupping therapy isn't a 'magic cure' for all ailments. The full benefits of cupping therapy are usually achieved after between 5 and 10 visits. Sometimes the benefits are noticed immediately but are short lived, in particular when dealing with emotional complaints or longstanding chronic problems. Ten sessions are considered to be one course of treatment. Patients less than 16 years of age normally require less treatment.

IS THE CUPPING MARKING A BRUISE OR AN ECCHYMOSIS?

There is an ongoing debate among cupping practitioners over whether we should call the subsequent cupping marks as such, or a 'bruise'? The *English Medical Dictionary* by Peter Collin (Collin, 1987) describes a bruise as: 'contusion or dark painful area on the skin, where blood has escaped under the skin following a blow'. The online MedicineNet.com dictionary gives the following description of bruising: 'a bruise is a traumatic injury of the soft tissues which results in breakage of the local capillaries and leakage of red blood cells. In the skin it can be seen as a reddish-purple discolouration that does not blanch when pressed upon.' A different explanation from the latter source is: 'a bruise is called a contusion and is typically a result of some degree of injury to the blood vessels in the skin. Local leakage of blood into the skin from the capillaries that occurs spontaneously and is flat is referred as ecchymosis.'

When we look at the various explanations above, it is clear that a bruise should have at least two characteristics: (1) contain a dark and painful area; and (2) be the result of a blow, injury or trauma. The noun 'ecchymosis', however, is explained as 'local leakage of blood into the skin from the capillaries that occurs spontaneously and is also painless'. Almost all blood thinning medications and treatments cause ecchymosis that is not painful but causes discoloration of the skin. All skin marks that are the result of cupping therapy, however dark they may appear, are not *painful*. There is no external or internal damage inflicted to the skin. Capillaries do not leak as result of 'injury or blow to blood vessels'. Also, all bruises will turn yellowy-green before totally fading away. With the exception of Strong cupping on the first two visits, all cupping marks will fade away without turning a yellowy-green colour. Even following the Strong cupping method, local pain will not accompany the cupping mark! Slight local sensitivity is the expected reaction immediately following the cupping application, and is usually much less tender over the next day or two. I personally prefer to call these effects 'cupping marks' as I find ecchymosis a rather technical term and too 'trendy' a word to use!

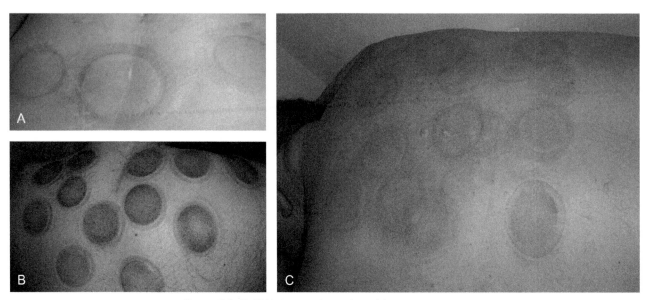

FIGURE 8-3 (A–C) Various cupping marks and their interpretation.

DIAGNOSIS THROUGH CUPPING MARKS

The general consensus amongst the cupping practitioners all around the world is: *the darker the cupping mark the more chronic is the stasis.* As the Blood and Qi circulations improve with subsequent visits so too does the cupping mark! Various degrees of cupping marks and their interpretation are illustrated in Figure 8-3.

REFERENCES

Collin, P.H., 1987. English Medical Dictionary. Peter Collin Publishing Ltd, Teddington, Middlesex.
MedicineNet.com Dictionary. Online. Available: www.MedicineNet.com.

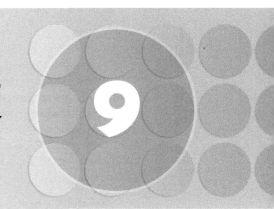

TWELVE METHODS OF CUPPING THERAPY

9

CHAPTER CONTENTS

WEAK (LIGHT) CUPPING (TONIFYING METHOD), 92

MEDIUM CUPPING (TONIFYING METHOD), 94

STRONG CUPPING (DRAINING METHOD), 95

MOVING CUPPING – TUI GUAN FA (DRAINING METHOD), 98

LIGHT-MOVING CUPPING (EVEN METHOD), 100

NEEDLE CUPPING (DRAINING METHOD), 102

HOT NEEDLE AND MOXA CUPPING – AI GUAN FA (TONIFYING METHOD), 104

EMPTY (FLASH) CUPPING – SHAN GUAN FA (TONIFYING METHOD), 106

BLEEDING/WET/FULL CUPPING – XUE GUAN FA (DRAINING METHOD), 109

HERBAL CUPPING – YAO GUAN FA (TONIFYING METHOD), 112

WATER CUPPING – SHUI GUAN FA (EVEN METHOD), 114

ICE CUPPING (COOLING) METHOD, 116

REFERENCES, 117

See online materials

As mentioned earlier, cupping has long been extensively practised within traditional Turkish communities, and I grew up in this environment, seeing the way it was practised and many times experiencing its benefits myself. I am convinced that cupping as practised today in most European countries is the legacy of the Ottoman Turks and their use of cupping in Hamams. The method my mother would generally use was straightforward and simple. She would oil our skin first and then apply up to six cups (or empty jam jars) for only 2 or 3 minutes, repeating the process several times. The cups were almost always applied on the back of the body (i.e. the upper part of the shoulder blade, or the lower back). This was the way I grew up to know and practise cupping, until I studied traditional Chinese medicine in 1983.

The first day at Professor Wong's clinic in Northcote, Melbourne, was, indeed, a memorable one for me. This was my first clinical practice day, having completed my studies. A senior practitioner was showing the novice what was expected during the first few weeks. The duties included preparing balls of cotton wool to be soaked in alcohol, sterilizing needles and other equipment, answering telephone calls and washing the cups used the previous day! To my colleagues, these strange-looking glass objects were the most fascinating tools of the trade, alongside the acupuncture needle. The principal of the academy, Professor Wong, was a great acupuncturist and herbalist, but above all he was a tactile therapist and a great believer in the healing power of massage and cupping. With almost every patient, his prescription would end with cupping or a massage treatment. I often volunteered to work at his Northcote clinic, where I learned the comprehensive use of cupping techniques. However, over the last 30 years in my own practice, and during my studies in China, I have developed some methods of my own and have been able to bring together 12 different cupping techniques (10 methods mentioned in the first edition of this book and 11 in the second). Over the last 13 years since the first book was published, I have received hundreds of letters and emails enquiring about the different techniques I mentioned in the book. Most readers described the cupping methods as 'intriguing', 'interesting' and 'fascinating'.

All 12 methods described below represents the most fundamental concept of this book: the cupping therapy and its organic association with Qi, Blood and the Wind element. All methods illustrated below therefore are designed to help the practitioner chose the cupping technique during the treatment protocol that is most appropriate to the patient's Qi/energetic condition. I am often asked by some patients to perform cupping treatment often unsuitable for their present energetic circumstances, such as Bleeding or Strong cupping methods, because of a magazine article they have seen or read! Like all other forms of medicine, cupping therapy is not a 'magic cure-all' but one that needs regular application, as well as the 'correct' technique most suitable to the individual's current condition.

Twelve Cupping Methods

- Weak (Light) cupping
- Medium cupping
- Strong cupping
- Moving cupping
- Light-moving cupping
- Needle cupping
- Hot Needle and Moxa cupping
- Empty (Flash) cupping
- Bleeding/Wet/Full cupping
- Herbal cupping
- Water cupping
- Ice cupping

WEAK (LIGHT) CUPPING (TONIFYING METHOD)

See *online materials*

Weak cupping is employed when Blood and Qi are sluggish, deficient (Xu) or stagnant, and a reversal of these conditions is desired. *The action of Weak cupping is intended to strengthen the Wei Qi, remove Wind, stagnation of Blood, Qi and Body Fluids and at the same time tonify the weak Qi and Blood,* and it is therefore termed a 'tonifying' method. The key factor in deciding when to apply Weak cupping is the present energetic state/condition of the patient. Pulse, tongue and visual diagnosis should all point to a deficiency.

Application

The patient and cups are prepared as described earlier, and the skin is moistened with oil. The practitioner should light the cotton wool and wait for a few seconds so that the fire is less intense when introduced into the cup. Remember, *the bigger the fire, the greater is the suction.* Apply the cups at the desired points until all have been used. At this point, the practitioner should take immediate note of the suction inside the cups. The amount of flesh drawn into the cups should be minimal and hardly raised. Should the initial suction be stronger than originally planned, the practitioner should press the edge of the cup with an index finger and let in some air to reduce the strength of the suction to the desired level. At no time should the patient feel an uncomfortable sensation of pulling or pain on the treatment area. If this happens, the practitioner should continue with the reducing technique until the patient feels comfortable. Weak cupping is the gentlest method of all and is particularly suitable for debilitated adults, elderly patients and young children, especially those under 7 years of age.

Light cupping can be applied almost anywhere on the body, and may cause a slight reddening of the skin, rather than a deep, dark cupping mark or blister. Therefore, the duration of Weak cupping can be as long as 30 minutes. When Light cupping is performed on hairy or very dry skin, the suction is likely to cease much earlier than planned. In this case, the practitioner should apply oil liberally and repeat the procedure. The gentle pulling action of this method stimulates the movement of Qi within the meridian system, bringing benefit to the patient and tonifying the Blood and Qi without the risk of further depleting energy in weak and frail patients (Colour Plate Figure 1, Fig. 9-1A, B).

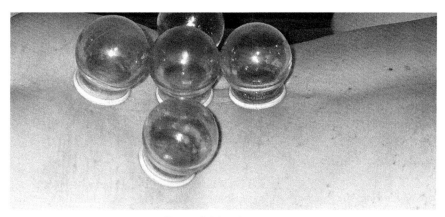

FIGURE 9-1 Weak cupping.

Conditions Most Suitable for Weak Cupping Method

- Common cold
- Sore throat
- Tonsillitis
- All abdominal and digestive complaints
- For people recovering from an illness or an operation
- All children under 16 years of age
- Asthma
- Anaemia
- Blood and Qi tonification
- Facial complaints including Wind-stroke (Bell's palsy) and cosmetic treatments
- Psychosomatic and emotional conditions
- Immune deficiency syndromes
- Fatigue
- ME sufferers
- Multiple sclerosis (MS) patients
- Cancer patients
- Expectant mothers.

CASE 9-1 Ms J – 36 Years Old and 6 Months' Pregnant (Restlessness with Poor Sleep)

Six months pregnant, Ms J, complaining of 'restlessness and poor sleep', came to see me. She already has 3 children all under 10 years old! She has not been able to have a 'quality sleep' for some time. She has a 'good home life' and follows a 'good diet'. Despite this, once she goes to bed, she tosses and turns and not being able to sleep makes her restless and moody, and the cycle continues until she gets exhausted and falls asleep. As a result she is getting up each morning feeling extremely tired and irritable.

Pulse. Rapid, weak at all levels.

Tongue. Red and dry body (sometimes gets sore tongue).

Medication. None.

Observation. Woman of medium build, reddish face, dry skin (all over the body) and dark circles under the eyes.

TCM Diagnosis. Chronic Kidney-Qi and Yin deficiency resulting in Heart Fire.

Treatment Principle. Tonify the Kidneys and the Lungs and Clear the pathogenic Heat.

Cupping Application. After 4 weeks of weekly cupping sessions, employing the Weak cupping method to the entire upper back of the body, she felt calmer and her sleep pattern returned to normal. Points concentrated on during the treatment were: Du-14 Dazhui, Du-12 Shenzhu, BL-13 Feishu, BL-15 Xinshu, BL-20 Pishu, BL-23 Shenshu and BL-42 Pohu.

Additional Therapy. Acupuncture.

CASE 9-2 A 25-year-old Woman with MS

Four years ago, Ms A had suffered a stroke-like lesion to the brain resulting in paralysis of the right side of her body and loss of speech. Within 2 months she recovered completely. Three years later, she had a similar attack but this time to the opposite side, which affected the left side of her body resulting in weakness of her left leg, left hand and poor speech. Her neurologist diagnosed it as an 'attack similar to multiple sclerosis'.

Medication. She was on steroids (but stopped by now) and Prozac.

Pulse. Even but weak, Liver pulse dominating (she gets frustrated and irritable quickly).

Tongue. Good body colour, trembling.

Observation. Thin, slightly on the pale side, likes to talk (speaking is an effort but perseveres) and has a sense of humour!

TCM Diagnosis. Blood and Qi deficiency with Wind pathogen invading the channels.

Treatment Principle. Tonify Blood and Qi and remove the invading pathogenic Wind.

Cupping Application. Weak cupping to the front and the back of the left leg and the entire upper back of the body. Cupping sessions were limited to 15 minutes with repeated applications to the same locations. After five sessions she reported 'feeling better'. The treatment is still ongoing.

Additional Therapy. Acupuncture, moxibustion and dietary.

Summary Points

- Tonifies Blood and Qi
- Strengthens the Wei Qi
- Removes pathogenic Wind
- Blood, Qi and Fluid stagnation
- Benefits children, adults recovering from illness, the elderly and the frail.

MEDIUM CUPPING (TONIFYING METHOD)

 See online materials

This is the most frequently used cupping method on patients with relatively strong Qi. *It manipulates the Wei Qi, Qi, Blood, lymphatic system and the external 'Wind' element (Wind-Heat and Wind-Cold).* Medium cupping can safely be administered to children over 7 years old, as well as to adults. With Medium cupping the suction is firmer but, as the patient's own Qi is also good, it will act as a tonifying method. However, there is a real danger of draining the patient's Qi if the cups are left on for longer than 30 minutes, leaving the patient lethargic. This is also the most effective method when dealing with the 'External Wind invading channels' pattern.

Application

To achieve a Medium suction the practitioner needs to use a bigger fire than with the Light method. The cups must also be held closer to the patient, to enable the practitioner to be quick in applying them; the suction will be firmer as the fire draws out the oxygen, thus creating a stronger vacuum. With this method the skin is pulled well into the cup, creating a slight redness as mentioned earlier (Fig. 9-2, Colour Plate Figure 2). If the cups are left on for longer, the redness will turn to dark red or purple, indicating a stronger application. If glass cups are used instead of the more traditional bamboo cups, the progress can be observed closely and early adjustment made if desired. Medium cupping can safely be applied anywhere on the body, including the face and abdomen.

Conditions Most Suitable for the Medium Cupping Method

In addition to the conditions mentioned above:

- Hot or Cold 'Bi' syndrome
- Stress-related conditions
- Headache
- Blood and Qi tonification
- Children's ailments
- Infertility complaints
- Sports injuries
- Musculoskeletal complaints
- Tremors and fits.

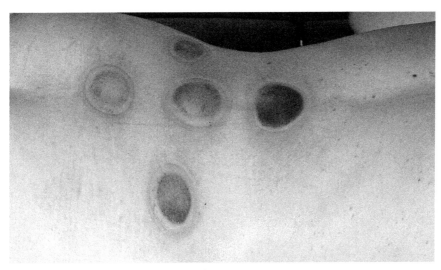

FIGURE 9-2 Medium cupping.

CASE 9-3 J – a 79-year-old Woman (Shingles with Lower Back and Shoulder Pain)

J had been suffering from shingles for over 4 months when she came to see me. She was waking up several times during the night owing to the pain. Lately she had also been complaining of lower back and shoulder pain. She also looks after her husband who is wheelchair bound, due to his severe respiratory condition.

Pulse. Slightly rapid, otherwise good.

Tongue. Red body proper, with thick yellow coating.

Medication. Blood pressure tablets, thyroxine and paracetamol.

Observation. She is well built and looks excellent for her age.

TCM Diagnosis. Wind-Heat attack with 'Hot Bi' syndrome.

Treatment Principle. Clear the pathogenic Heat and manage the 'Bi' syndrome.

Cupping Application. Weekly treatment to the upper back (avoiding the shingles area), and the lower back, employing Medium cupping technique for 5 weeks, helped to reduced her symptoms significantly. At the start of the treatment, two sessions of Bleeding cupping to Du-14 were also employed.

Additional Therapy. Acupuncture and herbal ointment.

Summary Points

- Tonify Blood and Qi
- Strengthen Wei Qi
- Elevate the Shen (Spirit)
- External Wind-Cold invading the channels
- Internal Wind-Heat
- External Wind-Heat
- Lymphatic drainage
- Benefits adults and children over 7 years old.

STRONG CUPPING (DRAINING METHOD)

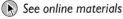 *See online materials*

Blood and the 'internal Wind' are the principal targets of this method. This is also one of the most draining techniques of all (Moving cupping is the other). Therefore, before deciding on Strong cupping the practitioner must ensure the suitability of the patient. Significant amounts of Blood and Qi are manipulated by this method, sometimes leaving the patient tired. Pulse, tongue and visual diagnosis should all emphasize an Excess, Full (Shi) condition. Defensive Qi (Wei Qi) is most affected and influenced by this method. The purpose of a Strong cupping treatment is to move Blood and Qi and eliminate internal/external pathogenic factors (internal Wind) and stagnation from patients with relatively strong Wei Qi. It is suitable for all forms of chronic musculoskeletal complaints and Blood stasis syndromes.

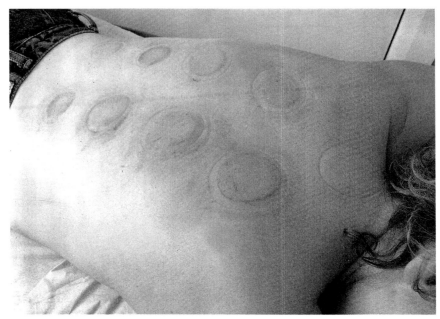

FIGURE 9-3 Strong cupping.

Application

The practitioner should prepare the patient and have the cups close at hand. For a Strong cupping technique a big fire is necessary in order to achieve a strong pulling action. For this reason, a rather large ball of cotton wool is taken, or two held together by forceps. On igniting the cotton wool, the fire is inserted into the cup without delay, and simultaneously the cup is turned onto the skin. A strong vacuum will be produced, giving a strong pulling sensation of the skin inside the cup. Because of the strong nature of the pulling action the skin will quickly turn red, and shortly after turn purple, inside the cup (Fig. 9-3). It is preferable to avoid the Strong method on a patient's first visit and introduce the treatment using a much weaker version, explaining that subsequent treatments will be slightly stronger. When using a Strong cupping method for the first time a very dark red cupping mark is inevitable; this can take up to 15–20 days to disappear completely. The cupping time should also be short: between 3 and 5 minutes during the first session. This can be increased up to 20 minutes in later applications. The dark-red cupping marks will become much lighter and the dispersal time much shorter, sometimes lasting only a day or two (Colour Plate Figure 3).

Following an acupuncture session, Strong cupping treatment may cause a small amount of blood to be drawn into the cup. This is quite acceptable given the strength of the suction applied by this method. Fine capillaries under the skin can also break relatively easily with strong suction, causing deeper and longer-lasting cupping marks. This is also the only method of cupping that can cause blisters to form rather quickly. Therefore, it is strongly advised that the practitioner should remain with the patient at all times during the treatment, observing the progress of the suction and, if necessary, removing the cups earlier than planned. One way of obtaining a Strong suction is to employ the wick method described in Chapter 7. When using the pistol handle cupping gun, three complete pulls also produces a Strong suction.

The Strong cupping method should be avoided on the face, stomach, abdomen, on children under the age of 16, the elderly and frail, and also during the entire period of the pregnancy.

Figure 9-4 shows the effect on the skin of the Weak, Medium and Strong cupping methods.

Conditions Most Suitable for Strong Cupping Method

- All excessive Heat conditions such as Stomach Heat, Liver Heat, Damp-Heat and febrile diseases
- Hypertension
- Headache

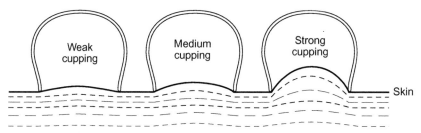

FIGURE 9-4 Section of the skin showing the effects of Weak, Medium and Strong cupping.

- Febrile diseases in adults
- Boils
- Skin complaints that are accompanied by Heat syndrome
- It is particularly beneficial in the treatment of Hot-type 'Bi' syndrome (see Chapter 12)
- Blood or Qi stagnation patterns
- Muscular cramps
- Sports injuries
- All musculoskeletal complaints including lower back ache and sciatica.

CASE 9-4 A 58-year-old Man (Paralysis and Pain on Both Shoulders, Accompanied by Constant Headaches)

Mr A was involved in a motorcycle accident 30 years ago (when he was 18 years old), which left him semi-paralysed in both legs. As a result he uses walking crutches to move about and to get in and out of his car. In the last few years he has undergone further spinal operations, which did not improve his condition, especially after the most recent operation to his cervical spine, which left him with weaker arms and a weaker grip in both hands. This has made him less active and more frustrated. As a direct result of his reduced mobility, he has gained weight and suffers from constant occipital headaches.

Pulse. Rapid and slippery.

Tongue. Red body proper, curling up.

Medication. Antidepressant and cocktail of painkillers.

Observation. Solid build, overweight, has good diet, likes talking, even temperament but can easily get depressed.

TCM Diagnosis. Distorted channels (due to numerous surgical interventions) with Damp-Heat dominating.

Treatment Principle. Restore the Blood and Qi circulation to the distorted channels and remove the Damp-Heat.

Cupping application. Strong cupping treatment applied for several months, concentrating on the entire upper back, including, neck and the shoulders, reduced the headaches considerably and returned strength to his arms and improved his grip. Because of his inability to climb onto a treatment couch I am unable to do cupping to his lower back. However, on a few occasions I have applied Strong cupping to his lower back while in a sitting position. He continues his booster treatment whenever he can manage to come to the clinic.

Additional Therapy. Acupuncture and massage.

CASE 9-5 A 55-year-old Woman (Frozen Shoulder Syndrome – Adhesive Capsulitis)

Mrs S suffered from 'frozen shoulder syndrome' to her left arm for over 4 months when she came to see me. She complained of 'stiffness and pain' when trying to move or lift her arm. She reported that the 'condition is getting worse with each day'.

Pulse. Rapid.

Tongue. Red and shiny, without any coating.

Medication. Blood pressure tablets and eight painkillers daily.

Observation. She is not able to remove her coat without help. Pain is clearly visible in her face when she attempts to lift her arm.

TCM Diagnosis. Yin deficiency is her general outlook, with Qi and Blood obstruction in the shoulder joint.

Treatment Principle. Remove obstruction and restore Blood and Qi circulation to the joint.

Cupping Application. First three visits, six cups using Light to Medium cupping technique were employed to the troubled shoulder with no benefit to the patient. Therefore, at follow-up visits I decided to increase the suction to Strong method and she agreed (I had to obtain her permission as this was going to cause darker cupping marks on her shoulder). After a further four treatments with Strong cupping technique, encircling the entire shoulder with six cups, her shoulder mobility improved and the shoulder pain was greatly reduced.

Additional therapy. Acupuncture, massage and Chirali Old Remedy®1 herbal ointment.

Summary Points

- Draining
- Influences the pathogenic internal Wind
- Blood and Qi manipulation
- Blood and Qi stasis
- Benefits Excess (Shi) conditions
- Can cause severe dark cupping marks that can last 2–3 weeks
- Can cause blisters
- Contraindicated for children, elderly and the frail.

MOVING CUPPING – TUI GUAN FA (DRAINING METHOD)

 See online materials

As mentioned earlier, Moving cupping is the second most draining of all the cupping methods. *This method manipulates more the Blood and to a lesser degree the Qi and the Fluids.* The object of this treatment technique is to apply Strong cupping therapy to a much larger area of the body by the moving/sliding action of the cup. Like the Strong cupping method, the patient should have strong Qi before Moving cupping is employed, in order to withstand the not-so-gentle pulling and moving action of the cup. Without any doubt this is the most painful cupping method that I know. For this reason alone, if the patient's Qi is deficient (Xu), and therefore weak, Moving cupping can only help to diminish it further. It is mostly applied to the Bladder channel on the back (about 1.5 and 3 inches [4–8 cm] either side of the spine; see Fig. 4.8), upper back, shoulders, upper and lower limbs and the abdomen (around the navel), especially when treating stagnation of any kind, excess Heat conditions, or some neurological conditions such as paralysis or post-stroke weaknesses (when treating post-stroke patients with Moving cupping one should always take into consideration the possibility of a local neuralgic pain that is sometimes associated with stroke patients).

Application

The practitioner should oil the skin liberally and apply a single medium-sized and medium-strength cup to the treatment area (Fig. 9-5). (The edges of the glass cup should be smooth and even, with no cuts or chips. This is one method in which bamboo cups are of no use, as their sharp edges make it impossible to move the cup once the suction takes hold.) The suction is controlled by gently moving the cup in any one direction. The cup should move freely and without a great deal of effort from the practitioner. If the suction is too strong, moving the cup will be difficult and any attempt to do so will result in extreme pain or a nasty bruise mark. The practitioner grips the cup with one hand while supporting the skin close to it with the other, then pulls and slides the cup alongside the meridian using long strokes. Short, up-and-down movements should be avoided as this may cause unnecessary pain. If there is difficulty in moving the cup this is an indication that the suction is too strong and needs to be reduced. The primary objective of Moving cupping is to resolve Blood stagnation/stasis, manipulate the excess pathogens and bring up the Heat to the surface of the skin. After only a few strokes pink/reddish cupping marks will appear alongside the line of movement (Fig. 9-5B). The more internal Heat that is present, the quicker the redness (Sha) will appear (Youbang & Liangyue, 1989). *This can also be used as a diagnostic tool as far as the Blood stasis and internal Heat are concerned; deep and darker cupping marks indicate a Full (Shi) condition, lighter cupping marks indicate deficient (Xu) conditions, requiring less vigorous treatment.* During the application of Moving cupping some air will almost always enter the cup, resulting in loss of suction. All that is necessary is to reapply the cup and continue with the movement. Rubber or silicon cups are also ideal for Moving cupping treatment.

One should avoid using the Moving method on an open wound or lesion, as the skin must be smooth and unbroken. The first session should not exceed 5 minutes, building up to a maximum of 20 minutes per session.

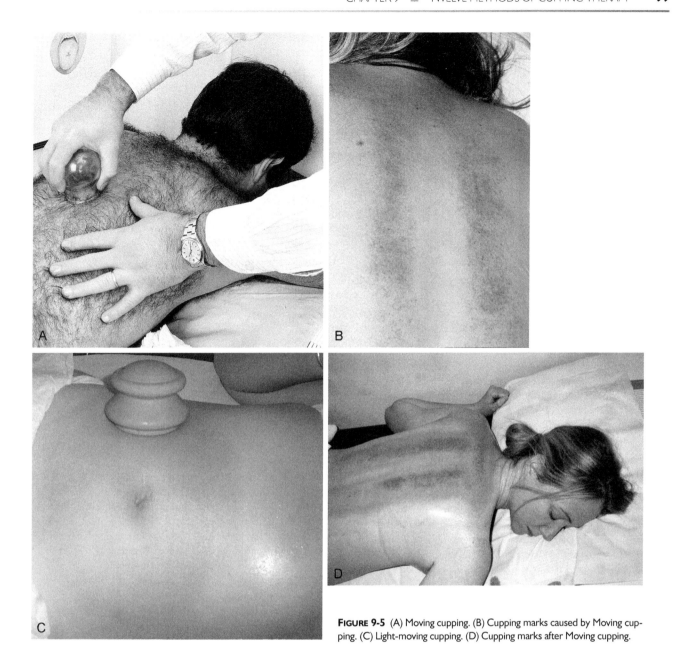

FIGURE 9-5 (A) Moving cupping. (B) Cupping marks caused by Moving cupping. (C) Light-moving cupping. (D) Cupping marks after Moving cupping.

Conditions Most Suitable for Moving Cupping Method

This treatment is not recommended for children under the age of 16, or for the frail and weak. For Hot skin conditions such as eczema, psoriasis and acne, or painful Hot 'Bi' syndrome, Moving cupping is most beneficial, though it is important to avoid direct application to lesions. This is also the most powerful method for manipulating the lymphatic circulation and, therefore, requires particular attention when dealing with any form of lymphoedema:

- Febrile diseases
- Musculoskeletal complaints
- Muscle or tendon relaxation
- Sports injuries
- All cosmetic cupping techniques including cellulite, facial, body toning and weight loss programmes.

CASE **9-6** A 35-year-old Woman (Breast Pain)

A 35-year-old female patient came to see me complaining from 'heavy pain' over her right breast. Previously she had seen her GP and was referred for numerous tests, which all came back negative. This kept her awake at night and mentally worried.

Pulse. Rapid, with Liver pulse prominent.

Tongue. Pale, shiny, wet with whitish coating.

Medication. Vitamins and painkillers (tramadol).

Observation. Tall and a good build, pale on the face, swims twice a week and works in an office. She gets more colds than her colleagues in the office (does not like her job!).

TCM Diagnosis. Wind-Cold dominating (particularly the Liver channel), accompanied by Liver-Qi stagnation.

Treatment Protocol. Remove the Wind-Cold and soothe the Liver-Qi.

Cupping Application. Moving Cupping was employed on both Bladder channels (the inner and the outer BL channel), employing Medium strength suction. To the front of body, Moving cupping was used with much less suction, to the area under the clavicle and following the breast contour, moving towards the breast bone and under the breast. Finally, a single large cup with Light suction was applied over the right nipple. The pain was reduced each week, and she recovered completely seven treatments later.

Additional Therapy. Acupuncture and herbal remedies.

CASE **9-7** A 70-year-old Man (Hip and Thigh Pain)

70-year-old Mr A came to see me complaining of a 'stabbing pain' that travelled from his left hip to the upper part of his left thigh. There was no pattern to the pain; it could appear any time of the day or night and last between a few seconds and a few minutes. This condition appeared almost a year after he had undergone 'successful hip replacement' surgery.

Pulse. Forceful at all levels.

Tongue. Good colour and body.

Medication. Simvastatin and aspirin (75 mg).

Observation. Mr A was a gentleman of slim build, who enjoyed his daily walks and good food. He has been taking cholesterol lowering statin medication for a number of years. My initial reaction was that the statin might be the cause of his stabbing pain. However, I was reassured that his GP ordered a 'full blood count' several months before and it was established that the cholesterol medication was not the cause of his complaint.

TCM Diagnosis. Blood stasis/stagnation due to his previous hip replacement surgery.

Treatment Principle. Remove the stagnation and open the channels to the front and the outer thigh (Stomach, Bladder and Gall Bladder).

Cupping Application. On each visit about 6–7 minutes of Medium strength, Moving cupping was applied to the Bladder, Gall Bladder and the Stomach meridians, taking the total treatment time to about 20 minutes each time, with cupping movements towards the knee. During the initial few sessions he often complained of 'feeling tender' during the cupping treatment, but after the third visit his tolerance level much improved. By the time he reached the sixth session, he reported that his pain was much less frequent and less severe. After having further six weekly treatments, he was completely pain free.

Additional Therapy. Acupuncture, massage and Chirali Old Remedy®1 herbal ointment.

Summary Points

- Draining
- It could be tender or even painful during the application
- Resolve Blood stasis
- Brings the internal pathogenic Heat to surface
- Avoid over the open wounds
- Avoid over the recent trauma
- Can cause blisters or dark cupping marks
- Contraindicated for children, elderly and the frail.

LIGHT-MOVING CUPPING (EVEN METHOD)

 See online materials

For many years I have practised and advocated Moving cupping only with patients with relatively 'Excess/Full' Qi or conditions. During recent years, however, I have practised Moving cupping on many patients outside this category with favourable results. This came about when I was treating a female patient with severe arthritic pains in her neck and shoulders. Following acupuncture treatment, 10 minutes of Light cupping were usually applied to the local area. On one occasion she described the pain as 'sharp and moving'. On hearing this description, I decided to employ Moving cupping on that particular day but with much-reduced suction power (see Fig. 9-5E), as she often complained of feeling 'tired and lethargic'. The following day she phoned to express her satisfaction as she had slept 'very well and comfortably' owing to the lack of pain and discomfort in her back and neck. On each subsequent visit she almost insisted on Light-moving cupping! The lymphatic system (Fluids) and the Qi are mostly manipulated by this method.

Application

The practitioner should prepare the patient as in Light cupping technique but use only a single cup. This can be glass, rubber or a silicon type cup. Oiling liberally the treatment location, the practitioner then applies a single Light strength cup, and without delay starts moving the cup to the desired direction with long strokes. At all times, one hand is moving the cup while the other is supporting the skin.

During the application of the Light-moving cupping method, slight pinkish cupping marks appear on the skin, normally following the direction and movement of the cup (see Fig. 9-5D). At no time should deep, dark red cupping marks be seen. All cupping marks should fade away within a day or two. The whole object of Light-moving cupping is to *disperse* stasis/stagnation without draining the patient. Energetically, it is an *even method, and effects mostly the Qi and, to a lesser extent, the Blood*. All Moving cupping techniques require special attention, particularly when there is a broken skin surface, where there are scratches, cuts, bruise marks, open wounds or when skin moles are present (avoid cupping over an open wound or over a mole).

Conditions Most Suitable for Light-Moving Cupping Method

- When treating children under 16 years old
- Old and frail patients
- Oedema; all conditions where oedema is present including the joints and the extremities
- Lymphoedema (opposite side of the body must be used)
- Stress release cupping–massage
- All cosmetic cupping procedures including facial and cellulite treatment
- Weight-loss programme
- Infertility
- Immune deficiency syndromes
- Cancer patients
- Multiple sclerosis patients.

CASE 9-8   A 30-year-old Woman (Facial Oedema)

Ms C for many years has been suffering from swollen/puffy eyes and face, especially during her period. She has no other health complaints.

Pulse. No significance.

Tongue. Pale and wet (almost dripping).

Medication. In the past she had taken diuretics but had since stopped.

Observation. Pale complexion, tall, slightly overweight.

TCM Diagnosis. Cold-Damp accumulating in the Upper Jiao.

Treatment Principle. Warm the Lungs, Spleen and Stomach and move the Fluids.

Cupping Application. *Medium strength warm cups* were first applied to the front and the Back-Shu points of the body; LU-1 Zhongfu, Ren-12 Zhongwan, Liv-13 Taichong, Ren-6 Qihai, Ren-4 Guanyuan, ST-25 Tianshu, BL-12 Fengmen, BL-13 Feishu, BL-20 Pishu and BL-23 Shenshu. This was followed by 15 minutes of Light-moving cupping to the face and the neck, moving the cups alongside the neck towards the clavicle. Ms C received a total of 14 treatments, after which her condition was moderately improved. She was also given dietary advice relating to her 'cold Stomach, Spleen and Lung' condition.

Additional Therapy. Acupuncture, moxibustion, dietary and herbal medicine.

CASE 9-9 An 8-year-old Boy (Stomach Pains and Poor Appetite)

An 8-year-old boy complaining from stomach pains and loss of appetite for 5 days was brought to me by his parents, who are also my patients.

Pulse. Rapid.

Tongue. Refused to show.

Medication. None.

Observation. His body weight to his height ratio is good; he does not look unwell. Clinging to his father, he does not answer my questions (gazing at the floor or looking to his father); his father is often on business trips abroad; he does not like going to school!

TCM Diagnosis. Liver-Qi stagnation pattern is the dominant feature. Resentment and anger towards his father, manifesting in stomach pains and loss of appetite.

Treatment Principle. Soothe the Liver-Qi.

Cupping Therapy. On the first two visits, I managed to massage his back and the stomach region only. On follow-up visits, using a silicon cup I applied Light-moving cupping (clockwise) circling the umbilicus. To the back of the body, I applied Light-moving cupping on the Bladder channel. Five minutes of cupping application to each side were applied. After three treatments the stomach pain was much reduced, he also felt better, and he stopped attending.

Additional Therapy. Moxibustion.

Summary Points

- Even method
- Benefits the lymphatic circulation
- Moves the Fluids
- Moves the Qi
- Treats oedema
- Suitable for all ages.

NEEDLE CUPPING (DRAINING METHOD)

 See online materials

(For acupuncture practitioners only.)

Needle cupping is mostly used for Re (Hot) types of painful 'Bi' syndrome – that is, red and painful muscular areas as well as the knee and elbow joints, where there is a need to stop the pain and remove the excess pathogenic Heat at the same time. The practitioner should administer the acupuncture treatment as intended under normal circumstances, leaving the needles in place as long as necessary. (One can reduce the acupuncture treatment time by 10–15 minutes if Needle cupping is intended to follow it.)

Application

Following the acupuncture treatment, the practitioner leaves the needles in position and applies oil to the surrounding skin. One should choose bamboo or large glass cups in order to accommodate the needles, and apply the cups over them (Fig. 9-6A). A Medium to Strong application is necessary if the

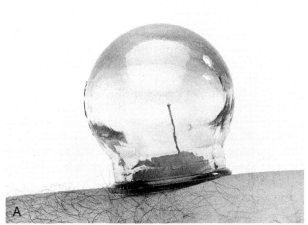
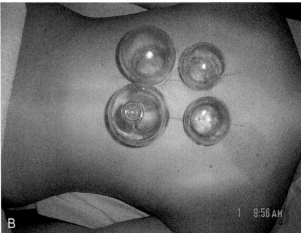

FIGURE 9-6 (A) Needle cupping: use a tall cup over the needle. (B) Through-and-through needle cupping.

treatment is over the joints and Weak to Medium if the treatment is over muscular areas, retaining the cups in position for 10–15 minutes. Some blood may be drawn into the cup through the needles; this is quite acceptable, especially if the suction is Strong. Needle cupping should be avoided on the Back-Shu points, as there is a real danger of the cup pushing the needle in deeper thereby causing a pneumothorax. To be on the safe side, short 0.5–1-inch (1.25–2.5 cm) needles are used during the treatment. This is one occasion when tall bamboo cups are preferable to the more rounded glass cups, as their height is ideal for needle clearance, making the application much safer. However, when cupping treatment is combined with the 'through and through needle technique' the application is quite safe (see Fig. 9-6B). This method is not recommended for children of any age.

Conditions Most Suitable for Needle Cupping Method

- 'Hot-Re' type 'Bi' syndromes
- Arthritis
- Rheumatoid arthritis complaints
- Osteoarthritis complaints
- Muscular stiffness, spasm or pain
- Sports injuries.

CASE 9-10 A 60-year-old Male (Swollen and Painful and Knee Joint)

60-year-old Mr M came to see me complaining of a swollen and painful knee joint. Eighteen months ago he had a fall while cycling, injuring his right knee. At the time he was referred for X-ray, which showed a degree of soft tissue damage and no broken bone. He was put on anti-inflammatory medication, which he took for 17 months (he stopped the medication because it caused stomach upsets).

Pulse. Rapid and forceful.

Tongue. Red body, no coating.

Medication. He has recently stopped taking diclofenac (anti-inflammatory).

Observation. The patient is well built, and likes activity (he swims, walks and cycles). Unfortunately, since his fall he has

stopped most of his activities and he is worried about putting on weight. The knee is looking reddish, swollen and painful and he is unable to bend it fully.

TCM Diagnosis. Blood and Fluid stagnation caused by the fall (Hot Bi).

Treatment Principle. Remove pathogenic Heat, disperse stagnation and restore the normal Blood–Fluid circulation to the joint.

Cupping Application. Needle cupping was applied to three points on the knee; both Xiyan (Extra points) and ST-34 Liangqiu. After eight visits, the redness and the swelling were much reduced and he was able to bend his knee fully.

Additional Therapy. Acupuncture and Chirali Old Remedy®1 herbal ointment.

CASE 9-11 A 45-year-old man (Stiff Neck with Pain)

Mr R developed a stiff and painful neck following a routine gardening chore 10 days previously. His neck complaint worsened a few days later and he decided to come to see me. He drives to work and describes the journey as 'almost impossible'.

Pulse. Nothing significant.

Tongue. Good body and colour.

Medication. Generic pain tablets.

Observation. Mr R, a keen gardener, had developed neck pain while practising his hobby 10 days' previously. He stands tall with a good posture. He sweats profusely when doing physical work, particularly when gardening.

TCM Diagnosis. Wind-Cold attack.

Treatment Principle. Remove the pathogenic Wind-Cold from the channels in the neck and relax the neck muscles.

Cupping Application. Needle cupping to the neck; 2-cun long needles are used to apply through and through needle technique to BL-10 Tianzhu, pointing towards BL-11 Dashu. Cupping is performed by using small-sized cups (number 1 or 2) to the middle of the neck, between the needles. Mr R received total of four treatments after which he was able to move his neck freely and drive without pain.

Additional Therapy. Acupuncture and Chirali Old Remedy®1 herbal ointment.

Summary Points

- Draining
- For acupuncture practitioners only
- 'Hot Bi' syndrome
- Disperses pathogenic Heat
- Treats joints
- Contraindicated for children of all ages.

HOT NEEDLE AND MOXA CUPPING – AI GUAN FA (TONIFYING METHOD)

See online materials

(For acupuncture practitioners only.)

Moxa *(Artemisia vulgaris)* is a great warming herb used by many practitioners for removing Wind-Cold and tonifying the Yang, Qi and Blood. It comes in many forms: the loose type, the smokeless charcoal type, the round, long, cigar-shaped dry type, and most recently the ready-cut form (smokeless or dry), which fits over the needle handle. It is the last type that is used during the Needle cupping treatment. Moxa rolls are divided further according to their strength (i.e. Medium-moxa, Hot-moxa and very Hot-moxa).

There are two versions of Hot cupping therapy: (a) Hot Needle cupping and (b) Moxa cupping (without the needle). Both the Hot Needle cupping and the Moxa cupping are used where Cold patterns are predominant as well as pain. Here, acupuncture can be used to move the channels open the obstruction and relieve the pain, and moxa is employed to heat the needle and transfer the heat to the acupuncture point in order to warm and tonify that particular energetic influence point. This method is particularly useful in the treatment of Yang deficiency patterns, especially when these are accompanied by Wind-Cold or Cold-type 'Bi' syndromes (see Chapter 12). Non-acupuncture practitioners wishing to use this warming method can do so by applying hot moxa with a piece of ginger placed on the skin and a loose or a piece of rolled moxa over a piece of ginger. A similar therapeutic effect will be achieved through this method.

Application

This technique also requires a great deal of care and patience. Use 1.5-inch (4 cm) needles to the desired points, cut about 0.5 inch (1 cm) of moxa roll and insert it on the coil of the needle. Place a small piece of fire-resistant paper or a piece of foil under the needle and on top of the skin to provide protection from falling ash. Light the moxa roll and wait until it burns out completely. This might take up to 10 minutes. At this stage, when the moxa roll is completely burnt out, the ash on top of the needle is cold or just warm. The needle, however, remains hot for a considerable length of time. Without touching the needle or the ash, apply the cup over the needle (Fig. 9-7A–C) (the same therapeutic effect can be achieved if the ash is tapped off the needle while retaining the needle in place). When the desired cupping time is over, remove the cup gently and, before removing the needle, shake off the ash by holding a tray under the needle and tapping gently on its base. For Moxa cupping only, cut a thick slice of fresh ginger and place it on the desired point. Cut about a quarter inch (0.5 cm) moxa from a moxa stick and place it over the ginger. Light the moxa and wait until the patient feels the warmth though the ginger on the skin. At this point apply a cup over the burning moxa. While the suction is taking place the heat from moxa should diminish. If, however, the moxa continues to get hot, remove the cup and the moxa from the skin without further delay.

Conditions Most Suitable for Hot Needle Cupping Method

- Hot Needle cupping is especially beneficial in the treatment of Wind-Cold Bi syndromes of the joints as well as muscular complaints
- Spleen or Stomach 'Cold-type' patterns
- Asthma

FIGURE 9-7 (A) Moxa cupping: light the moxa and wait until it is completely burnt out before applying the cup over it. (B) Although the moxa is burnt out, the needle is still very hot and continues transferring heat to the acupuncture point. (C) After Moxa cupping.

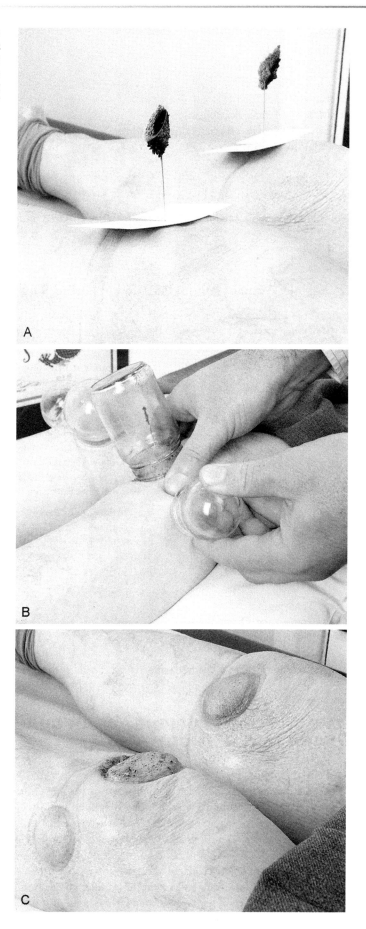

- Cough
- Anaemia
- Yang Xu (deficiency)
- Qi Xu (deficiency)
- Blood Xu (deficiency)
- Male and female infertility
- Lower back ache especially due to Kidney-Yang deficiencies
- Adult incontinence
- Impotence
- Frigidity
- Dysmenorrhoea (painful periods).

(Hot Needle cupping treatment is not suitable for children under the age of 16.)

CASE **9-12** **A 42-year-old Woman (Painful Periods and Feeling Tired)**

Mrs S has for some years been suffering from severe periods pains (worse on the first 2 days), so much so that she has to stay in bed wrapped up with hot water bottle on her stomach and back. Her arms are painful with loss of strength in her grip. She is a hairdresser and stands on her feet all day. Most days she also feels 'totally exhausted' before the day is out.

Pulse. Faint at all levels (difficult to feel the pulse, almost non-existent).

Tongue. Thin, wet and pale.

Medication. Multivitamins.

Observation. Mrs S is a slightly built woman with two small children and a business to run, looks tired and pale. She works 6 days a week, mostly standing on a concrete shop floor.

TCM Diagnosis. Chronic Yang deficiency with Cold Bi pattern dominating (she has drawn the pathogenic Cold through her feet to the abdomen).

Treatment Principle. Tonify the Lungs, Spleen and Kidney-Yang and warm the channels.

Cupping Application. A total of 12 sessions of Empty cupping were given, to the Front-Mu and the Back-Shu, Lung, Spleen, Stomach and the Kidney points. Also, Hot Needle cupping was applied to LI-15 Jianyu, LI-11 Quichi, ST-29 Guilai, Ren-4 Guanyuan and Ren-6 Qihai. Towards the end of her course her pains were much reduced and her energy returned so she no longer felt exhausted but 'a little tired at the end of the day'.

Additional Therapy. Acupuncture and moxibustion.

Summary Points

- Tonifying
- Tonify Yang, Qi and Blood
- Treats Wind-Cold (internal/external)
- Cold Bi
- Contraindicated for children under 16 years old.

EMPTY (FLASH) CUPPING – SHAN GUAN FA (TONIFYING METHOD)

 See online materials

Empty cupping is also called Flash cupping for its speed during the application. This is actually a Medium to Strong cupping method, but is applied rapidly and the cups remain in place for a very short time (i.e. less than 30 seconds). *It is mainly used to stimulate and strengthen the Wei Qi, also in lesser degree to move the Blood and Qi in the weak and frail.* The rather short duration is enough to stimulate the Wei Qi, Qi and Blood, but not enough to drain. It is therefore a tonifying as well as dispersing technique, particularly when dealing with acute onset of Wind-Cold or Wind-Heat invasion, in the weak and frail, and in children under the age of 16. Flash cupping also has an especial uplifting effect on the Heart-Qi, particularly when emotions are involved that may cause Heart-Qi stagnation.

Application

Empty cupping is applied on the back as well as the front of the body, and the technique is simple. The practitioner should oil the area to be cupped, place up to 12 cups near at hand, light a large cotton-wool ball and apply the cups simultaneously (Fig. 9-8). Once all the cups are in place, one must start removing them without delay, beginning with the first to be applied, then, when all have been removed, reapply them immediately in different positions. This can be repeated for between 5 and 10 minutes. Slight pinkish cupping marks will appear all over the back (Fig. 9-9), but these will fade away within a day or two.

Conditions Most Suitable for Flash (Empty) Cupping Method

- This is a favourite cupping method for children
- All stress and emotional-related conditions
- Tiredness
- Low fevers in children or the elderly
- Common cold
- Feeling of cold or fever
- Digestion complaints
- Gastrointestinal problems.

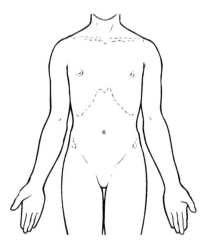

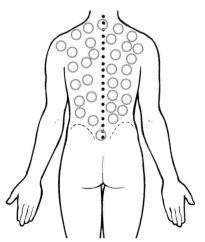

FIGURE 9-8 Empty cupping method: during this method of treatment up to 10 cups can be employed at the same time.

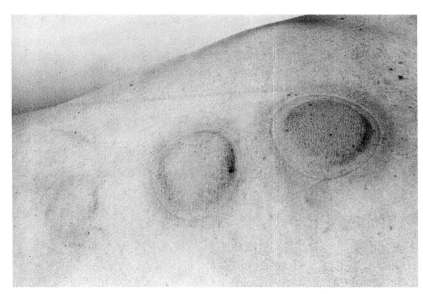

FIGURE 9-9 Following the Empty cupping treatment, no significant cupping marks should appear on the skin.

CASE 9-13 A 52-year-old Man (Lung Cancer with Cough and Phlegm)

52-year-old Mr R had been diagnosed with lung cancer, a year and half ago. During the last 14 months he received radiotherapy and chemotherapy treatments. He now feels quite tired and has a persistent cough with phlegm.

Pulse. Forceful at the superficial and empty on the deeper levels.

Tongue. Dry, red body colour with thick yellow coating.

Medication. Generic cough syrup.

Observation. Mr R, a well-built gentleman, reported that in the last 12 months he also lost a lot of weight, and his appetite diminished too. He also gets wheezy and tired easily, especially when he is engaged in conversation for more than few minutes.

TCM Diagnosis. Lung-Qi empty, due to cancer of the lungs, accompanied by Stomach and Spleen Yin deficiency.

Treatment Principle. Tonify the Kidney-Yang, Spleen and the Stomach-Yin and strengthen the Lung-Qi.

Cupping Application. Flash cupping application to the Front-Mu points of the Lungs, Stomach, Spleen and the Liver. To the back of the body; the Back-Shu points of the Lungs, Liver, Spleen, Stomach and the Kidneys were employed. Six treatments later his phlegm and cough were much reduced. Unfortunately he took a bad turn due to a brain metastasis and died soon after.

Additional Therapy. Acupuncture and herbal medicine.

CASE 9-14 A 28-year-old Woman (Emotional, Feeling Low and Tearful)

Ms M, a 28-year-old teacher has been feeling tearful and emotional for number of months ('low and tearful, I can easily stay home all day'). This condition is affecting her professional career as well her home life. She reports that this condition appeared without any warning, 'it just came about quite suddenly', which can happen any time of the day, while at work or at home. Her sleep pattern also changed and she often wakes up during the night. She has no particular dream pattern.

Pulse. Faint at all levels.

Tongue. Thin, pale and no coating.

Medication. Over the counter iron tablets and herbal medicine.

Observation. Softly spoken and slim-built professional woman with a 3-year-old child. Bringing up her child, and her teaching, have allowed her energies to fade away and diminish completely. In the past she has been diagnosed as 'anaemic'. Alongside her soft voice (ant-like), her movements also appeared to be in slow motion.

TCM Diagnosis. Chronic Blood and Qi deficiency resulting in Heart-Blood deficiency and disturbed Shen.

Treatment Principle. Tonify the Spleen, Stomach, Lungs, Liver, and the Kidneys and calm the Shen.

Cupping Application. Empty cupping treatment, covering the entire upper and the lower abdomen, including the Ren-8 Shenque, was applied to the front of the body. To the back of the body, Empty cupping treatment was applied to the entire upper and lower back, making sure that each cupping session did not exceed 15 minutes, on each side of the body. At around the seventh visit she reported feeling 'better and brighter'. She had a further 12 visits and now comes for a booster treatment once a month.

Additional Therapy. Extensive moxibustion, acupuncture, herbal medicine, and dietary advice.

Summary Points

- Tonifying
- Stress- and emotional-related complaints
- External Wind-Cold
- External Wind-Heat
- Benefits children, elderly and the frail adults.

BLEEDING/WET/FULL CUPPING – XUE GUAN FA (DRAINING METHOD)

 See online materials

Wet cupping mostly affects the Blood and the 'internal Wind'. This was the most favoured and practised cupping method of all by the early practitioners, who, particularly in Europe and Middle Eastern countries, employed the Bleeding cupping technique in order to purge foul blood, which was considered the source of disease, from the body. Leeches were also widely used for the same purpose. Today this method is used in the treatment of a sudden increase in blood pressure, high fevers, Blood stasis, and in discharging pus from boils and furuncles which represents Excess, with Blood Heat, Blood-Poison and stagnation. Bleeding cupping is also administered to treat a variety of sports injuries. A renowned expert in Chinese sports medicine and martial arts expert Tom Bisio in his book *A Tooth from the Tiger's Mouth* (Bisio, 2004, pp. 164–172) describes in detail the application and the effectiveness of Bleeding cupping when treating sports injuries, in particular acute sprains and strains (see Chapter 14). From the above description it can be seen that this method is suitable only for adults with strong, Excess (Shi) Qi, and not for children or the elderly. Most Middle Eastern patients almost *insist* on having Bleeding cupping when visiting my clinic; some I refuse to bleed because of their inappropriate current energetic constitution. To a great extent the majority of Middle Eastern countries still practise Bleeding cupping as the only method, sometimes compromising the health of the patient. However, it is quite interesting when we look at Chapter 16 (Evidence-Based Cupping Research) where the authors Hui-juan Cao and Jian-ping Liu underline Wet/Bleeding cupping technique as the most effective cupping therapy method!

Application

The acupuncture point Dazhui (Du-14) on the first thoracic vertebra is the point that is empirically bled during most treatments. Bleeding Du-14 has multifunctional properties; as well as removing the excess Heat from the Blood level it also tonifies the Du channel. However, other Blood stasis syndromes in different parts of the body can also be bled. The practitioner should have the patient sitting on a chair, resting and supporting his head on a pillow in front of him. The Dazhui point is first sterilized with alcohol and a very small incision (0.5 cm or the length of a rice grain) is made with a surgical blade or, using a plum-blossom needle, the point firmly tapped for a short time to cause bleeding (Fig. 9-10AB). I normally use the latter technique. Once the point is bled, a Strong cupping method is applied to it using a large cup (size 4 or 5). The blood will quite quickly be observed being drawn slowly into the cup (Fig. 9-11, Colour Plate Figure 4AB). If the incision is adequate, between 20 and 100 mL of blood can be drawn into the cup. However, if the patient is taking any form of anticoagulant drug this may result in more bleeding.

Removing the cup also requires attention and care; the practitioner should refrain from hurrying as this may cause the blood to spill or spray from the cup. Within a maximum of 5 minutes the bleeding should stop. If the bleeding continues, finger pressure is applied on the cut for a few minutes. Most of the blood in the cup will be only semi-coagulated and therefore still quite fluid. Before removing the cup, the practitioner should wear disposable surgical gloves on both hands, providing protection from direct contact with the blood. If the patient is in a prone position, ask them to sit upright and place a large paper towel under the cup with one hand. While pressing the upper edge of the cup with the other hand, remove the cup in an upward motion, making sure that the mouth of the cup remains covered with the paper towel at all times. Alternatively, ask the patient to roll over to one side, lifting one shoulder off the pillow. Once in this position the practitioner can easily remove the cup without any spillage of blood (Fig. 9-12). Once the cup is removed cover the cut with a plaster. It is not recommended to bleed more frequently than once a month, and no more than 100 mL of blood should be drawn at any

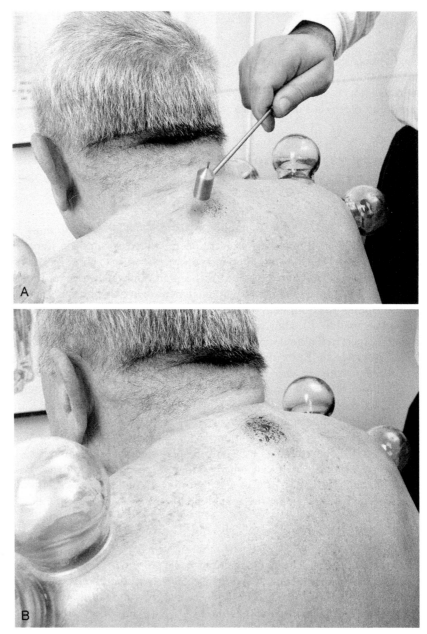

FIGURE 9-10 (A, B) Bleeding cupping: before the cupping application, bleed the point using a plum-blossom needle or a blade and nip a small, 0.25 cm cut.

one time. The colour of the blood extracted also has a diagnostic value: the darker the colour the longer the stasis/stagnation has been present, and the opposite is true for lighter-coloured blood.

Conditions Most Suitable for Bleeding/Wet/Full Cupping Method

- Acute hypertension
- Sports injuries with Blood stasis
- High fevers (only where excess pattern is present. Avoid Bleeding cupping on patients with High fevers who accompany Deficiency syndromes)
- Boils and furuncles
- Blood-Poison
- Blood stasis
- Skin condition (psoriasis)
- Removing toxins and poison from bites and stings
- Insect bites.

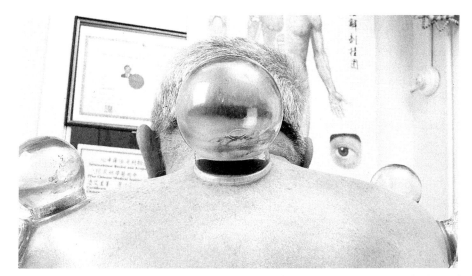

FIGURE 9-11 Application of a cup over the bleeding point: up to 100 mL of blood can be extracted by this method.

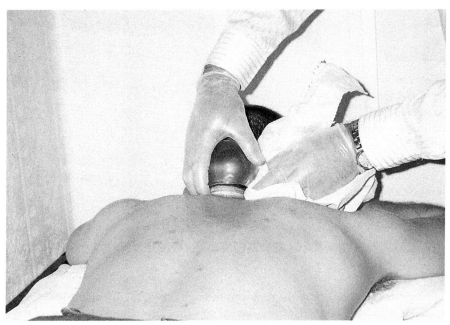

FIGURE 9-12 Removal of the cup: wear surgical gloves and hold extra paper towels to the mouth of the cup before gently removing it.

CASE 9-15 A 25-year-old Woman (Repetitive Strain Injury [RSI])

25 years old Ms E came to see me complaining of a painful right wrist and elbow. The pain appeared 3 weeks ago after some heavy gardening, which involved digging as well as weeding. The pain gets worse when lifting heavy objects and when rotating the arm.

Pulse. Nothing significant.

Tongue. Good body colour and shape.

Medication. Painkillers when needed.

Observation. Both, the wrist and elbow are slightly red and swollen with pain when palpating. She is a strong athletic-looking lady with good posture, who likes being busy. She works in an office and her elbow and the wrist pain get worse towards the end of the day. She is also right-handed.

TCM Diagnosis. 'Hot Bi' caused by repetitive use of the joints (RSI).

Treatment Principle. Remove the pathogenic Heat and open the channels.

Cupping Application. After four sessions of Bleeding cupping to the wrist and her elbow, using plum-blossom needle technique, her pains were much reduced and the redness of the joints had almost disappeared.
Note: Using plum-blossom needle technique on the bony joints may be painful. Therefore, much care and attention are necessary when treating bony joints with this technique.

Additional Therapy. Acupuncture.

CASE **9-16** **35-year-old Woman (Skin Condition – Psoriasis)**

35-year-old Ms A had been suffering from the skin condition 'psoriasis' for as long as she can remember. The red skin patches covered with scales were mostly concentrated on both legs and nowhere else. If scratched the patches would bleed easily. This condition affected her confidence, and prevented Ms A taking part in outdoor activities, in particular during the summer season.

Pulse. Normal.

Tongue. Red body proper slightly swelled with no coating.

Medication. In the past, she had used hydrocortisone creams extensively but has now stopped.

Observation. Ms A, of Indian origin and an accountant by profession, reported that the patches sometimes shrink but never disappear completely.

TCM Diagnosis. Yin deficiency dominating, Heat-Poison accumulating in the Lower Jiao.

Treatment principle. Treat Yin deficiency, nourish the skin and clear the Heat-Poison.

Cupping Application. On each visit the treatment would commence with Moving cupping for about 7 minutes, to the Bladder channel on the back of the body. This would always be followed with Bleeding cupping to Du-14 Dazhui. Further Bleeding cupping applications to the psoriasis patches were applied, choosing a different lesion on each visit. *The local bleeding method helps disperse the Heat-Poison and the Blood stasis as well as allowing fresh blood to replace the stagnant Blood within the lesion.* Five months of weekly treatment improved the skin texture, eliminated the scales and returned the skin to a pinkish colour, compared with its red-purple colour before.

Additional Therapy. Acupuncture and herbal medicine.

Summary Points

- Draining
- Treats Blood and 'internal Wind'
- Excess conditions
- Disperses pathogenic Blood Heat
- Blood stasis
- Sports injuries
- Skin conditions
- Contraindicated for children, elderly and the frail.

HERBAL CUPPING – YAO GUAN FA (TONIFYING METHOD)

See online materials

Herbal cupping offers dual benefit to the recipient, through simultaneous application of cupping therapy accompanied with herbal prescription. A herbal decoction, its nature depending on the condition of the patient, is prepared and applied directly on the relevant points as described below. The warm herbal prescription is expected to be absorbed through the skin adding its healing powers to that of the cupping therapy.

Application

There are two varieties of Herbal cupping technique: (a) the *Bamboo boiling method* and (b) the *Herbs in the cup* method.

(a) The Bamboo Boiling Method

A few bamboo cups are required, plus a relatively deep pan, water, metal clamps, some form of fire, and herbs in a prescription based on the treatment.

Put the herbs and the bamboo cups into the deep pan and cover them with water (glass cups become too hot and are therefore not suitable for this method). Bring the water to the boil and simmer for 30 minutes (Fig. 9-13). Prepare the patient in the normal way, and expose the part to be cupped. When practitioner and patient are both ready, lift one cup at a time out of the pan with a metal clamp (Fig. 9-14). Wait briefly to ensure that the bamboo cup is not too hot or that boiling water is not falling on the patient, and then apply the cup in the normal fashion using fire and cotton wool. Once again, extra caution must be observed not to cause burns or blisters with hot cups

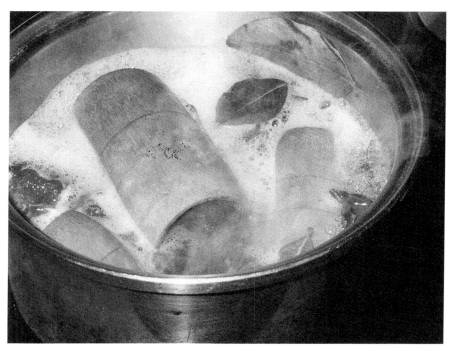

FIGURE 9-13 Herbal cupping: herbs, according to prescription, are boiled together with bamboo cups.

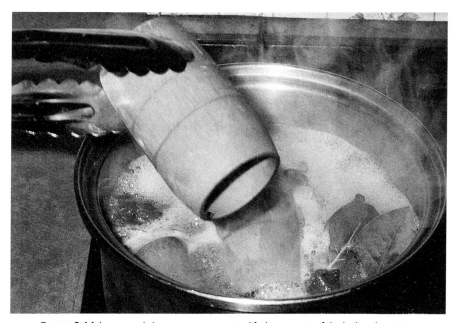

FIGURE 9-14 Long metal clamps are necessary to lift the cups out of the boiling decoction.

or hot water dripping onto the skin. The best precaution is to try the cups on your own skin before applying them to the patient. The herbs are absorbed by the bamboo cups, which in turn transfer their healing properties to the patient. This method is usually employed when external pathogens such as Cold, Damp and Wind attack the body, causing stiffness and aching, particularly in the neck and shoulders (common cold, asthma and cough). Although this treatment is not recommended for children of any age, it is particularly beneficial for the elderly and the frail with Blood and Qi deficiency that is accompanied with Cold or Wind pathogens. Cups can be left on for between 10 and 20 minutes.

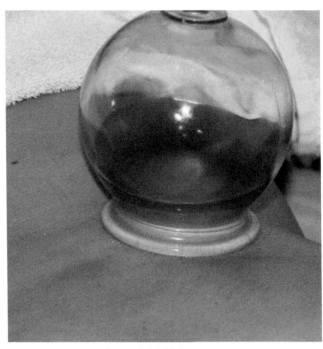

FIGURE 9-15 Herbs in a cup

(b)Herbs in the Cup Method

The herbal prescription is prepared separately and left to cool to a tepid temperature. The lukewarm herbal prescription is then poured into a bamboo, glass, or a vacuum-operated cup (quarter filled) (Fig. 9-15AB). If a vacuum-operated cup is used, once the quarter-filled cup is turned on the skin the air inside the cup is withdrawn and suction is achieved. If the fire cupping method is used, fire is briefly and quickly introduced into the cup and turned on the skin. The suction should be Medium to Strong method, but pay attention not to cause blisters on the skin.

Conditions Most Suitable for Herbal Cupping Method

- Asthma
- Emphysema
- Cough
- Digestive complaints
- Gastrointestinal complaints
- Bed-wetting in children
- Incontinence in adults
- Male and female infertility
- Qi deficiency syndromes
- Blood deficiency syndromes.

Summary Points

- Tonifying method
- Prepare herbal prescription in advance
- Apply only when the herbal prescription is lukewarm (tepid).

WATER CUPPING – SHUI GUAN FA (EVEN METHOD)

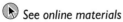 *See online materials*

As far as I am aware this is one of the least used and practised cupping methods. First, the practitioner needs to be quite experienced and fast to use this particular method; secondly, it can be quite messy if not correctly applied at the first attempt. The Water cupping technique disperses the inhibited (subdued) Lung-Qi, regulates the Lung-Qi and resolves Phlegm (Youbang & Liangyue, 1989).

Application

The technique involves filling a glass or bamboo cup one-third full with warm water and employing the cupping process in a rather quick fashion. Hold the cup close to the patient with one hand, bring it close to the point to be cupped and insert the burning cotton wool, swiftly and simultaneously turning the cup onto the skin. When performed properly, no water spillage occurs. If the application is performed slowly some water spillage is inevitable. This should, however, present no problem as the water used is only warm and will cause no harm.

A pistol-handle cupping apparatus is also suitable for this method. Quarter-fill the cup with warm water and place it on the desired location. Extract the air by using the pistol pump. Although removing the cup may cause anxiety with some practitioners, when the removal technique is followed correctly there is no need for apprehension or panic! First, make sure that the skin is oiled liberally with massage oil before employing Water cupping. When the desired cupping time is over, hold the cup with one hand while supporting the skin close to the cup with the other. Start sliding the cup towards the outer aspect of the body (i.e. over the shoulder). In this way the cup can be removed without getting the patient wet (Fig. 9-16A, B).

Water cupping is especially beneficial for asthma sufferers. It is particularly beneficial in the treatment of dry cough and asthmatic conditions with thick and sticky phlegm that is difficult to bring up. This technique is used to treat children as well as the adults. Water cupping is mostly employed on BL-13 (Feishu). There are usually no dark cupping marks left with this method.

Conditions Most Suitable for Watercupping Method

- Dry-type asthma
- Dry-skin conditions

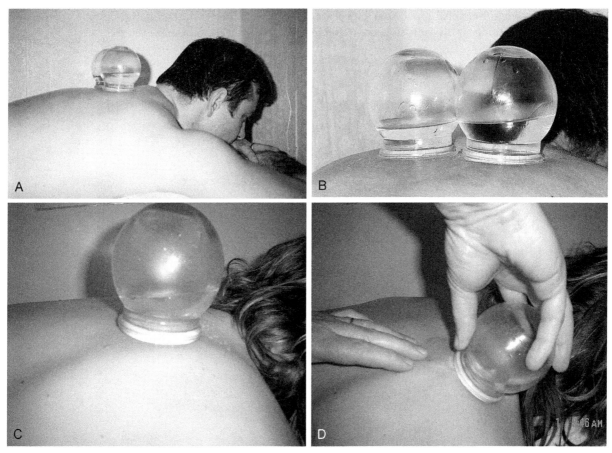

FIGURE 9-16 (A–C) Water cupping. (D) Sliding the water up over the shoulder.

Summary Points

- Even method
- Disperses inhibited (subdued) Lung-Qi
- Dry-type asthma
- Dry-type cough
- Dry-skin conditions
- Requires rapid application technique.

ICE CUPPING (COOLING) METHOD

Ice cupping was first introduced to me by a physiotherapist while I was in Poland, who also explained that this technique is often used to treat acute as well as chronic muscular pains and swellings in the hospital's physiotherapy department where she worked. This method of cupping is mostly employed when the cause of the stagnation is a pathogenic Heat that needs to be dispersed. Therefore, Ice cupping is considered a 'cooling' method. Energetically speaking, it appears to go against all TCM teaching – even the term '*ice or cold*' signifies death! However, many physiotherapists around the world employ alternating Heat and Cold applications for the purpose of dispersing stagnation, reducing pain and swelling. But this is an example of where the diversity of cultures can be seen in action, by practitioners employing opposite techniques to treat similar conditions!

I also feel that a technique that has been successfully used in hospitals for many years in different parts of the world deserves a mention. For many hundreds of years when treating sprains and strains Western-trained doctors and physiotherapists have employed ice therapy as the emergency 'first-aid tool'. This is because ice application on the skin tissue produces a temporary anti-inflammatory action, resulting in a local reduction of swelling. It must also be kept in mind though that ice application may cause Qi as well as Blood and channel blockage. The Ice cupping technique has a multifunctional application: it cools the tissue, which causes the shrinking action in order to reduce swelling, at the same time the movement of the cup helps to disperse the stagnation (Fig. 9-17).

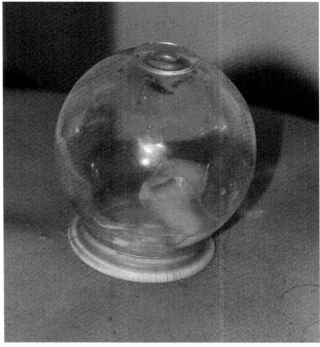

FIGURE 9-17 Ice cupping.

Application

The application is very simple: an ice cube is inserted into the cup and a vacuum is obtained in the usual manner. (Rubber, silicon, fire or pump action cups can all be employed.) Usually a Medium cupping strength is obtained while the cup is constantly moved over the lesion.

Caution: Ice burn can occur on the skin if the ice cube is not moved constantly and it is left on a dormant position. This can happen even after as short a period such as 2–3 minutes!

Conditions Most Suitable for Ice Cupping Method

- Acute or chronic muscular pains accompanied by Heat patterns
- Acute or chronic joint complaints accompanied by Heat pattern
- Acute or chronic muscular spasm
- All Heat patterns and chronic sports injuries.

Summary Points

- Cooling
- Cooling and dispersing
- Brings the pathogenic Heat to surface
- Sport injuries.

REFERENCES

Bisio, T., 2004. A Tooth from the Tiger's Mouth. Fireside, New York.

Youbang, C., Liangyue, D., 1989. Essentials of Contemporary Chinese Acupuncturists' Clinical Experiences. Foreign Languages Press, Beijing, p. 166.

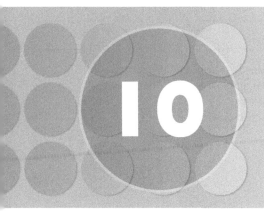

10 CUPPING THERAPY ON CHILDREN AND ADULTS

CHAPTER CONTENTS

CUPPING THERAPY ON ADULTS, 120

HOW OFTEN CAN CUPPING BE APPLIED?, 121

HOW MANY CUPS ARE USED IN ONE SESSION?, 121

CHILDHOOD DISEASES, 122

REFERENCES, 122

Treatment with cupping therapy of the children's ailments are discussed in Chapters 12 and 13.

From the very first week of opening my practice in Melbourne, Australia, I have been treating children with both acupuncture and cupping. However, it was not until I studied paediatric acupuncture in England, with Julian Scott, who is a prominent acupuncturist and a teacher on the subject, that I discovered the full potential of Chinese medicine in the management and treatment of children's diseases.

Children in general respond well and do not mind cupping therapy (Fig. 10-1, Colour Plate Figure 5A-H). They certainly prefer it to acupuncture! Children under the age of 7 require just a little extra care and patience during treatment, as at this age they are quite unpredictable; one minute they appear quite calm and relaxed, and the next, with little warning, they can turn into quite the opposite: weepy, angry and restless. It should also be remembered that the skin of a child of this age is extremely sensitive and vulnerable. I would certainly not recommend any method of cupping for children under the age of 4 years unless the practitioner is quite experienced in treating the very young. It is also worth bearing in mind that some children are afraid of fire. Before the treatment proceeds, therefore, the accompanying parent should be given a full explanation of the cupping procedure so as to gain their cooperation. If necessary, apply a small cup to the inside of the parent's arm, and let the child touch and feel the cup. Distraction of any kind by the parent will help to relax the child, inspire confidence and divert the child's attention from the practitioner during the application.

Small glass cups (size 1–2) are the most suitable for children under 7; sizes 2 and 3 can be used for children under 16. The golden rule to follow when treating children under 7 is that the maximum treatment time allowed is just 3 to 5 minutes, and for those between 7 and 16 years old 5 to 10 minutes. The strength of the cups should also be Empty, Weak or Medium cupping method; Strong, Moving, Needle, Moxa or Full cupping methods should *never* be employed on children under the age of 14 years old. For those practitioners who have limited experience of treating children, I would strongly recommend the use of cupping apparatus that does not require fire (i.e. rubber, silicon, pistol-handle cupping sets and screw-top cupping sets). Children also mark and blister easily, and a close watch is consequently needed at all times. A gentle massage after the cupping treatment will take away the apprehension and relax the child, and at the same time build a good rapport for future treatment.

Cupping treatment on children particularly in Europe was very common practice until the early 1900s. In an English medical publication *Aids to Paediatric Nursing* (Duncombe, 1962), cupping therapy is mentioned as one of the methods used to treat pleurisy resulting from 'complication of tuberculosis'. In Chinese clinics, cupping treatment is employed daily, and ten treatments constitute a single course. In the West, as with acupuncture, treatment once weekly is considered normal. However, treatment up to three times a week is possible when dealing with acute conditions such as fever or Wind-Cold attack. Bamboo cups are contraindicated during the treatment of children's conditions owing to their

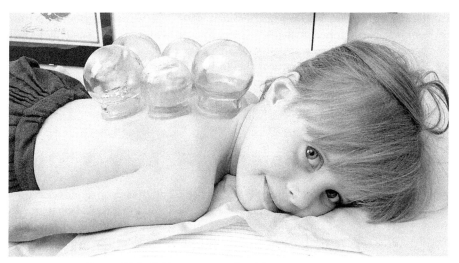

FIGURE 10-1 Children are quite relaxed during cupping treatment.

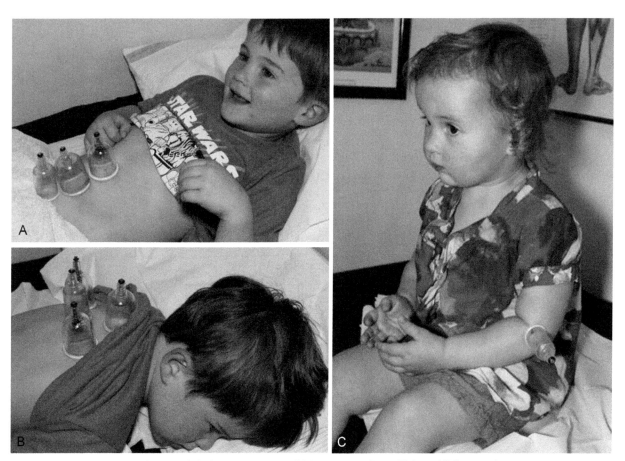

FIGURE 10-2 Cupping in children: (A) digestive complaints; (B) fever; (C) fever.

sharp edges, which may cause a cut on delicate skin, and the inability of the practitioner to monitor the condition of the skin during the process.

Usually the Back-Shu, local and the abdominal points are cupped. For a more comprehensive study on children's treatment with Chinese medicine, see Scott & Barlow (1999). In my clinics I regularly employ cupping treatment to treat children's conditions, sometimes on its own and sometimes to supplement the acupuncture treatment. My recommendation is: as we are not sure when the complete meridian system is fully developed in children (some sources indicate this as being by 5 years old and some by the age of 7), rather than concentrating on the specific acupuncture point treatment a more generalized, non-specific treatment protocol should be followed when dealing with children under 7 years old. A prominent TCM practitioner and teacher Stephen Birch, in his book *Shonishin. Japanese Pediatric Acupuncture* (Birch, 2011), also prescribes cupping (Kyukaku) in the treatment of a large variety of children's conditions (Fig. 10-2).

CUPPING THERAPY ON ADULTS

When cupping therapy is employed on adults it is extremely difficult to categorize and select the treatment modality using age alone as a guide. I cannot think of a general formula that could be put into practice according to age. Therefore, almost always, observation, listening, tongue and pulse diagnosis should be used to determine the correct cupping method and duration for each particular patient. No matter how strong or healthy the patient may appear to be, the above precautions will ensure the correct cupping application. In this way the patient receives the full benefit, instead of their existing Qi possibly being depleted as a result of the wrong method being chosen. Avoid performing unnecessarily long sessions of cupping, especially during the first and second visits, as this can also deplete Qi. Also, during the first and second visits, use Weak to Medium methods in preference to the more draining methods detailed in Chapter 9.

A 'dizzy' or 'light-headed' feeling after treatment is a common complaint among patients over 60 years of age. To prevent this, help the patient to get up from the couch when the session is over, and a few minutes before they need to get dressed. Generally speaking, patients under the age of 60 tolerate cupping quite well. Once or twice weekly treatment can safely be administered (with the exception of

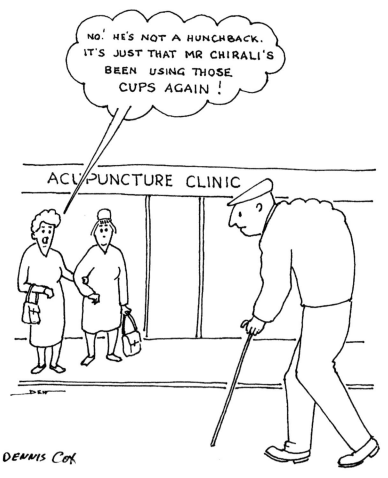

FIGURE 10-3 An artist patient's impression of the cupping treatment!

Bleeding cupping). When treating patients over the age of 60, and in particular over the age of 70, more attention has to be directed towards the skin condition. This is the age where skin becomes dehydrated and subcutaneous fat content much reduced, causing the skin to become emaciated and fragile. It is also common to observe bruising marks under the skin, sometimes caused by a knock or the medication patients are on. Avoid direct cupping therapy on such bruises. Never, ever, apply Strong or Moving cupping over such dehydrated skin. Cupping marks will also take longer to dissipate and vanish completely.

HOW OFTEN CAN CUPPING BE APPLIED?

In Far Eastern countries such as China, Vietnam and Korea, and in particular in Chinese hospitals, cupping is applied every day until the patient gets better. Children and adults are treated similarly. Ten sessions are considered as one course, and a week of rest is given between courses. In the West, however, once a week is considered the normal frequency. The concept of pain differs considerably between East and West. The expectations are also quite different. Where Eastern patients generally have a higher pain threshold, the reaction of Westerners is just the opposite. Maybe the saying 'no pain, no gain' is appropriate here!

When treating children under the age of 14, once-a-week treatment is considered an acceptable frequency. Adults under the age of 60 can be treated as much as twice a week (with the exception of Bleeding cupping). For adults over the age of 70, once-a-week treatment is sufficient. However, as mentioned earlier, during the 'acute' stage of disease, three times a week or even treatment once every other day can be given with favourable results. Similarly, in all age groups, when Light, Empty or Light-moving cupping is employed the treatment frequency can be increased to as much as once every other day. This is because Blood, Qi and the lymphatic fluids are gently stimulated rather than forcefully manipulated, which overtaxes the whole energetic and metabolic system.

HOW MANY CUPS ARE USED IN ONE SESSION?

This very much depends on the geographical location where the treatment is taking place (Fig. 10-4); in Far Eastern countries, for instance, I have seen as many as 50 cups being applied during the same session! In these countries the patients receiving the treatment also expect this amount of cups, otherwise they may get disappointed and will let you know! Also the only two methods usually employed

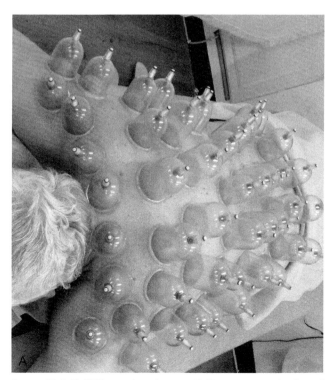
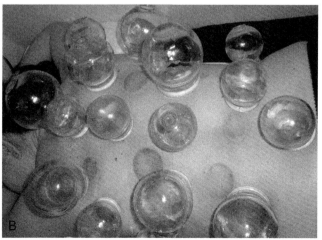

FIGURE 10-4 (A, B) The number of cups applied in treatment varies depending on local tradition – treatment of back points using different numbers of cups.

are Strong and the Bleeding cupping methods. There is normally nothing in between! In the West, however, it is more usual for practitioners to use between 6 and 12 cups during one session. In our household, both my grandmother and my mother used two cups at a time, and I too grew up practising cupping with fewer cups rather than a great number. My personal advice to the practitioners wishing to employ 20 cups or more is to avoid using the Strong suction method and to limit the suction strength to Light or Medium technique for a short period of time (i.e. less than 15 minutes).

CHILDHOOD DISEASES

(See Chapters 12 and 13.)

REFERENCES

Birch, S., 2011. Shonishin: Japanese Pediatric Acupuncture. Thieme, Stuttgard.
Duncombe, M.A., 1962. Aids to Paediatric Nursing. Baillere, Tindall & Cox, London.
Scott, J., Barlow, T., 1999. Acupuncture in the Treatment of Children. Eastland Press, Seattle WA.

COSMETIC CUPPING THERAPY

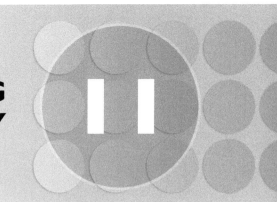

11

CHAPTER CONTENTS

PREPARATION, 123
APPLICATION, 124
ARTERIES AND VEINS OF WHICH THE COSMETIC CUPPING THERAPIST SHOULD BE AWARE, 125
WHAT TO EXPECT DURING AND AFTER THE COSMETIC CUPPING APPLICATION, 126
FACIAL CUPPING FOR A CLEARER COMPLEXION, 126
BREAST ENHANCEMENT, 128

CELLULITE CUPPING THERAPY, 130
WEIGHT LOSS CUPPING PROGRAMME, 130
ABDOMINAL CUPPING, 132
HEAVY LEG SYNDROME, 132
BODY TONING – TREATING SELECTIVE PARTS OF THE BODY, 133
FREQUENTLY ASKED QUESTIONS (FAQ), 142
REFERENCES, 143

Cupping therapy in the cosmetic field is a relatively new concept. Both the application and benefits are fast gaining acceptance throughout the acupuncture world as well as among the cosmetic profession. Over the last few years several versions of electrical as well as manual cupping suction pumps have been introduced to the cosmetic sector, especially in those beauty salons and spas that offer a 'natural facelift' or 'body toning'. However, I am not entirely persuaded by the training in human physiology and anatomy given to the cosmetic business sector, particularly in the field of cupping application techniques. This chapter will hopefully help address some of these concerns, allowing it to be a 'reference chapter' for beauty therapists who wish to add cupping therapy to their current skills.

I would like to think that the contemporary beauty therapist is sufficiently trained in the skills of skin care procedures, as well as recognizing the most common skin conditions. All the precautions and contraindications mentioned in Chapter 17 are therefore relevant and rigorously applicable.

PREPARATION

Before commencing with the cupping application, each client's medical history, including any medication taken, should be recorded in the client's treatment card/record. All make-up and related products covering the treatment area are removed from the skin by following the standard cleansing protocol. The skin texture should be good (warm and smooth to touch, with a good skin colour, and not dull and rough). If the skin appears to be dehydrated extra moisturizing oil should be applied before the cupping application and the client/patient advised to increase their fluid intake. When drinking the daily recommended amount of fluids our skin rehydrates quite fast, sometimes within the same day! The client is prepared for cupping by warming the skin area with a warm towel (Fig. 11-1), or by gently massaging the area. The hand cupping technique (see Fig. 5-1) is a wonderful way to warm up the body, except for the face.

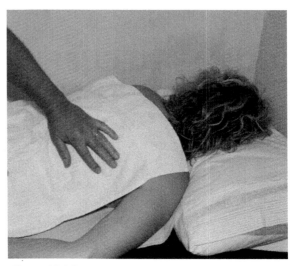

FIGURE 11-1 Preparing the area for cupping with warm towels.

APPLICATION

Selection of the right cup size is one of the most important factors when performing cosmetic cupping therapy. For instance, *smaller-sized* cups are preferred for facial cupping, whereas *larger cups* can be employed while working on the arms and legs. If glass cups are used, make sure that the edges of the cups are smooth, do not contain cracks or are uneven. Choose the right-sized cups to be used and have them placed close to you. Silicon, rubber or - clear Perspex cups are ideal for cosmetic cupping applications (Fig. 11-2). Get the client/patient into a comfortable position, and position yourself so that, if required during the treatment, you can reach out for more cups or massage oil comfortably; either sit behind the client if treating the face, or stand by the side of the client during cellulite treatment sessions (Fig. 11-3). Apply massage oil generously and moisturize the treatment area. During the cosmetic cupping sessions Empty, Light or Light-moving cupping techniques are mostly employed.

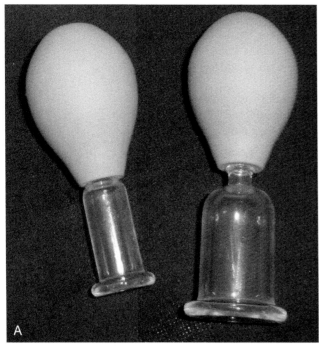

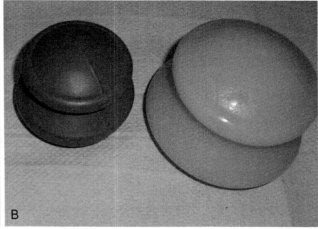

FIGURE 11-2 (A) Clear Perspex or (B) silicon or rubber cups are ideal for cosmetic cupping applications.

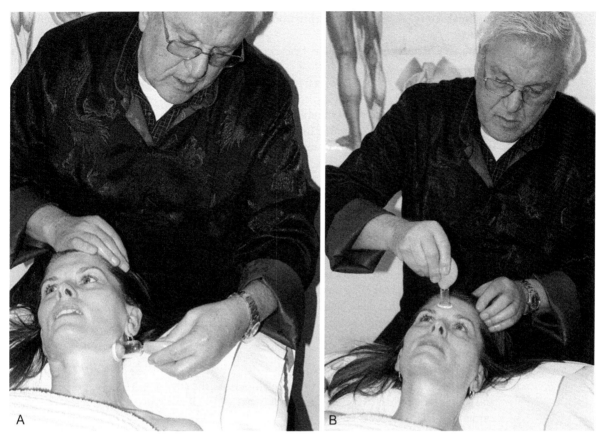

FIGURE 11-3 (A, B) Positioning for cosmetic cupping sessions to the head and neck: Empty, Light or Light-moving cupping techniques are mostly employed.

ARTERIES AND VEINS OF WHICH THE COSMETIC CUPPING THERAPIST SHOULD BE AWARE

Artery: Blood vessel taking blood from the heart to the tissues of the body
   arcuate artery – curved artery in the foot or kidney
   axillary artery – artery leading from the subclavian artery at the armpit
   basilar artery – artery that lies at the base of the brain
   brachial artery – artery running down the arm from the axillary artery to the elbow, where it divides into the radial and ulnar arteries
   cerebral arteries – main arteries taking blood into the brain
   common carotid artery – main artery leading up each side of the lower part of the neck
   communicating arteries – arteries that connect the blood supply from each side of the brain, forming part of the circle of Willis
   coronary arteries – arteries that supply blood to the heart muscle
   femoral artery – continuation of the external iliac artery, which runs down the front of the thigh and then crosses to the back
   hepatic artery – artery that takes blood to the liver
   common iliac artery – one of the two arteries that branch from the aorta in the abdomen and divide into the internal and external iliac arteries
   ileocolic artery – branch of the superior mesenteric artery
   innominate artery – largest branch from the aortic arch, which continues as the right common carotid and right subclavian arteries
   interlobar artery – artery running towards the cortex on each side of a renal pyramid
   interlobular arteries – arteries that run to the glomeruli of the kidneys
   lingual – artery that supplies the tongue
   lumbar artery – one of four arteries that supply the back muscles and skin

      popliteal artery – artery that branches from the femoral artery at the knee and leads into the tibial arteries

      pulmonary arteries – arteries that take deoxygenated blood from the heart to the lungs to be oxygenated

      radial artery – artery that branches from the brachial artery, starting at the elbow and ending in the palm of the hand

      renal arteries – pair of arteries running from the abdominal aorta to the kidneys

      subclavian artery – artery running from the aorta to the axillary artery in each arm

      tibial arteries – two arteries that run down the front and back of the lower leg

      ulnar artery – artery that branches from the brachial artery at the elbow and joins the radial artery in the palm of the hand

Vein: Blood vessel that takes deoxygenated blood containing waste carbon dioxide from the tissues back to the heart

      azygos vein – vein that brings blood back to the heart from the abdomen

      basilic vein – vein in the arm, running from the hand along the forearm to the elbow

      deep vein – vein that is deep in tissue, near the bone

      hepatic vein – vein that carries blood from the liver to the vena cava

      lingual vein – vein that takes blood away from the tongue

      portal vein – vein that takes blood from the stomach, pancreas, intestines and spleen to the liver

      pulmonary vein – vein that carries oxygenated blood from the lungs back to the left atrium of the heart (it is the only vein that carries oxygenated blood)

      superficial vein – vein that is near the surface of the skin

Venous bleeding: Bleeding from a vein

Venous blood: Deoxygenated blood, from which most of the oxygen has been removed by the tissues and so it is darker than oxygenated blood (it is carried by all veins except the pulmonary vein, which carries oxygenated blood)

Venous thrombosis: Blocking of a vein by a blood clot

Venous ulcer: Ulcer in the leg, caused by varicose veins or by a blood clot

WHAT TO EXPECT DURING AND AFTER THE COSMETIC CUPPING APPLICATION

During the cupping application the client / patient is expected to feel a firm-pulling sensation over the skin; this should not be a painful sensation! During the treatment the surface of the skin is expected to appear warm with pink / reddish colour (Fig. 11-4A). Following cosmetic cupping application it is quite common to see some cupping marks remaining on the skin due to the pulling action of the cups, or if the cups are left in situ for a long time (i.e. for more than 2 minutes) (Fig. 11-4B). Therefore avoid Strong methods, particularly when working on the face. The practitioner must monitor the skin texture / colour continuously, and also should avoid leaving the cups in situ for more than 2–3 minutes at a time. As continuously and repeated advocated throughout this book, one should begin the first few sessions with Empty or Light-cupping method and increase the suction strength as the treatment progresses in the pursuing days and weeks. After explaining to the patient the benefits, expectations and contraindications of cupping therapy, a written patient consent form is highly recommended before starting the cosmetic cupping treatment.

FACIAL CUPPING FOR A CLEARER COMPLEXION

To the traditional Chinese medicine practitioner, facial features are quite important particularly during the diagnosis stage. Looking and observing the facial skin colour, texture, lines, puffiness, ears, eyes and the tongue all help to formulate the correct TCM diagnosis. Emotional states such as happiness, joy, contentment, sadness, frustration and anger are all reflected on the face too. Unfortunately, urban dwellers can't completely avoid one of the major aging factors, which is air pollution. Poor air quality, particularly when it is loaded with heavy metals, not only damages our lungs but also clogs the pores of our skin resulting in an unhealthy and dull complexion. Of course the situation is far worse if the individual is also a smoker. All the main 14 meridians (see Chapter 4) either have a direct

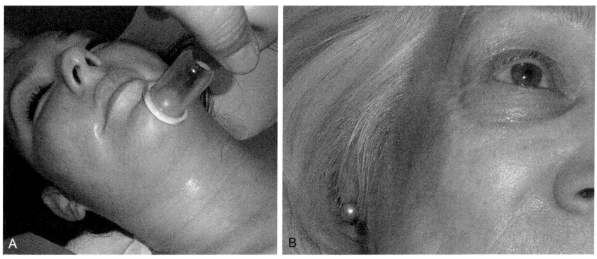

FIGURE 11-4 (A) During treatment the surface of the skin is expected to appear warm with pink/reddish colour. (B) A cupping mark as a result of 3 minutes' cupping to the face.

acupuncture point located on the face or are connected to the face by internal connecting channels. As far as Chinese medicine is concerned, malnutrition and deficiencies in Fluids (Yin and Blood deficiency, or Xu) and 'Qi' are considered to be the main culprits in poor skin appearance. Dehydrated skin with many deep lines (wrinkles) is particularly attributed to Fluid deficiency (Yin Xu). Dull, colourless and tired looking facial features are attributed to Qi or Blood deficiency. Of course, for a more successful outcome the underlined patterns mentioned above should all be identified and addressed by a qualified therapist.

Facelift

Is cupping therapy facial application a facelift? I think this terminology is not the most correct term to describe cupping treatment applied to the face. My preferred description for the facial cupping procedure is as a *'facial energizing'* or *'facial rejuvenation'* programme, because this is exactly what is happening during the cupping treatment: *oxygen-rich blood* is forced to the face, fluid circulation is encouraged and, most importantly, the lymphatic system is activated resulting in healthier and livelier looking skin. The skin is literally energized and rejuvenated through the power of cupping therapy. Also, during cupping the production of collagen and elastin may be stimulated, resulting in firmer skin texture, erasure of fine lines and reduction of deeper lines. Cupping also promotes Qi and Blood circulation; this increased circulation nourishes the skin, which helps it look fresher and younger. In the cosmetic field the facial rejuvenation programme is by far the most popular cosmetic treatment demanded by patients/clients, particularly female clients. Cupping therapy to the face is very effective and the result can be seen around the sixth visit (one course of treatment is ten sessions), which is a relatively short time when compared with other hands-on techniques, but of course for some not quick enough!

Cupping on the face needs particular attention. This is because the facial skin is the thinnest and finest particularly around the eyes (0.1 mm) and can be sensitive to external stimulation and manipulation. Prepare the patient and apply cups as directed in the above section. For a facial cupping treatment, silicon, rubber or the more recent Perspex suction cups are more suitable. Working in harmony with the facial contour, apply between five and seven long strokes, starting from the forehead, then on each side of the face, under the eyes, the sides of the nose, around the mouth/lips, the front of the ear (jaw bone) and, finally, behind the ear, over and under the chin, neck and the upper chest (décolletage).

Eyes

Cupping around the eyes directs the Qi towards the eyes and gets rid of eye tension and the 'tired look' in the eyes. Cupping also helps to disperse the fluid accumulation around the eyes. Small-sized rubber-top glass suction cups are normally applied around the eyes, employing a Light-moving technique.

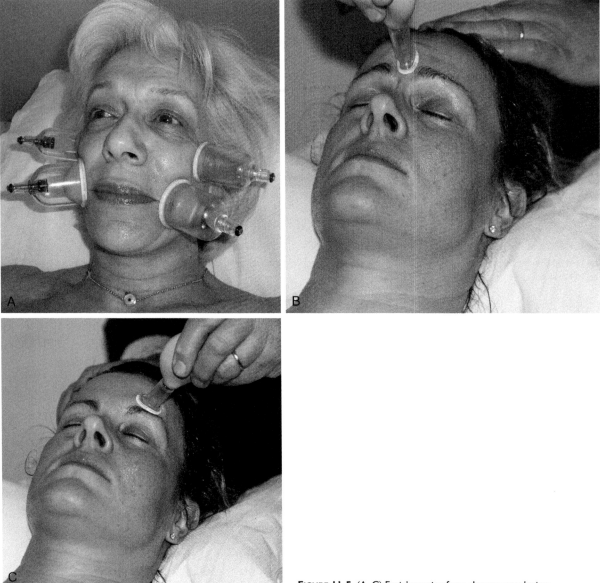

FIGURE 11-5 (A–C) Facial cupping for a clearer complexion.

Treatment should start just above the eyebrow from the middle of the forehead and the cup moved towards the outer aspect of the eye (the Taiyang point). From Taiyang, continue the movement of the cup aiming under the eyes and towards the nose (inner canthus of the eye). This action can be repeated 15 to 20 times on each visit.

Cupping applied twice a week for the period of 6 weeks is most effective. After the initial 6 weeks' treatment period is completed, a maintenance course of once a week or fortnightly treatment is recommended (Fig. 11-5).

BREAST ENHANCEMENT

The female breasts fully develop during the young adulthood years of 18–20. Breasts evolved for breast feeding; as breast tissue development is hormonally linked, they do not complete this process until pregnancy, when they produce breast milk in response to hormonal signals (Lawrence & Harrison 1983).

From time to time I have seen patients who complained that their breasts were 'too small for my body'. In most of these cases I declined to treat them because to me they looked quite normal size for their body weight/height proportion; consequently, such change is not to be expected from cupping. I have, however, treated about a dozen cases of extremely flat-chested patients, all aged between 15 and 20, as detailed below.

Cupping Application

Breast cupping therapy was employed in conjunction with acupuncture points (GB-21 Jianjing, ST-15 Wuyi, directing downward towards the nipple, and ST-18 Rugen directing upward towards the nipple). In all cases, large cups were applied in order to envelop the whole of the breast (Fig. 11-6). It is imperative that the cupping treatment begins with Light to Medium cupping and increases to Strong cupping only in later sessions, beginning with 5 minutes and increasing to up to 20 minutes on each visit. Each course consisted of between 20 and 30 sessions. During the treatment, five patients achieved more than a 50% increase in their breast size, four achieved a 20% increase, and in three no change was observed. No follow-up study has been undertaken. Cupping on inverted nipples produced temporary results.

Since the publication of the previous edition, I have treated several more patients with a similar complaint. As a result I have come to the conclusion that two major factors influence the outcome of breast enhancement treatment: one is age, and the other is the body mass index (BMI) of the patient. Patients who are over the age of 20 and patients who are severely underweight in relation to their height have a poor prognosis.

When to Avoid Breast Cupping?

Below is a list of conditions where cupping therapy on the breast should be altogether avoided:

- Individuals under 15 years of age
- When any sign of inflammation or swelling is present
- When pain, tenderness or discharge is present from the nipple
- When there are size or colour abnormalities between the two breasts
- When there are lumps or skin texture irregularities on or near the breasts.

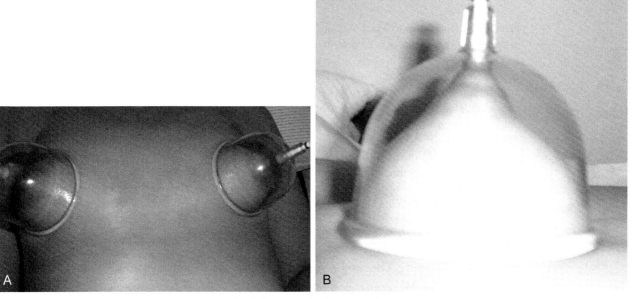

FIGURE 11-6 (A, B) Cupping for breast enhancement.

CELLULITE CUPPING THERAPY

The orange-peel appearance of cellulite under the skin is mostly seen in women. It is generally the result of poor lymphatic circulation coupled with lipid accumulation and stagnation of fluids leading to swollen fat cells, which form the cellulite beneath the skin. However, the medical profession still isn't entirely sure how cellulite forms. Many factors contribute to its formation, ranging from pregnancy to birth control pills and irregular eating habits to poor digestion, a sluggish elimination mechanism and hormonal activity (this may explain why women have more problems with cellulite than men). Excessive consumption of sugar, salt, smoking and lack of regular exercise are also believed to be contributory factors.

Over the years I have used cupping therapy for the treatment and management of cellulite quite successfully. I can almost guarantee the results to be 'satisfactory' following 3 months of therapy! In conjunction with the cupping, a daily regimen of walking for between 30 and 50 minutes, increasing the fluid intake up to 2.5 litres per day and reducing salt consumption (salt encourages the cells to retain fluid) are also recommended both during and after the cupping therapy programme.

Cupping Application

TO THE BACK OF THE BODY. Place the patient/client in a prone position. Apply oil liberally to both legs, starting from below the calf muscle to the iliac crest. Warm the treatment location as described above. For the first few visits, apply Empty or Light-moving cupping for 10 minutes to each leg, starting from the calf muscle (gastrocnemius) and working upwards to the thigh (hamstrings) and to the buttock (gluteus maximus), terminating at the top of the hipbone (iliac crest). Increase the treatment duration by 5–7 minutes on each visit to up to 30 minutes' application to each leg.

TO THE FRONT OF THE BODY. Place the patient in a supine position. Apply massage oil to the front of the legs, starting from the knee to thigh (quadriceps), sides (tensor fascia clatae) and the groin region. Before staring the cupping therapy, warm the treatment area as described above. Then apply the cups using only the Empty or Light-moving methods. *A word of caution: the inner areas of the legs are extremely sensitive, which can cause undesirable pain if Strong cupping manipulation is applied.*

The direction of the cupping movement should always be aimed towards the lymph glands, (i.e. towards the groin). This action promotes the lymphatic system, helps with the lipid metabolism, encourages fluid, Blood and Qi circulation, increases the flow of nutrients to the skin, bone and the muscle mass, as well as helping to remove waste matter such as toxins from the skin, resulting in the reduction of swollen fat cells (Fig. 11-7).

WEIGHT LOSS CUPPING PROGRAMME

During my recent trip to Taichung and Taipei in Taiwan, I have visited several cupping clinics, offering cupping therapy as part of their weight loss programme. Most treatment protocols were similar. In each session, which is every other day and sometimes every day, a different part of the body is targeted for the treatment. Once the area to be treated is decided upon (mostly the abdomen, thighs and the buttock area), that area is then covered with several large electroacupuncture adhesive pads and stimulated for around 30 minutes, applying medium- to low-frequency stimulation. This is believed to hasten the breakdown of fat tissue and tone the muscle mass. Local stimulation apart, no other acupuncture points are used. Following the removal of the adhesive electroacupuncture pads and, depending on the area to be treated, around 20 Medium to Strong cups are applied and left in situ for up to 15 minutes. In order to minimize the cupping marks over the treatment area the cups are removed and reapplied several times during this period. Thereafter, starting with Medium cupping technique and leaving the cups in position for 5 minutes, gradually increasing the duration and the strength of the cups at each visit. Moving cupping is also applied for a short duration (up to 10 minutes) (Fig. 11-8).

How Does Cupping Therapy Assist in Weight Loss Programmes?

The dual action of the cupping application *(massage, friction and suction)* activates the venous microcirculation as well as lymphatic drainage. This increased metabolic activity helps to break down fat tissue and encourages the elimination of excess fluids and toxins from the body. Furthermore, cupping is known to help the elasticity of the skin by increasing local microcirculation. One of the most

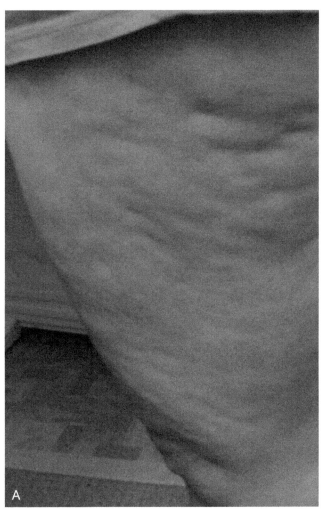
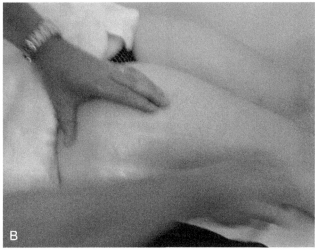

FIGURE 11-7 (A, B) Treating cellulite.

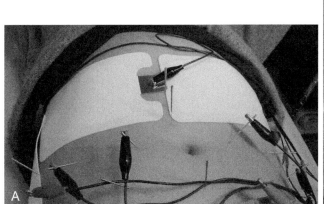
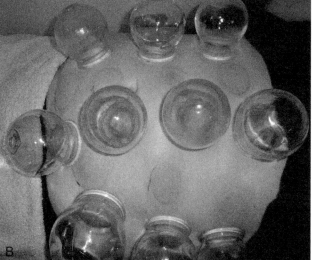

FIGURE 11-8 (A, B) Cupping for weight loss.

desirable outcomes of cupping therapy is its ability to enhance the metabolic rate; cupping applied to the skin, especially when applying Moving cupping, creates heat and this results in the increased rate. My personal view is that cupping therapy should be offered as part of a comprehensive weight loss programme that includes a dietary advice and a sensible exercise regimen suitable to the individual.

During the treatment period, the person should also increase the fluid intake by drinking more water or teas (between 1.5 and 2.5 L per day). My personal favourite antioxidant and cleansing drinks are artichoke, thyme, dandelion and green tea. Four to six glasses of warm tea are taken daily, between the meals.

ABDOMINAL CUPPING

The abdominal area covers the space in front of the body between the thorax (chest) and the pelvis. Before commencing the treatment, the practitioner should make sure that the client/patient's stomach is neither full nor completely empty (i.e. the person is fasting). For the abdominal cupping procedure both these situations are contraindicated. The practitioner should advise the patient to have something light to eat 2 hours prior to the treatment.

Place the patient in a supine position, apply massage oil liberally and warm up the abdominal area as described earlier. For the first 10 minutes, randomly apply around 50 cups targeting the entire abdominal area, employing only the Empty cupping technique only. After 10 minutes, choose a single cup and continue the treatment applying long strokes with the Light-moving cupping technique for a further 10 minutes. The treatment sequence should start from the top, under the breastbone (sternum) and moving the cup towards the outer aspect of the body, circling the umbilicus clockwise and expanding the circle before finishing the treatment. For follow-up visits, the treatment time can be increased to as much as 50 minutes a session (Fig. 11-9).

HEAVY LEG SYNDROME

In TCM, 'heavy leg syndrome' is considered to be 'Accumulation of Phlegm and sluggish Fluid metabolism in the Lower Jiao' (lower part of the body). The term 'Phlegm' in this context does not literally mean phlegm as 'mucus' but rather the fluids in the lymphatic circulation becoming 'thick and sticky' and not flowing freely around the body (normal body fluids are clear and runny). When this condition occurs, the fluid circulation naturally slows down, resulting in heavy limbs that can be quite uncomfortable. If the circulation is really poor it will cause heaviness of the limbs as well as fluid accumulation (oedema).

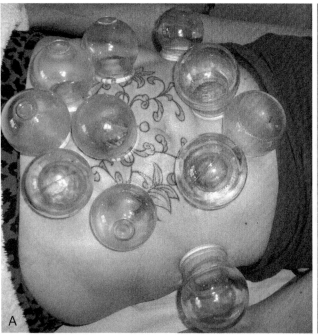
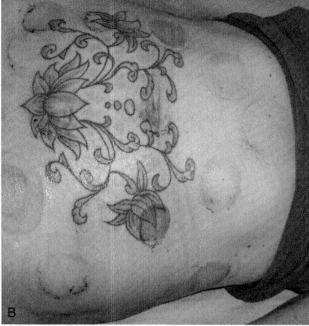

FIGURE 11-9 (A, B) Abdominal cupping.

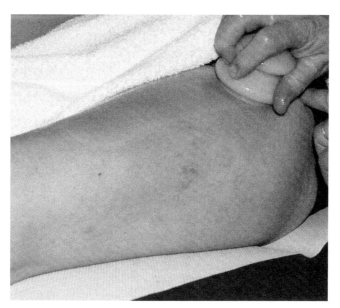

FIGURE 11-10 Cupping for heavy leg syndrome.

Cupping Application

Have the patient lie back in a supine position, with both legs elevated (place several pillows under the feet). Oil the skin well, covering the area from toe to groin. Using rubber or silicon cups, apply Light-moving cupping technique to the legs, always starting from the ankle and working towards the groin. After 15 minutes of treatment to the front, ask the patient to turn face down in a prone position and repeat the same treatment for a further 15 minutes, starting from just below the calf muscle and working toward the buttocks (Fig. 11-10). Alongside the cupping therapy, some dietary advice is also given; such as avoiding cold food and drinks as well as dairy produce – all of which contribute to Phlegm production.

BODY TONING – TREATING SELECTIVE PARTS OF THE BODY

Cupping therapy on a regular interval (once or twice a week) to a selective area of the body is possible. This will help to increase the local metabolism rate, resulting in a healthier, brighter, and firmer skin. The most suitable cupping technique to use is the Moving cupping technique. When correctly administered, it can get rid of stagnant fluids, assist in toxin elimination and help the lipid metabolism through increased blood and lymphatic activity.

CUPPING APPLICATION. Select the area to be treated and apply massage oil liberally. For the first few minutes, warm the area to be treated with a gentle massage or a hand-cupping technique. Proceed with Empty or Light-moving cupping until the location turns pink or slightly reddish in colour (never allow skin to turn dark red or purple colour during the treatment as this is the indication of a 'Strong cupping' technique, which is not a desirable method for cosmetic cupping). Continue the treatment for 5–10 minutes to each area. Once the desired time is up or the skin becomes sensitive, move the treatment to a different area and continue the treatment with the same technique. *For maximum benefit and the smooth flow of the cup, always follow the contour of the muscle mass directly under the skin* (Fig. 11-11, Fig. 11-12).

Neck

Precaution: Cupping over the neck requires particular attention, as the skin tissue over the neck in particular the front of the neck is quite thin and is likely to mark easily.

CUPPING APPLICATION. Employ Light-moving technique, starting from the clavicle and moving along the neck towards the chin (Fig. 11-13). Five to seven strokes alongside the neck and under the chin using a single silicon cup are the most effective.

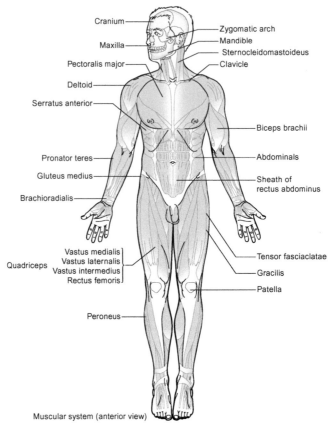

Muscular system (anterior view)

FIGURE 11-11 Muscular system (anterior view). *(After Lawrence & Harrison 1983 Massageworks. Perigee Books, with permission.)*

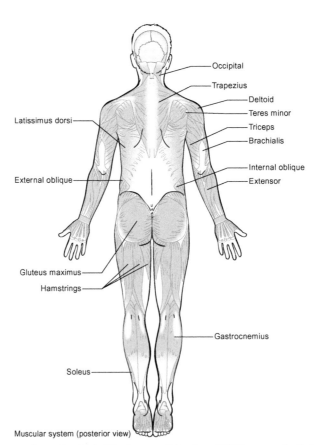

Muscular system (posterior view)

FIGURE 11-12 Muscular system (posterior view). *(After Lawrence & Harrison 1983 Massageworks. Perigee Books, with permission.)*

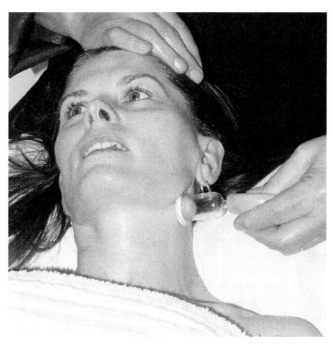

FIGURE 11-13 Cupping the neck.

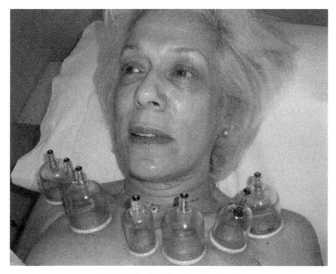

FIGURE 11-14 Cupping the chest.

Chest

CUPPING APPLICATION. Using a Perspex pistol-handled or a silicon cupping set, apply Light to Medium strength moving technique, starting from the middle of the chest bone (sternum) and moving the cup over the chest muscle (maxilla) towards the shoulders (Fig. 11-14).

Shoulder and Arm

CUPPING APPLICATION. Using a silicon or glass cup, apply Medium strength moving cupping to the deltoid muscle, constantly moving the cup from the tip of the clavicle over the deltoid muscle towards the biceps brachii and triceps brachii down to the elbow. *Word of caution:* the arm (i.e. the segment between the shoulder and the elbow) is in many people quite a sensitive area when palpated or rubbed. Therefore particular attention is needed during a moving cupping application. In full collaboration with the patient/client, the practitioner should be able to determine the most appropriate suction strength and treat accordingly. Otherwise, the standing cupping (Light to Medium cupping) technique with 10 to 12 cups can be used on the arm for up to 10 minutes at a time (Fig. 11-15).

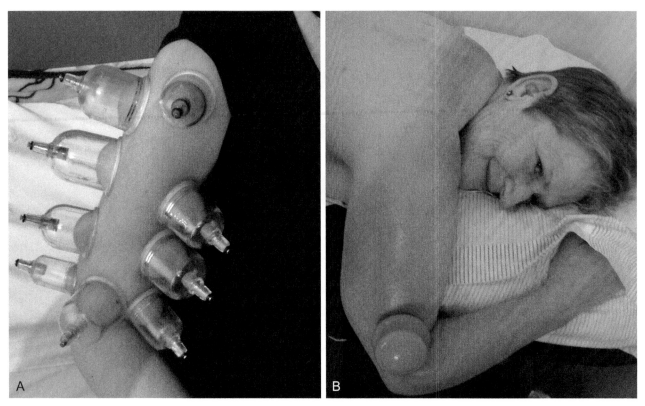

FIGURE 11-15 (A, B) Cupping the shoulder and arm.

Forearm

CUPPING APPLICATION. Using a single silicon or glass cup, apply Medium strength moving cupping, starting from the elbow crease (pronator teres muscle) and sliding/moving the cup towards the wrist. Repeat the same movement to the back of the arm, similarly starting from the tip of the elbow and working towards the wrist (Fig. 11-16).

Hypochondriac Regions

The hypochondriac region is also a sensitive area owing to its lack of protective muscular mass under the skin. The skin tissue is almost glued to the ribs, causing sensitivity when palpated or friction is applied.

CUPPING APPLICATION. The best position for this treatment is to have the patient lie on their back and bring the arms over the head, which exposes the entire hypochondriac region. Using a silicon cup, apply Light to Medium strength moving cupping, starting from the midline of the body and working laterally towards the outer aspect on the serratus anterior muscle (Fig. 11-17).

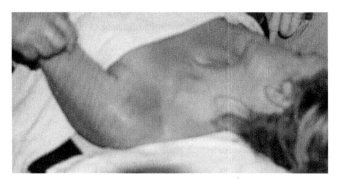

FIGURE 11-16 Cupping the forearm.

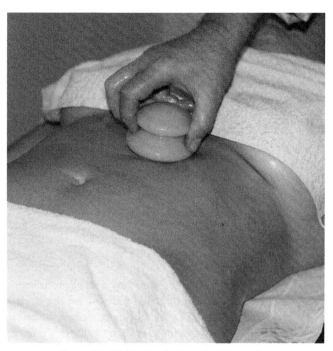

FIGURE 11-17 Cupping the hypochondriac region.

Diaphragm

CUPPING APPLICATION. Using a single silicon or glass cup, apply Light to Medium strength moving cupping on the diaphragm muscle, starting from the tip of the xiphoid process and working laterally towards the outer aspect of the body. As you perform the diaphragm cupping, ask the patient to breathe in when you bring the cup to the midline and to breathe out when sliding the cup from the middle to outer aspect of the body. This enables the diaphragm muscle to expand and contract in synchronization with the cupping application (Fig. 11-18).

Stomach

The stomach region is the space in front of the body below the diaphragm and above the pelvis. In most people, this area of the body is well covered with fat tissue over the important organs, which lie underneath the abdominal wall:

Right upper quadrant: Right lobe of liver, gall bladder, right kidney, portions of small and large intestines

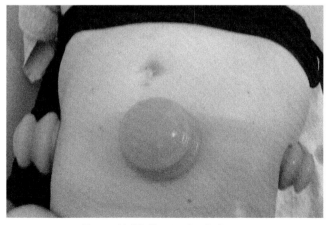

FIGURE 11-18 Cupping the diaphragm.

Right lower quadrant: Cecum, appendix, portions of small and large intestines, reproductive organs (right ovary in female and right spermatic cord in male) and right urethra

Left upper quadrant: Left lobe of liver, stomach, pancreas, left kidney, spleen, portions of small and large intestines

Left lower quadrant: Most of small intestine, portions of large intestine, left urethra and reproductive organs (left ovary in female and left spermatic cord in male).

CUPPING APPLICATION. When cupping the stomach region, one must pay special attention to the sensitivity and the reaction coming from the patient. Flash cupping, Light, Medium and Light-moving techniques all can be employed to the stomach region. This can be done by using a single cup or up to 20 cups. If a moving technique is required, a single cup (glass or silicon) will do. If more static versions are required, then the Flash cupping, Light and Medium techniques are employed (Fig. 11-19).

Thighs

When cupping the inside upper thighs, extra care is needed as this area is one of the most sensitive anatomical locations on the body.

CUPPING APPLICATION. Light, Medium, Strong and moving cupping techniques all can be employed. From a single to 20 cups can be placed on the thighs, depending on the treatment modality chosen. The muscle structures of the legs tolerate cupping therapy quite well, with the exception of the gracilis muscle (which runs down the inside of the leg from the top of the leg down to the top of the tibia), the quadriceps, tensor fasciae, and hamstrings (Fig. 11-20).

Legs

CUPPING APPLICATION. Using a single cup, apply Light to Medium moving technique starting from the knee joint and moving the cup towards the feet. The peroneal muscles (brevis, longus and tertius) on the outside of the lower leg are less sensitive compared with the gastrocnemius (large calf muscle on the back of the leg) (Fig. 11-21).

Feet

CUPPING APPLICATION. A single cup to apply moving cupping to under the feet can be employed, as well as various static cupping techniques (Fig. 11-22).

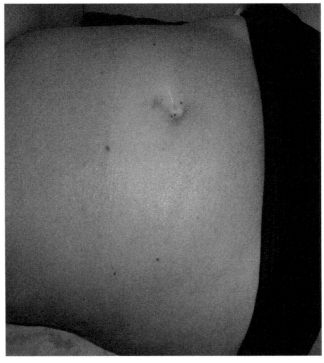

FIGURE 11-19 Cupping the stomach.

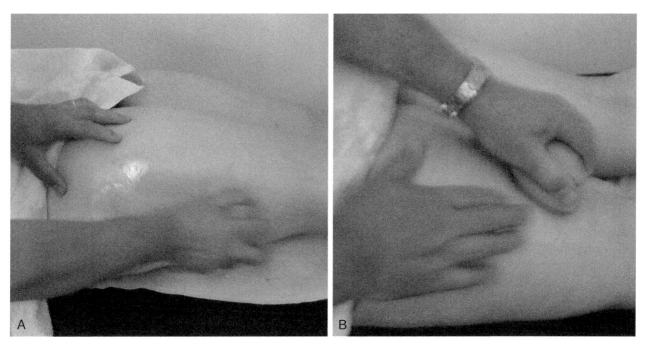

FIGURE 11-20 (A, B) Cupping the thighs.

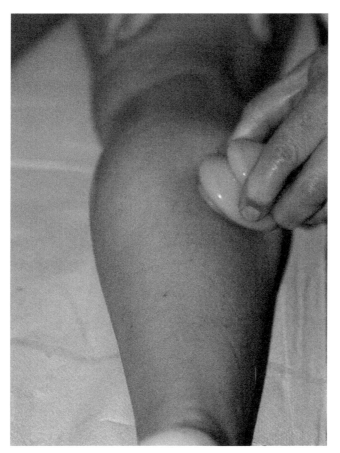

FIGURE 11-21 Cupping the legs.

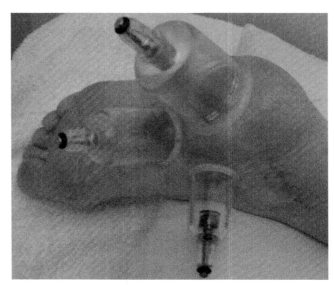

FIGURE 11-22 Cupping the feet.

Buttocks

Humans are genetically designed to store fat tissue, as a source of energy when in need, around the buttocks.

CUPPING APPLICATION. Moving, Medium and Strong cupping methods are tolerated well on the buttock region. Two specific movements are employed during this treatment: *circular* and *long strokes*. A circular movement is used, starting from the outer lower buttock (gluteus medius) down towards the upper thigh and from here making a U-turn up towards the middle of the buttock (gluteus maximus) and terminating at the mid flank (lower back). The second movement on the buttock is a long stroke movement – again using a single cup and starting from the middle of the flank. Move the cup laterally over the gluteus maximus to terminate at the hip joint (Fig. 11-23).

Lower Back

This is the area directly opposite the umbilicus extending to the buttocks and the hips, where excessive abdominal fat tissue also gathers ('apple shape' type).

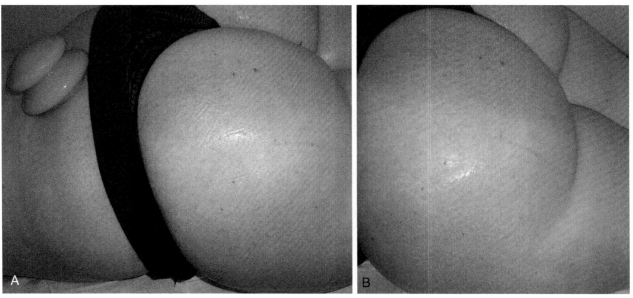

FIGURE 11-23 (A, B) Cupping the buttocks.

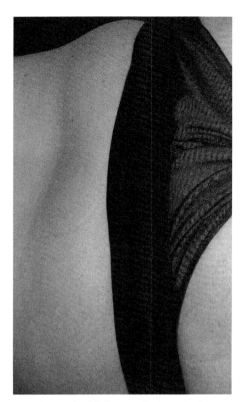

FIGURE 11-24 Cupping the lower back.

CUPPING APPLICATION. Light to Medium moving cupping, using a single cup to as many as 20 cups, can be applied to the lower back. If moving cupping is the preferred method, commence on the midline and move the cup laterally towards the front of the body (Fig. 11-24).

Middle and Upper Back

Most of this area is protected by the rib cage and houses the vital organs such as the kidneys (located in the middle of the back with one on each side of the spine, lying just below the rib cage), the heart and the lungs (in the upper chest). The upper back is dominated by a large superficial trapezius muscle, which extends longitudinally from the occipital bone to the lower thoracic vertebrae and laterally to the scapula (shoulder blade). Fat tissue mostly gathers at the base of the neck (the first thoracic vertebrae) and under the arms.

CUPPING APPLICATION. Flash, Light, Medium, Strong cupping as well as Medium to Light-moving cupping methods all can be employed to this region of the body. Use a single cup for moving method or as many as 20 cups for the standing cupping techniques (Fig. 11-25, Fig. 11-26).

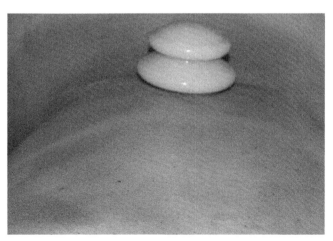

FIGURE 11-25 Cupping the middle back.

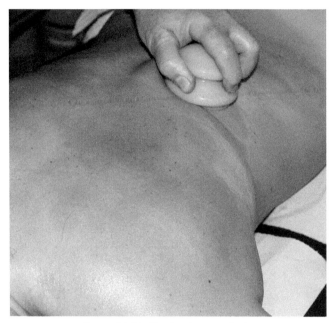

FIGURE 11-26 Cupping the upper back.

FREQUENTLY ASKED QUESTIONS (FAQ)

What Causes Dehydration?

ANSWER. The term 'dehydrated skin' is used to describe the appearance of a dry and lifeless skin. It is caused by not drinking enough fluid. Also, losing more fluid than you take in can result in dehydration. Activities such as physical hard work and exercise, which can cause excessive sweating, prolonged exposure to hot environment and excessive alcohol consumption can all lead to dehydration. Medical conditions such as high fever, vomiting, diarrhoea and diabetes can also cause it.

What are the Symptoms of Dehydration?

ANSWER
The following:

- Skin that returns slowly into position when pinched up (this is also called the 'dehydration skin test')
- Feeling tired
- Dry eyes
- Dry mouth
- Dry lips
- Not passing urine for 6 hours or more
- Low blood pressure
- Headache.

What do you Mean by 'Good Skin Texture'?

ANSWER. Healthy skin 'has a good texture'. This terminology is mostly used to describe warm, soft, smooth and hydrated skin.

How Long Should Each Cupping Session Last?

ANSWER. The first few sessions should not exceed 10 minutes to each chosen area. Over the following sessions, cupping therapy is gradually increased to up to 30 minutes.

How do I Deal With Hairy Skin?

ANSWER. In order to obtain good suction with hairy skin, apply extra oil or use non-flammable water-based gel.

How do I Know If the Client's Qi/energy is low?

ANSWER. A good indicator of Qi is the colour of the tongue proper, facial complexion and the voice. A dry and pale coloured tongue almost always indicates Qi deficiency; so does a dull facial complexion with the eyes wandering around the room and avoiding direct eye contact. During conversation if the vocal tone is weak and hard to comprehend this also is an indicator of poor Qi.

Are Dark Cupping Marks Normal?

ANSWER. A dark or purple cupping mark is an indication of prolonged use of Strong cupping method to the same location and should be avoided. This normally occurs in the beginning of the treatment or if the cup is applied to a sensitive location. This is easily avoidable if the proper cupping procedure is followed as described above.

Should I Bleed from the Cupping Location?

ANSWER. Apart from in relation to the Bleeding cupping technique, no blood or any form of bleeding should take place during or after the cupping session. However, there is an exception: a few drops of blood may form inside the cup if the cupping treatment takes place immediately following an acupuncture treatment. Even this amount is limited to one to three drops of blood. Therefore, with the exception of the method mentioned above, no form of bleeding to the cupping location is expected. Should bleeding take place the patient should seek further advice.

Should I Feel Dizzy Following the Treatment?

ANSWER. Some patients (around 10%) feel slightly light-headed or even dizzy following a cupping session. This is quite a normal situation, is due to the Qi and Blood stimulation and should not lead to panic. If this happens, the patient should be offered a warm drink and few minutes' rest before discharge from the clinic.

How Frequently can One Have Cosmetic Cupping Therapy?

ANSWER. At hospitals and clinics in the Far East, including China and Taiwan, daily treatment is quite common. However, in the West once or twice a week is the norm. Most cosmetic conditions will respond well to sessions twice a week.

What If the Treatment is too Painful for the Client?

ANSWER. Cupping therapy is normally well tolerated despite some degree of pulling sensation and friction on the skin that occurs during the treatment. However, some people's pain threshold is low. In such a case, reduce the suction strength and try again until a comfortable and acceptable level of suction is obtained. If the treatment continues to be intolerable or painful, stop and terminate the treatment without further delay, as this method of treatment may not be suitable for that particular patient.

Can I Cup Over Skin Moles?

ANSWER. No, avoid all forms of cupping therapy over a mole.

How Quickly Should I See a Result?

ANSWER. In most cases the skin texture will show some form of improvement after the sixth session.

What are the Contraindications for Cupping Therapy?

ANSWER. See the conditions mentioned in chapter 17.

REFERENCES

Lawrence, D.B., Harrison, L., 1983. Massage works: A practical encyclopedia of massage techniques. Putnam Publishing (Perigee Books), New York.

12

CUPPING THERAPY IN THE TREATMENT OF COMMON DISORDERS

CHAPTER CONTENTS

INTRODUCTION, 144
ABDOMINAL PAIN, 145
ANAEMIA, 149
ASTHMA, 150
ATROPHY SYNDROME, 154
ATTENTION DEFICIENCY DISORDER (ADD)
AND ATTENTION-DEFICIT HYPERACTIVITY
DISORDER (ADHD), 155
BACK PAIN AND SEXUAL
COMPLAINTS, 156
BED-WETTING (NOCTURNAL
ENURESIS), 159
BOIL/CARBUNCLE, 161
CHEST PAIN, 162
COMMON COLD AND INFLUENZA, 163
CONSTIPATION, 165

COUGH, 166
DYSMENORRHOEA, 168
FEVERS, 170
GROWING PAINS, 171
HYPERTENSION, 171
LARYNGITIS, 173
MUSCULOSKELETAL PAIN
('BI' SYNDROME), 173
SKIN COMPLAINTS, 176
STROKE (WIND-STROKE) BELL'S
PALSY – FACIAL PARALYSIS, 177
TIREDNESS, 179
VEINS (VARICOSE/BROKEN), 181
WEAK/POOR CONSTITUTION, 182
ENDNOTES, 182
REFERENCES, 183

INTRODUCTION

The treatment of diseases by cupping has long been practised by eminent English surgeons. Samuel Bayfield, in 1823, gave a detailed list of conditions and cupping sites to his readers:

The Scalp: hair must be shaved off, and a small mouthed Glass will generally be required; the Occiput; the Temple; the Nape of the Neck; behind the Ears to promote Sleep; the Lower Jaw; the Trachea; the Trapezius and Deltoid Muscles; the Chest, the Abdomen; the Back, Loins and Nates; the Thigh and Leg; the Perineum; on the Dorsum ilii and each side of the Knee Joint.

In this chapter, some disorders and the treatment methods employed are discussed in the context of patient history, as they are presented in a clinical situation. The main therapies practised in my clinics are traditional Chinese medicine acupuncture and Chinese herbal medicine. Therefore, the use of acupuncture points together with the aetiology and pathology of the disorder will be discussed in most cases. The therapies and remedies offered are based on my own clinical experience. The therapy of cupping is, therefore, integrated with acupuncture treatment in as many as 80% of clinical cases, except in Chapter 14 (Sports injuries) and Chapter 15 (Myofascial trigger points cupping therapy), sections where only the cupping therapy application is detailed. Case histories will be discussed alongside the various disorders.

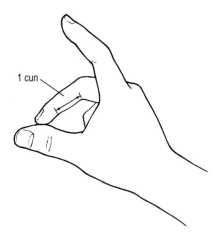

FIGURE 12-1 Cun calculations are made according to the patient's size and not the practitioner's.

When giving the location of cupping points, body landmarks and their proximities are used with supporting drawings and pictures. The Pinyin acupuncture nomenclature, with traditional cun measurements, is also included. The locations of the acupuncture points are explained in the Glossary section. The anatomical locations are described with help from the following texts: *Essentials of Chinese Acupuncture* (Chen & Deng, 1980), *Illustrated Dictionary of Chinese Acupuncture* (Zhang & Wu, 1986), *Anatomical Atlas of Chinese Acupuncture Points* (Chen, 1982), *The Foundations of Chinese Medicine* (Maciocia, 1989), *Grasping the Wind* (Ellis et al, 1989) and *Chinese Herbal Medicine Formulas and Strategies* (Bensky & Barolet, 1990).

Cupping treatment is usually employed on bilateral acupuncture points (i.e. on both sides of the Bladder channel, the BL-23 Shenshu points) unless indicated otherwise.

Therapists who do not use acupuncture and wish to activate the prescribed acupuncture points can do so by stimulating them using cupping, massage, acupressure, shiatsu or other tactile techniques.

The cun is a Chinese measuring unit of approximately 1 inch (when the middle finger is flexed, the distance between the two interphalangeal joint creases is measured as 1 cun); each person's cun measurement is therefore unique (Fig. 12-1).

ABDOMINAL PAIN

Abdominal pain is pain around and below the umbilical region. It is a very commonly seen condition, especially in children.

Aetiology and Pathology

Abdominal pain may be either due to a digestive problem, or perhaps of gynaecological origin. In children it is usually caused by overeating, or overconsumption of cold food and drink. The rule of thumb is: if the onset of pain follows the consumption of food or a drink, or is accompanied by diarrhoea or constipation, it is most likely to be digestive in origin. Abdominal pain associated with menstrual cycle disorders, such as dysmenorrhoea or irregular periods, indicates the probability of gynaecological dysfunction.

Treatment

Digestive Origin

TREATMENT PRINCIPLE. Regulate the Spleen and the Stomach, remove Food obstruction or Cold (if Cold is present it causes contractions manifested by pain, especially in children).

CUPPING APPLICATION

Cupping therapy. Medium to Weak cupping on Ren-12 (CV-12) Zhongwan, Liv-13 Zhangmen and BL-20 Pishu. Reported additional cupping points in the treatment of digestive diseases

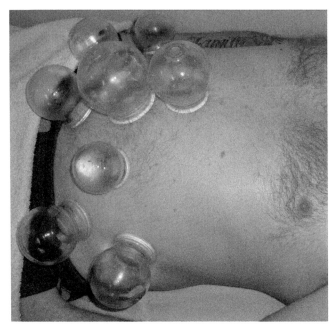

FIGURE 12-2 Treatment of abdominal pain of digestive origin.

(Cui & Zhang, 1989) include: 45 cases of *acute dysentery* treated by cupping after diagonal needling and bloodletting around the umbilicus; *acute and chronic gastroenteritis* with cupping of ST-19 Burong, ST-22 Guanmen, ST-25 Tianshu and ST-24 Huaroumen as the main points and supplemented with Ren-4 Guanyuan, ST-36 Zusanli and BL-21 Weishu, with very good results (Fig. 12-2).

Children's Digestive Disorders

Forty-five cases of simple *uncomplicated indigestion* have been reported (Cui & Zhang, 1989) to have been cured with cupping of BL-25 Dachangshu with up to five treatments. For *childhood diarrhoea*, cupping of Ren-8 Shenque, BL-20 Pishu, BL-21 Weishu, BL-25 Dachangshu and BL-17 Geshu can be used, with optional bleeding of Sifeng Extra. For *chronic childhood diarrhoea*, cupping of Du-1 Guiwei (Changqiang) or Ren-8 Shenque, Ren-6 Qihai, ST-25 Tianshu and Du-1 Changqiang is useful (personal communication, Chen Bin, 1995).

Cupping Duration
Children

- **Under 5 years:** 2–3 minutes, Empty or Light cupping
- **5–7 years:** Up to 10 minutes, Empty or Light cupping
- **7–14 years:** Up to 15 minutes, Light or Medium cupping.

Adults

- **Young adults:** Medium cupping, up to 20 minutes
- **The weak and frail:** Weak or Empty cupping, up to 10 minutes.

Gynaecological Origin

TREATMENT PRINCIPLE. Move Qi and Blood; remove stagnation or Cold if present.

CUPPING APPLICATION

Cupping Therapy. Medium to Weak cupping on Liv-13 Zhangmen; Medium to Weak cupping on the points of ST-29 Guilai and BL-32 Ciliao.

Cupping Duration. For all ages not more than 15 minutes (Fig. 12-3).

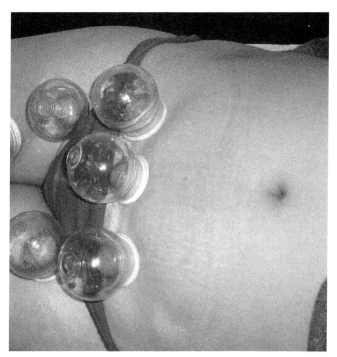

FIGURE 12-3 Treatment of abdominal pain of gynaecological origin.

PRECAUTION

Because the abdominal region is fleshy and very sensitive, even Light or Medium strength cupping is enough to cause hyperaemia (cupping marks) and blistering when administered for long periods of time. One should also note that suction applied to the abdomen will draw more flesh into the cup than anywhere else on the body. This should, however, present no problem, as the strength should be only Light or Medium.

Cupping is also applicable during the menstrual period.

CASE 12-1 Male Patient Aged 45 (Abdominal Pain)

Complaint. Stomach pain and tiredness, suffered for over 10 years.

Present Medication. Nothing now, but he has taken various medications for many years with little or no effect.

Pulse. Faint, at all levels.

Tongue. Pale, with a thin white coating (he was scraping his tongue daily). In some cultures, especially on the Indian continent, most people scrape the coating from their tongue first thing in the morning as part of their oral hygiene.

Observation. He is of a good build, working as a store manager; he exercises three times a week, and plays golf at weekends; he likes beer, drinking 8–10 pints a week, and eats irregularly.

Diagnosis

This is a deficiency condition, caused by excessive consumption of cold drinks and irregular eating habit; the Stomach/Spleen Yang-Qi is injured. Cold Spleen also fails to nourish the Blood, hence the tiredness.

Treatment Principle. Warm the Middle and remove the Cold, regulate the Spleen/Stomach and stop the pain.

Cupping Application. Ren-12 Zhongwan, Liv-13 Zhangmen and BL-20 Pishu, all Light to Medium cupping, for 10–15 minutes on each visit.

Conclusion and Additional Recommendations. The patient was advised to reduce the amount he drank and to eat more regular meals, to introduce fresh ginger into his diet (he did not like ginger), eat warm soup before his meals, and to wear more clothes while at work (he wore only a T-shirt while working because he felt hot). After ten treatments the Stomach pain disappeared but he still felt tired; he was still drinking as heavily as before. More treatment was necessary, but he could not afford to continue.

Conclusion. The continuous drinking was damaging the patient's Spleen- and Stomach-Yang, but he refused to acknowledge this. The persistent tiredness was the result of a heavy working schedule, many sporting activities and overconsumption of cold beer.

CASE 12-2 Female Patient Aged 32 (Abdominal Pain)

Complaint. Lower abdominal pain before periods, lower back pain most of the time, nasal blockage and feeling cold, even during the summer, for over 2 years.

Present Medication. She takes the contraceptive pill, and also various vitamin supplements.

Pulse. Faint, at all levels.

Tongue. Swollen and extremely pale, no coating.

Observation. The patient is over 6 feet tall with a good body weight. She works long hours on the Stock Exchange floor, and is on her feet for 8–10 hours a day. She swims and exercises up to three times a week. She eats healthy food, except for her lunch break, when she has a sandwich or just a drink. She likes socializing and is out almost every night until late. A very intelligent and mentally alert person, she is aware that she is 'burning the candle at both ends' but cannot help it!

Diagnosis. Kidney-Yang deficiency.

Treatment Principle. Tonify the Kidney-Yang, warm the Middle and clear Phlegm.

Cupping Application. Ren-4 Guanyuan, ST-29 Guilai and BL-23 Shenshu, Light cupping for 10 minutes at each visit (Fig. 12-4).

Conclusion. The patient received 10 weekly treatments followed by 4 weeks of rest, continuing with bi-weekly treatments for a further 3 months. Her period pains ceased and she stopped feeling the cold so much. Her nasal congestion is much reduced but not completely cleared.

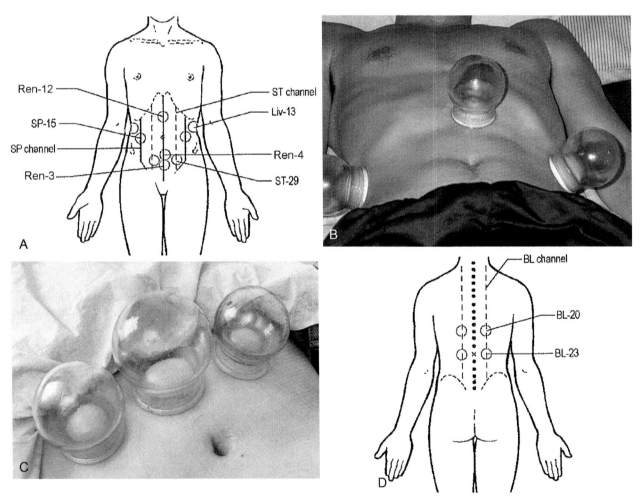

FIGURE 12-4 (A) The most-used abdominal points during cupping treatment for abdominal complaints. (B) Treating abdominal pain of digestive origin. (C) Treatment abdominal pain of gynaecological origin. (D) Two of the most-used points on the back, the Back-Shu points of BL-20 and BL-23.

ANAEMIA

This is a Blood disorder characterized by a reduction in the number of red blood cells in the circulation. The normal haemoglobin values for men are 8.7–11.2 mmol/L, and for women 7.8–10.5 mmol/L. The lower values in women are the result of monthly blood loss during menstruation.

Aetiology and Pathology

The patient appears pale and lethargic, often complaining of headaches, dizziness, tiredness on the slightest exertion, and loss of appetite. Lack of iron, folic acid or vitamin B_{12} is the main cause of anaemia according to Western medicine. The treatment is therefore to identify the missing agent and replace it (e.g. by prescribing iron supplements). In TCM, however, this condition is clearly seen as a deficiency of the Spleen- and Stomach-Qi, as Blood is produced by the Spleen from the food we eat. Therefore, the Spleen and Stomach are the cardinal organs in Blood production.

Treatment

TREATMENT PRINCIPLE. Tonify the Spleen and Stomach.

CUPPING APPLICATION

Cupping Therapy. Weak to Medium strength cupping on Ren-12 Zhongwan, Liv-13 Zhangmen, BL-17 Geshu and BL-21 Weishu, followed by Empty cupping to the whole of the back, in the prone position (Fig. 12-5).

Cupping Duration. The maximum cupping time permissible in all cases is 5 minutes during each visit. As mentioned earlier, this is a deficiency syndrome, therefore long sessions of cupping should be avoided.

PRECAUTION

The patient may feel slightly dizzy or disorientated for a few minutes after treatment, and should not be discharged quickly if·this occurs. A cup of warm herbal tea and a few minutes' rest is all that is needed.

CASE 12-3 Female Patient Aged 30 (Anaemia)

Complaint. Feeling tired and dizzy since giving birth to twins 6 months ago.

Present Medication. She has been taking iron tablets for the last 6 months, but complains of constipation and still feels extremely tired and light-headed most of the time.

Pulse. Faint, at all levels, almost imperceptible at the Kidney pulse.

Tongue. Pale body, no coating.

Observation. The delivery of the twins was difficult and fraught with complications; she nearly lost both children. A very slim-built lady, she has a 7-year-old, very active daughter. The twins are not sleeping particularly well and wake up between three and five times a night. She has no help at home, and her husband goes to work early and comes home late. Her appetite is good but she always eats in a hurry and while on the go, seldom sitting at the table for more than 5 minutes before she has to get up again. She also has a constant fear that something horrible is going to happen to the children; therefore she feels the need to be with them and watch over them all the time. This in particular results in her being both physically and mentally very tired and restless.

Diagnosis. A deficiency of the Kidney-Qi and Blood, failing to nourish the Heart. The complications and the blood loss during the delivery of the twins have left her Blood and Qi deficient. Also, lack of sleep and having to take her 7-year-old daughter to school daily have depleted her Kidney energy.

Treatment Principle. Tonify the Blood and the Kidney-Qi, and nourish the Heart.

Cupping Application. Light to Medium cupping for 10 minutes, on Ren-12 Zhongwan, Liv-13 Zhangmen, Ren-6 Qihai, BL-20 Pishu and BL-23 Shenshu, followed by Empty cupping on the whole of the back, for 5 minutes only (See Fig. 9-8).

Conclusion. The patient has completed one course of 10 visits and feels much more energetic, with fewer dizzy spells. The irrational fears continue to bother her, however, especially when she hears or reads particularly bad news. She continued with monthly booster treatments for a further 8 months, and now feels more in control and has less fear. She has recently discontinued her treatment, as she felt completely better.

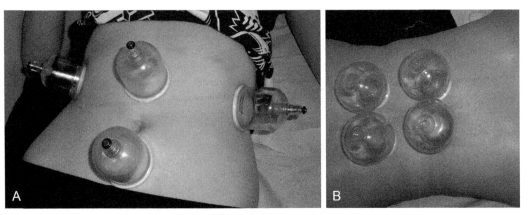

FIGURE 12-5 (A, B) Treatment of anaemia.

ASTHMA

One of the most commonly seen complaints in the clinic is the respiratory condition of asthma, which seems to be increasing especially in children. I am particularly pleased that parents take their children to alternative practitioners much earlier than we have seen in the past. The most common clinical manifestation of asthma is a severe shortness of breath, which is very distressing. An allergy, for example to food, dust, air pollution, particular perfumes, house mites, cat or dog hair, or stress, can be responsible for the actual attack, but it is not always possible to identify the culprit. Most asthmatic children grow out of it by the time they reach their teens. In adulthood late-onset asthma is very common, especially after retirement age.

Aetiology and Pathology

In TCM 'wheezing' is looked upon as the first indication of asthma. During sleep, at rest or on exertion, wheezing, which is often accompanied by coughing or shortness of breath, is a clear indication of Lung-Qi deficiency. In general there are two types of asthma: the Deficient (Empty) type, and the Excessive (Full) type. In the Excessive type the Lung-Qi is exhausted as a result of invasion by Wind-Cold or Wind-Heat, and the onset is usually sudden. In the Deficient type the Lung-Qi deficiency is also accompanied by Kidney-Qi deficiency, and the manifestation is more of a chronic nature. In my own experience it is very rare that an alternative practitioner will see an asthmatic patient during the actual attack. The treatment is therefore mainly concentrated between the attacks, or is of a preventive nature.

In Deficient-type asthma the clinical manifestations are wheezing, shortness of breath, pallor, tiredness, a feeble continuous cough and cold extremities.

The clinical manifestations of Excessive-type asthma are a raised temperature with a red face and cheeks, wheezing, an intense cough, stuffy chest with exuberant, thick yellowy phlegm and shortness of breath. Children often suffer from the Excessive type of asthma because their Protective Qi (Wei Qi) is underdeveloped. According to Julian Scott (Scott & Barlow, 1999), weaknesses in children's digestive organs, such as 'Spleen and Stomach deficiency' and excessive consumption of 'rich food', are a major contributory factor to the production of Phlegm, which causes a blockage in the lungs resulting in shortness of breath.

There are two deficient patterns: Lung and Kidney-Yin deficiency, and Lung-Qi with Kidney-Yang deficiency. Lung and Kidney-Yin deficiency manifests itself as a chronic long-term condition, with more frequent night attacks. The patient feels restless and hot and, because of the Fluid (Yin) deficiency, thirst, dry throat and night sweats accompany the wheezing and shortness of breath. The Lung-Qi and Kidney-Yang deficiency pattern also presents as a long-term condition, with more Cold features, such as cold limbs, curling up in bed, backache and frequent urination, accompanied by wheezing and shortness of breath. The patient's abdomen and lower back are extremely cold to the touch.

Treatment

Deficient Asthma – Lung and Kidney-Yin Deficiency

TREATMENT PRINCIPLE. Remove the external pathogen, nourish the Lungs, tonify the Stomach / Spleen and the Kidneys, resolve Phlegm and stop the coughing.

CUPPING APPLICATION

Cupping Therapy. Light to Medium cupping on Ren-12 Zhongwan, Liv-13 Zhangmen, Dingchuan Extra, BL-13 Feishu, BL-20 Pishu and BL-23 Shenshu; use the Empty method on the Back-Shu points if the patient is listless and lethargic (Fig. 12-6, Fig. 12-7).

Reported Additional Cupping Points in the Treatment of Asthma. Chronic bronchitis was treated with cupping to Du-14 Dazhui, Du-12 Shenzhu, BL-11 Dashu, Dingchuan Extra, BL-13 Feishu, BL-12 Fengmen, BL-14 Jueyinshu, BL-15 Xinshu, Ren-22 Tiantu, Ren-17 Shanzhong, Ren-20 Huagai and LU-1 Zhongfu, cupping alternately the front and the back points (Sherwood, 1992). Cupping was more effective for a tickling sensation in the throat, expectoration and coughing, but less effective in the treatment of tight chest and shortness of breath. A different prescription for asthma is cupping of the area between Du-14 Dazhui and BL-13 Feishu, after needling Du-14 Dazhui, BL-12 Fengmen and BL-13 Feishu. Several asthmatic patients at Yuzhong, Gansu Province, were treated with Water cupping on BL-13 Feishu and ST-15 Wuyi (Chen & Deng, 1989: 166).

Cupping Duration
Children

- **Under 5 years:** 2–3 minutes of Weak or Empty cupping
- **5–7 years:** Up to 10 minutes of Weak or Empty cupping
- **7–14 years:** Up to 15 minutes of Weak or Medium cupping.

  Adults

- **Young adults:** Medium to Strong cupping, up to 20 minutes
- **The weak and the frail:** Weak or Empty cupping, up to 10 minutes.

Deficient Asthma – Lung-Qi with Kidney-Yang Deficiency

TREATMENT PRINCIPLE. Remove the external pathogen, warm and tonify the Lungs, Stomach / Spleen and Kidneys, stop the coughing and calm the wheezing.

CUPPING APPLICATION

Cupping Therapy. Light to Medium cupping to the same points as in the section above.

Full (Excessive) Type Asthma

TREATMENT PRINCIPLE. Clear Heat from the Lungs, tonify Stomach / Spleen, open bowels, resolve Phlegm, stop the coughing and calm the wheezing.

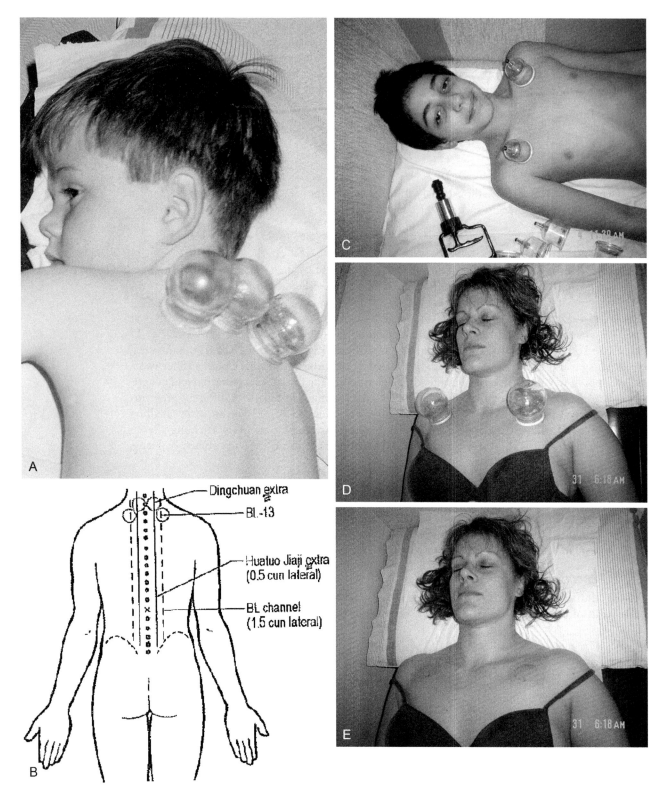

FIGURE 12-6 (A) Treating asthma with cupping is very effective, especially in children. (B) Treating asthma with the points of Dingchuan Extra and BL-13 Feishu, also the Extra channel of Huatuo Jiaji (0.5 cun lateral to each side of the spine. Notice the Bladder channel, which is 1.5 cun lateral to the spine). (C–E) Treating asthma with Front-Mu points.

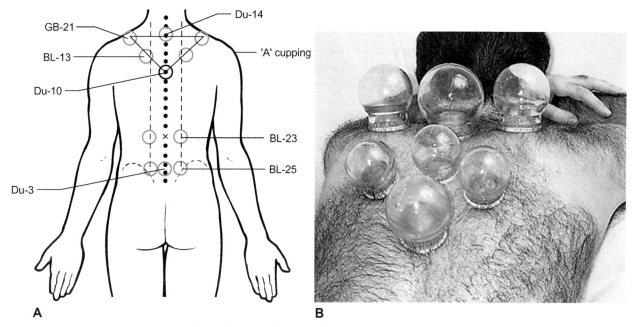

FIGURE 12-7 (A) Asthma (and back pain) back treatment points; (B) 'A' cupping.

CUPPING APPLICATION

Cupping Therapy. Strong cupping on LU-1 Zhongfu, Du-14 Dazhui, Dingchuan Extra and BL-13 Feishu.

Cupping Duration

Children

- **Under 5 years:** 2–3 minutes, Empty or Light cupping
- **5–7 years:** Up to 10 minutes, Empty or Light cupping
- **7–14 years:** Up to 15 minutes, Light or Medium cupping.

Adults

- **Young adults:** Strong or Moving cupping, up to 20 minutes
- **The weak and frail:** Weak or Empty cupping, up to 10 minutes.

CASE 12-4 Male Patient Aged 7 (Asthma)

Complaint. Asthmatic since the age of 1 year, during the last 5 weeks he has developed a bad cough and wheezing; there is no phlegm.

Present Medication. Prophylactic beclometasone dipropionate (Becotide).

Pulse. Nothing significant.

Tongue. Slightly red tip, otherwise good.

Observation. He is talkative, has a pronounced white forehead, poor appetite, and is sleeping poorly owing to his coughing bouts. Normally he comes for his treatment after school, and so

by this time he is quite tired. He is happy to have the treatment and stay in the clinic for a rest afterwards.

Diagnosis. Deficient type of asthma, Lung-Qi and Kidney-Yang Xu (deficiency). Pulse and tongue diagnosis often contradicts the symptoms when corticosteroid drugs are used (my own observation).

Treatment Principle. Tonify the Lungs and Kidneys, arrest the wheezing and stop the coughing.

Cupping Application. Light cupping on Dingchuan Extra and BL-15 Feishu, on each visit; asthma points Dingchuan Extra and BL-13 Feishu (see Fig. 12.6, Fig. 12.7).

ATROPHY SYNDROME

This condition is characterized by weakness and numbness of the limbs, wasting or reducing in the size of a limb, eventually leading to paralysis. It has been my own observation at the clinic that patients suffering from this and similar conditions usually do not seek alternative therapies at an early stage of their diagnosis.

Aetiology and Pathology

In the healthy state, the muscles, tendons and bones are nourished by fluid (Yin) and Qi (Yang). In atrophy syndrome, however, the muscles, tendons and bones are weak, indicating deficiency – of Blood and Qi – leading to malnourishment of muscles, tendons and bones. The Spleen-Qi nourishes the tendons, while the Lung-Qi tonifies and nourishes the Skin; the Liver is the 'master' of the Blood, and Kidneys are 'master' of the bones. As far as the clinical indications are concerned, multiple sclerosis and muscular dystrophy can also be included in this category.

Treatment

TREATMENT PRINCIPLE. Remove obstruction (Wind, Heat, Phlegm or Damp) from the channels, tonify Qi and Blood, and nourish the muscles and tendons.

CUPPING APPLICATION: UPPER LIMB

Cupping Therapy. Medium cupping to LI-14 Binao, LI-15 Jianyu, Jianneiling (Jianqian) Extra, GB-21 Jianjing, BL-12 Fengmen and Du-14 Dazhui. Also use Moving cupping on the Bladder channel on the back of the body.

APPLICATION: LOWER LIMB

Cupping Therapy. Medium cupping to BL-26 Guanyuanshu, GB-30 Huantiao, GB-31 Fengshi and ST-31 Biguan. Light-pressure Moving cupping can be applied on the channel between ST-31 and ST-34 Liangqiu, and the Gall Bladder channel between GB-30 and GB-33 Xiyangguan (Fig. 12-8).

Cupping Duration

Children

- **Under 14 years old:** 10 minutes, Light cupping only.

Adults

- **Young adults:** Medium or Moving cupping, up to 20 minutes
- **The weak and frail:** Weak, Empty or Moving cupping, up to 10 minutes only.

General Cupping or Acupuncture Points to be used in All Cases of Atrophy Syndrome. LU-5 Chize clears Lung Heat and benefits the sinews. Ren-6 Qihai resolves Dampness and benefits the entire energy of the body. Ren-12 Zhongwan (Front-Mu point of the Stomach) tonifies the Spleen and Stomach. Liv-13 Zhangmen (Front-Mu point of the Spleen) tonifies the Spleen and helps disperse the Liver-Qi. SP-10 Xuehai tonifies and moves the Blood. BL-12 Fengmen expels pathogenic Wind, releases the Exterior and regulates the Nutritive and Wei Qi. BL-20 Pishu (Back-Shu point of the Spleen)

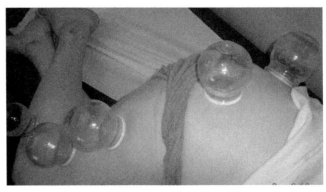

FIGURE 12-8 Treatment of atrophy syndrome.

tonifies the Stomach and Spleen and benefits Blood. BL-23 Shenshu (Back-Shu point of the Kidneys) tonifies the Kidney-Qi, nourishes Blood and strengthens the lower back. GB-34 Yanglingquan benefits the sinews and removes obstruction from the legs. GB-39 Xuanzhong is a special influence point for the marrow (Colour Plate Figure 7AB).

PRECAUTION

In many cases the patient's sensory feelings are impaired, therefore extra care is needed during cupping. Do not allow the skin to over-mark or bleed, or it may take rather a long time to heal, causing a postponement of future treatment.

CASE 12-5 Female Patient Aged 32 (Atrophy Syndrome)

Complaint. Paraplegia over the last 6 months.

Present Medication. Propantheline bromide 15 mg, three times a day (causes constipation). Imipramine 25 mg, 4 tablets before going to bed.

Pulse. Faint, at all levels.

Tongue. Pale, with a thin body.

Observation. The patient lost the use of her legs as a result of a fall and injury to the spinal cord at the level of the 10th thoracic vertebra. She spent 6 months in hospital following the accident. No operation was performed and physiotherapy was the only treatment used. Her sleep and appetite are good, but bowel movements are possible only with pressure applied to the lower abdomen. She is susceptible to bladder infections, which are controlled by antibiotics. Her self-esteem and morale were low. She has two children, 7 and 10 years old. Her husband is extremely supportive and also helpful around the house. She had a pale complexion, a low voice, and did not enjoy conversation. She has lost some weight, in particular her leg muscles, where muscular atrophy was observed.

I was called to see whether anything could be done to get her back on her feet again. We discussed the hospital report, which said that she would remain paraplegic for the rest of her life, owing to the severity of the spinal cord injury. I explained that acupuncture and cupping therapy would help her Energy and Blood circulation, and perhaps stop the muscular atrophy. If this can be achieved, muscle tone will return. As far as reversing the paraplegia were concerned, no promises or high hopes were raised.

Diagnosis. Injury to the Governing Vessel (Du Mai), hence injury to the Yang-Qi, resulting in paralysis and muscular atrophy to the lower parts of the body and the legs.

Treatment Principle. Remove the stagnation from the Du Mai, tonify Qi and Blood, and nourish the muscles and the tendons of the lower extremities.

Cupping Application. Moving cupping on the Huatuo Jiaji Extra channel, bilaterally (see Fig. 12-6B).

Conclusion. Five years on, this patient still continues with the treatment, twice weekly. The paraplegic condition is unchanged, but she exercises on the parallel bars and drives her car with confidence. The muscle tone in both the legs and buttocks has returned to normal and bladder control is very good. Recently she has been complaining of flatulence and constipation.

ATTENTION DEFICIENCY DISORDER (ADD) AND ATTENTION-DEFICIT HYPERACTIVITY DISORDER (ADHD)

Both conditions are relatively 'new diseases' that have appeared in the last 20 years. It is mostly seen in the Western developed countries with overcrowded cities, where children are perhaps not always allowed or permitted to enjoy being children! It is almost unheard of in the Far East, Middle East and most Mediterranean countries, where children still enjoy a relative freedom and have strong family ties and relationships. Both conditions were formally identified in the new *Diagnostic and Statistical Manual of Mental Disorder, Fourth Edition* (American Psychiatric Association, 1994). Both conditions have overlapping characteristics such as having difficulty in paying attention, being easily distracted, hyperactive, impulsive, suffering from forgetfulness and tiredness. But the unfortunate and sad reality is that both conditions are described under the heading of 'mental disorders'. Consequently the orthodox approach to treating both conditions is dietary advice supported with drug therapy (Scott & Barlow, 1999).

Aetiology and Pathology

Excess Heat and Phlegm patterns are considered to be the main two culprits (there are four patterns) according to Scott & Barlow (1999); 'These children are hot and restless!' observes Julian Scott. Pathogenic Heat rises up to the heart and the head resulting in restlessness, a poor sleep pattern, daytime hyperactivity and such children also enjoy being noisy and destructive. In TCM pathogenesis excessive Heat also contributes to the 'internal Wind', which in turn contributes to even more behavioural turbulence. Children with Phlegm and Heat have the same behaviour as above; in addition they may also be obese and even more destructive.

Treatment

TREATMENT PRINCIPLE

1. **Heat type:** Clear the Heat and calm the Heart (Shen/spirit)
2. **Heat and Phlegm:** Resolve the phlegm, clear the Heat and calm the Heart.

CUPPING APPLICATION

1. Apply between 3 to 5 minutes of Empty/Flash cupping, for 6 to 10 weeks, twice a week if possible, targeting the upper back, covering the area from BL-15 Xinshu to GB-21 Jiangjing, including the Du-14 Dazhui point.
2. Apply between 3 and 5 minutes of Empty/Flash cupping for six to ten weeks, twice a week if possible, to the entire back covering the area from the lower Bladder points BL-52 Zhishi and BL-23 Shenshu to the upper shoulders points GB-21 Jiangjing and not forgetting the Du-14 Dazhui point.

EXPLANATION. Empty/Flash cupping on children is quite easy especially when you don a playful approach to cupping therapy! As indicated earlier on, demonstrate the technique on the parent's arm first and then on to the child. On each application make sure that the suction strength is never strong but always a Weak or a Medium strength. Repeated Flash cupping to the above points cools the Blood, regulates the flow the Qi, brings the Blood from the deeper levels to the more superficial level. Also dredges the Governing Vessel and the Bladder channel helping to eliminate the internal Wind.

BACK PAIN AND SEXUAL COMPLAINTS

Back pain is one of the most commonly seen complaints in the clinic. I am fairly sure that this applies to most pain clinics and general practitioners' surgeries all over the country. Back pain can be caused by prolonged bad posture or through a sudden movement or lifting (not necessarily even a heavy load), which may result in dislocation of a vertebra or injury to the associated muscles or ligaments. Engaging in work that one is not used to, such as painting, decorating or gardening, can also cause back muscle and ligament contraction, resulting in cramping pains.

Upper Back Pain – Aetiology and Pathology

Upper back pain is pain in the neck, shoulders and upper trunk (cervical and thoracic vertebrae). This part of the body is most vulnerable to attacks of external pathogens such as Wind-Cold, Wind-Heat and Damp, but especially Wind-Cold. When Wind-Cold enters the channels (Bladder and Gall Bladder) on the neck or head it moves under the skin and penetrates to deeper muscular levels. One of the characteristics of this type of attack is its onset and location. Usually onset is sudden and is not fixed at any one point, instead moving alongside the channel, especially the Gall Bladder channel. Most of the time the patient goes to bed and wakes up in the morning with a stiff or painful neck.

Treatment

TREATMENT PRINCIPLE. Remove the pathogenic factors, i.e. Cold, Damp or Wind-Cold, open the channels and stop the pain.

CUPPING APPLICATION
  Cupping Therapy. 'A' cupping (see Fig. 12-7), or to GB-21 Jianjing, Du-14 Dazhui, BL-12 Fengmen and SI-11 Tianzong (Fig. 12-9).

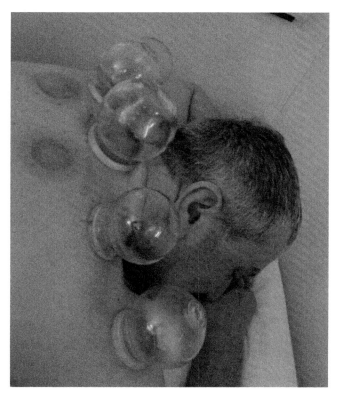

FIGURE 12-9 Treatment of upper back pain.

Reported Additional Cupping Points (Cui & Zhang, 1989). For shoulder pain, SI-14 Jianwaishu and SI-11 Tianzong. For spondylosis, cupping followed by needling the tender points of the spinous process as the main treatment, supplemented by SI-11 Tianzong and SI-9 Jianzhen.

Cupping Duration
Children

- **Under 5 years:** 2–3 minutes, Empty cupping
- **5–7 years:** Up to 10 minutes, Empty or Light cupping
- **7–14 years:** Up to 15 minutes, Light or Medium cupping.

Adults

- **Young adults:** Medium, Strong or Moving cupping, up to 20 minutes
- **The weak and frail:** Weak or Empty cupping, up to 10 minutes.

Lower Back Pain, Sciatica and Sexual Complaints – Aetiology and Pathology

Excessive overwork, standing for long periods of time, multiple pregnancy and childbirth, excessive sexual activity and external pathogenic factors such as Cold and Damp, all injure the Kidney-Qi and deplete Kidney-Yang. The clinical manifestations are chronic, dull backache, worsening as the day progresses, tiredness, impotence and pain travelling down to the leg (lumbar vertebrae, sacrum and coccyx). The lower back is very much influenced by the Kidney-Qi, rather than Wind-Cold. This part of the body is usually well covered, unlike the neck and chest. Kidney-Qi (especially the Kidney-Yang Qi) is considered to be the 'master' and the 'ruler' of the lower back by all the ancient and contemporary Chinese Medicine scholars. Consequently, when treating lower back conditions, Kidney-Qi is the primary focus of the treatment protocol.

Sexual complaints and lower back pain are closely interrelated. TCM considers Kidney-Yang Qi as the 'ruler' of the lower back, especially the reproductive organs, in men and women alike. Therefore, all the above Kidney-Qi deficiency syndromes will have a profound negative effect on the sexual mechanism, such as prolapsed internal organs, loss of libido, tiredness, dryness, pain during intercourse and impotence.

Treatment

TREATMENT PRINCIPLE. Tonify the Kidney-Qi, particularly the Kidney-Yang, remove pathogenic factors and relieve stagnation of Qi and Blood.

CUPPING APPLICATION

Cupping Therapy. Du-3 Yaoyangguan, Du-4 Mingmen, BL-23 Shenshu, BL-25 Dachangshu and BL-54 Zhibian or GB-30 Huantiao. Hot Needle cupping on Ren-4 Guanyuan, Du-4 Mingmen and BL-23 Shenshu when the patient presents a Wind-Cold or Wind-Damp syndrome. Cupping therapy is extremely effective in treating lower back pain (Fig. 12-10).

Reported Additional Cupping Points (Cui & Zhang, 1989). For pain in the loins: BL-23 Shenshu, BL-26 Guanyuanshu and BL-24 Qihaishu. Sciatica: acupuncture to GB-30 Huantiao, BL-49 Zhibian, GB-34 Yanglingquan and BL-23 Shenshu, followed by moxibustion and cupping to the local points.

Cupping Duration
Children

⊚ **Under 14 years:** up to 10 minutes, Empty or Medium cupping.

Adults

⊚ **Young adults:** Medium, Strong or Moving cupping, up to 20 minutes
⊚ **The weak and frail:** Empty or Medium cupping, up to 10 minutes.

Cupping and its Effect on the Sex Mechanism. Cupping on Du-3 Yaoyangguan and Du-4 Mingmen removes the obstruction, relaxes the muscle and improves the Qi and Blood circulation to the second, third and fourth lumbar vertebrae, which has a particular influence on the nerves supplying the sexual organs, according to Dr Paul Sherwood (1992) who states:

The sex act involves a complex interlinking of nerves and mini-brains which are situated at the lower end of the spinal cord. These are activated by both the brain itself and by sensory nerves that emanate from various erotic centres in the body. The most important of these by far are the cluster of nerves in the clitoris and parts of the vagina in women, and the tip of the penis in men. When stimulated, these nerve centres send impulses along the parasympathetic nerves to activate the sex organs. In the lumbar region the parasympathetic nerves pass through the spinal nerve canal along the second, third and fourth lumbar nerve roots.

CASE 12-6 Female Patient Aged 45 (Back Pain)

Complaint. Recurrent lower back pain in the lumbar region, with a feeling of heaviness in the leg muscles.

Present Medication. None.

Pulse. Slow (she is a marathon runner), weak Kidney pulse.

Tongue. Pale, with a thin white coating.

Observation. The patient is a physical education teacher and spends most of her days in the swimming pool, teaching swimming. Her hobby is running marathons, and she takes part in at least two serious marathons a year. She trains almost every weekend, between 10 and 20 miles at a time. She has muscular pains from time to time but recovers quickly. She is tall, and has good muscle structure.

Diagnosis. Kidney-Yang deficiency, with Damp-Cold invading the channels. Spending long hours in the pool is causing

Damp-Cold invasion of the channels. This results in tiredness and pain in the joints and muscles. Excessive exercise injures the Blood and depletes the Kidney-Yang, resulting in general body pains, particularly in the lower back.

Treatment Principle. Remove Damp-Cold and tonify the Kidney-Yang.

Cupping Application. Medium strength cupping on BL-23 Shenshu, BL-25 Dachangshu and Du-3 Yaoyangguan (see Fig. 12-7A).

Conclusion. Response to the treatment was very rapid, and the patient returned to her weekly running routine after 2 weeks. She was advised to slow down and perhaps take up a more gentle sport, more suitable for her age. However, she enjoys what she is doing and shows no intention of slowing down or giving it up.

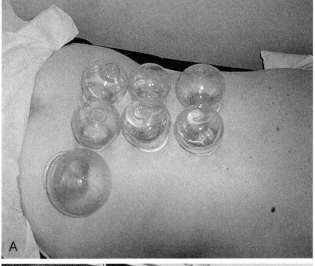

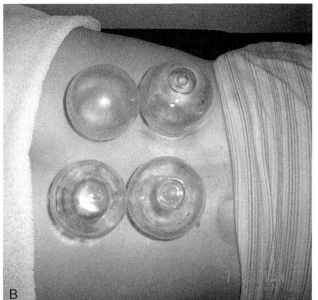

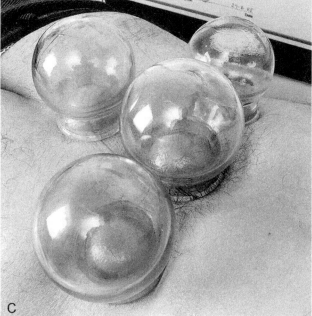

FIGURE 12-10 (A–C) Often-used lower back points for the treatment of back pain and sexual complaints.

BED-WETTING (NOCTURNAL ENURESIS)

Bed-wetting after the age of 3 years is considered to be a problem and one that needs to be treated. This is one childhood problem that Western medicine fails to treat effectively. Chinese Medicine, however, is highly successful, especially when combined with cupping. The majority of nocturnal enuresis cases seen in the clinic are between 7 and 12 years old. The parents of younger children are not particularly worried. Once the child reaches the age of 7 and trips away with school are inevitable, the problem is then highlighted and treatment is pursued.

Aetiology and Pathology

Bed-wetting is primarily a deficiency syndrome: deficiency of Kidney-Yang (seen more in children) and deficiency of Qi of the Lung and Spleen (seen more in the elderly). The Kidney-Qi governs the Bladder, therefore a strong Bladder is dependent on a strong Kidney-Qi, especially the Kidney-Yang

Qi. When deficient Kidney-Yang fails to control the Bladder and also to warm the Triple Burner, copious water runs downwards to fill the Bladder, resulting in nocturnal enuresis. Usually in children a deep sleep pattern is also observed. Excessive mental or physical activity weakens the body Qi, which results in near exhaustion and deep sleep. A hereditary weak constitution is another factor in Kidney-Yang deficiency syndrome. Cold is also a prevalent factor in nocturnal enuresis. Cold, especially in the lower back and abdomen, prevents the Kidney-Yang Qi reaching and controlling the Bladder, thereby giving rise to nocturnal enuresis. Qi deficiency in the Lung and Spleen is mostly associated with the natural ebbing of the body's Qi.

Treatment

TREATMENT PRINCIPLE. Warm and tonify the Kidneys; strengthen the Bladder.

CUPPING APPLICATION

Cupping Therapy. Medium cupping on Ren-3 Zhongji, Ren-6 Qihai, Du-4 Mingmen, BL-23 Shenshu and BL-28 Pangguangshu (see Figs 12-4, 12-7A, Colour Plate Figures 28 and 29).

Additional Cupping Points in the Treatment of Enuresis (Cui & Zhang, 1989). Enuresis due to neurological dysfunction was treated with cupping after needling over the sacral region. This restored the function of the central nervous system, enabling better Bladder control.

Cupping Duration

Children

- **Under 5 years:** 2–3 minutes, Empty or Light cupping
- **5–7 years:** Up to 10 minutes, Empty or Light cupping
- **7–14 years:** Up to 15 minutes, Light or Medium cupping
- **14–16 years:** Up to 20 minutes, Medium cupping.

CASE 12-7 Male Patient Aged 14 (Nocturnal Enuresis)

Complaint. He has been bed-wetting since very young.

Present Medication. None.

Pulse. Faint, at all levels.

Tongue. Very thin body and pale in colour.

Observations. This patient has come to the clinic with both of his parents, who were quite concerned about his persistent bed-wetting. It is now particularly worrying because he wants to join his classmates on school trips, which can sometimes last several days. Several visits to their local doctor have produced no result. His height was the first noticeable diagnostic tool: he is almost 6 feet tall at the age of 14! An intelligent boy, he also takes part in many school sporting activities, some of them at quite a serious level. He speaks very softly and, before answering a question, always looks for his parents' approval. He has no interest in food – in fact, during one of his rare unaccompanied visits to the clinic he has confided that, for him, eating is a waste of time. On questioning he also admits to suffering from long-term painful knees and legs. According to his parents his sleep is like death – once he puts his head on the pillow, he is fast asleep and no amount of noise will wake him. Mornings are also a problem: he refuses to wake up for school until the last minute, consequently most of the time he misses his breakfast.

Diagnosis. Hereditary constitutional deficiency, coupled with a rapid growth in height, preventing the Kidney-Qi 'catching up'. Both parents are quite tall and of slim build. The mother has a long-term Kidney function problem: only one of her kidneys is functioning properly. The patient's low voice and painful knees and legs all indicate Kidney-Yang deficiency. In this case the Kidney-Essence is also inadequate to nourish the fast-growing bones, thus making them painful, especially on exertion. The boy's poor appetite only serves to exacerbate his symptoms.

Treatment Principle. Tonify the Kidney-Yang and nourish the Qi and Blood.

Cupping Application. Light to Medium strength cupping was regularly applied to Ren-3 Zhongji, ST-29 Guilai and BL-28 Pangguangshu (see Figs 12-4 and 2-8).

Conclusion. This patient received weekly and sometimes bi-weekly treatments for about 6 months. His nocturnal enuresis has greatly improved but not completely stopped. Meanwhile he has grown another few inches. Reluctantly he has given up playing rugby, but continues to do other activities and refuses to rest during the day. His eating habit – or rather the lack of it – is a major concern to his parents; he, on the other hand, is not worried. He now has some good weeks and some bad weeks, when he is mostly tired. He now goes on outings for up to a week.

BOIL/CARBUNCLE

These are bacterial infections and inflammation of a hair follicle or sebaceous gland, seldom seen in Western clinics as a result of improved living conditions and the widespread use of antibiotics. They are, however, a very common occurrence, especially among children, in developing countries. Poor hygiene, poor dict and a lack of proper sanitation facilities, coupled with spitting habits, further weaken the already deficient Wei Qi, making it difficult for the body to repel infections. A boil initially appears as a small, red, hard and painful nodule that then fills with pus (yellow fluid composed of blood serum, dead tissue, white blood cells and bacteria, produced by the body in response to infection) and enlarges. Once the pus appears to collect and accumulate inside the boil, the skin over it becomes quite sensitive, thin and shiny. Only at this stage is the boil considered 'ripe' and ready to be discharged. Boils are extremely contagious and should not be squeezed, as this causes the infection to spread and damages the skin of the surrounding tissues. A carbuncle is larger than a boil and has several openings for discharge. Both are equally painful to touch, particularly when pus is collecting and accumulating. Skin boils usually appear on the face, scalp, shoulders and buttocks. Stress (particularly during exam periods in students), allergy, diabetes and a compromised immune system can also cause boils to appear.

Aetiology and Pathology

Pathogenic factors such as Turbid Phlegm, toxins accumulating in the Blood, and Heat, cause stagnation of Qi and Blood.

Treatment

TREATMENT PRINCIPLE. Clear the Heat/Poison, invigorate Qi and Blood, and tonify Qi.

PRECAUTION

Surgical gloves must be worn at all times during this therapy.

CUPPING APPLICATION

Cupping Therapy. Use a Strong or Bleeding cupping method on Du-14 Dazhui and Du-10 Lingtai. Pierce the top of the ripe boil (see Fig. 12-11A) and apply a Strong cup over it, allowing pus and some blood to exude; for this purpose choose a large cup – number 4 or 5. Remove the cup when the discharge stops and dress the boil in a normal fashion, using an antiseptic cream or a crushed fresh

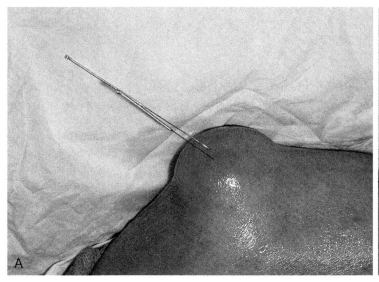
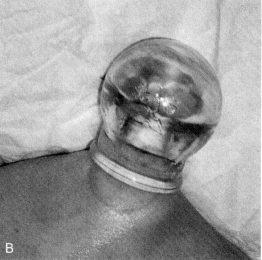

FIGURE 12-11 (A) Boil on the elbow: an acupuncture needle is inserted to cause bleeding. (B) Cupping over the ripe boil discharges pus.

dandelion (*Taraxaci mongolici*) poultice. Pistol-handle cupping apparatus is particularly effective for drawing the pus out of the boil.

Reported Additional Cupping Points (Cui & Zhang, 1989). The technique described in this report is to bleed the boil (with or without pus) and apply a large cup over it. Local and distal points were reported to be cupped together with acupuncture on Du-10 Lingtai. Bleeding cupping is also used on Du-14 Dazhui as well as cupping over the boil.

CASE **Female Patient Aged 78 (Boil/Carbuncle)**

Complaint. Carbuncle on the right elbow.

Present Medication. Gaviscon liquid.

Pulse. Faint and rapid.

Tongue. Red body with horizontal cracks.

Observation. She is an existing patient who attends the clinic for her arthritic condition. The carbuncle had appeared as a small nodule and grew to the size of a golf ball within 4 weeks. With her permission I decided to treat it.

Treatment Principle. Discharge the Blood-poison.

Cupping Application. Strong cupping application with a small (number 3) glass cup over the boil (Fig. 12-11).

Conclusion. On the application of a Strong cup some blood mixed with pus was discharged. On the second visit a week later, the size of the boil was greatly reduced and no treatment was given. On the subsequent visit it had completely disappeared, leaving a slight red mark on the skin.

CASE **Male Patient Aged 70 (Boil/Carbuncle)**

Complaint. Large painful boil located on the left lower back of the body.

Present Medication. Aspirin.

Pulse. Rapid.

Tongue. Slightly dry body, normal colour.

Observation. Boil appears to be very red, full of pus and painful to touch. It has been exuding bloody pus for over a week. Patient has become restless and is unable to sit or lie on his back.

Treatment Principle. Discharge the Blood-poison.

Cupping Application. Applied using pistol-handle cupping apparatus.

Conclusion. A total of three (once a week) applications of Bleeding cupping were administered before the discharge of pus completely stopped. Subsequently, the patient was able to go on to his pre-booked holiday!

CHEST PAIN

Chest pain can be the result or indication of numerous internal or external pathogens: Wind-Cold attacking the exterior, Phlegm with cough obstructing the Lung and causing Lung-Qi deficiency, heart-related pain such as angina or coronary heart disease, or sometimes pain that has nothing to do with the lungs or heart, such as indigestion or wind. Most patients with chest pain visiting my clinic have initially visited their doctor or hospital, and most of them have been diagnosed as having 'non-cardiac-related unspecified pain'. This particular category forms the subject of this section.

Aetiology and Pathology

External pathogenic factors such as Damp or Wind-Cold invade the Upper Jiao, causing stagnation of Qi. This leads to channel obstruction and pain. The most vulnerable time is between the changes of seasons, when people are inappropriately dressed. During the warmer seasons the body perspires more frequently, allowing the external pathogens to penetrate and invade the channels through open sweat pores.

Clinical Manifestations of Wind-Cold

A stabbing pain around the heart, behind the sternum or radiating to the back between the shoulder blades; usually the pain is worse on inhaling, and better on exhaling or when heat is administered. Cough and phlegm may accompany the pain. Sometimes this type of pain can last for several months with varying intensity.

Treatment

TREATMENT PRINCIPLE. Release the external pathogen, move Qi, open the channels and remove obstruction from the chest, and stop the pain.

CUPPING APPLICATION

   Cupping Therapy. Medium to Strong cupping on LU-1 Zhongfu, K-25 Shencang, BL-12 Fengmen, GB-21 Jiangjing, BL-15 Xinshu, SI-12 Bingfeng and BL-17 Geshu. Alternatively, use Medium to Strong 'A' cupping (see Fig. 12-7).

   Reported Additional Cupping Points. Intercostal neuralgia (Cui & Zhang, 1989) was treated first by acupuncture to P-6 Neiguan and SP-9 Yinlingquan through GB-34 Yanglingquan, followed by cupping to the local painful regions. Angina pectoris (Chen & Deng, 1989: 23) and coronary heart disease were treated with Bleeding cupping to BL-23 Shenshu, BL-15 Xinshu and BL-14 Jueyinshu. The pain was gradually relieved after only one treatment.

   Cupping Duration
   Children

⊚ This condition does not apply to children under 14.

   Adults

⊚ **Young adults:** Medium to Strong cupping, up to 20 minutes
⊚ **The weak and the frail:** Weak or Empty cupping, up to 10 minutes.

CASE (12-10) Male Patient Aged 50 (Chest Pain)

Complaint. He had collapsed with severe chest and neck pain in the left side of the body while driving home from work. His wife was in the car with him, and was able to drive him to the nearest hospital, where tests were carried out for a possible coronary problem. Diagnosis was negative and he was sent home with a painkiller.

Present Medication. None.

Pulse. Strong and floating.

Tongue. Red body, with thin white coating.

Diagnosis. As it was summer the patient had been working bare-chested in front of a cloth-presser, all day, for the entire week. He also perspires profusely. Air-conditioning had recently been installed at the factory and, at his request, one outlet was placed above his head. Consequently, Wind-Cold had entered the channels via the sweat pores, causing spasm and pain in the chest muscles.

Treatment Principle. Remove the Wind-Cold, relax the chest muscles and stop the pain.

Cupping Application. Strong 'A' cupping method was applied on each visit (see Fig. 12-7).

COMMON COLD AND INFLUENZA

Folklore remedies in many cultures will certainly include cupping as their main treatment for the common cold. In the clinical situation I also personally favour cupping to all other therapies when treating the chest for a Cold-related disorder.

Aetiology and Pathology

In TCM the common cold and influenza are considered to be external pathogenic factors of Wind-Cold or Wind-Heat invading the body externally. In Western medicine, however, they are seen as a viral infection of the chest. Both of these assumptions are, of course, correct in their own pathologies.

Let us take a closer look at the clinical manifestations and differentiation of the two patterns mentioned above, in TCM terms:

1. **Wind-Cold:** Fever with no sweating, pain and stiffness in the head and neck and a general body aching. Usually a lingering, ongoing condition, aversion to cold and wind, and a preference for warm drinks. Pain is usually reduced after applying heat. No swelling, usually a feeling of cold all over the body with pain.
2. **Wind-Heat:** A sudden onset with fever and some sweating, sore throat and thirst with headaches, aversion to heat, a preference for cold drinks, pain worse when heat is applied, redness with swelling and pain.

Treatment

Wind-Cold

TREATMENT PRINCIPLE. Remove the external pathogen, induce sweating and keep the patient warm.

CUPPING APPLICATION

Cupping Therapy. Apply Light to Medium 'A' cupping technique (see Fig. 12-7). After removing the cups, immediately reapply to the following points: LU-1 Zhongfu, BL-12 Fengmen, BL-43 Gaohuangshu and BL-23 Shenshu (Fig. 12.12).

Cupping Duration

Children

- **Under 5 years:** 2–3 minutes, Empty or Light cupping
- **5–7 years:** Up to 10 minutes, Empty or Light cupping
- **7–14 years:** Up to 15 minutes, Light or Medium cupping.

Adults

- **Young adults:** Medium or Strong cupping, up to 20 minutes
- **The weak and frail:** Empty or Weak cupping, up to 10 minutes.

Wind-Heat

TREATMENT PRINCIPLE. Remove the pathogen Wind-Heat, reduce fever and stop the coughing.

CUPPING APPLICATION

Cupping Therapy. Strong cupping method on Du-14 Dazhui, BL-12 Fengmen, BL-13 Feishu and BL-43 Gaohuangshu, followed by a Strong 'A' cupping (see Fig. 12-7) or Moving cupping on the Bladder channel bilaterally.

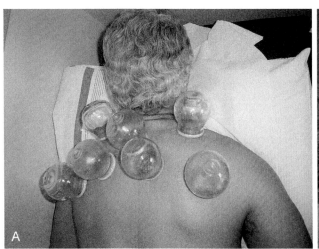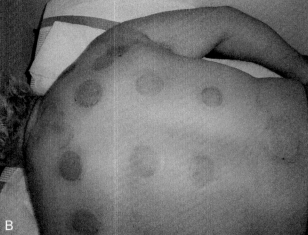

FIGURE 12-12 (A, B) Treating the common cold and influenza.

Cupping Duration
Children

- **Under 5 years:** 2–3 minutes, Empty or Weak cupping
- **5–7 years:** Up to 10 minutes, Empty or Weak cupping
- **7–14 years:** Up to 15 minutes, Weak or Medium cupping.

Adults

- **Young adults:** Strong or Moving cupping, up to 20 minutes
- **The weak and frail:** Light to Medium cupping, up to 10 minutes.

CASE 12-11 Female Patient Aged 13 (Common Cold)

Complaint. Continuous sneezing, with a runny nose.

Present Medication. None.

Pulse. Rapid and floating.

Tongue. Slightly red body, no coating.

Observation. She is a student and also likes partying. According to her father, 'she wears very little' when she goes out. Being an only child she has her own way a good deal. She is also extremely pale, constantly feels tired and prefers to stay in bed, especially in the mornings. Her attitude is that of a 19-year-old girl. Despite the fact that it is winter, she wears a very light dress with no jumper.

Diagnosis. Qi Xu (energy deficiency) with Wind-Cold invasion. Owing to her excessive activities and lack of rest she has depleted her energies, leaving her Wei Qi (defensive energy) in very poor condition. The fact that she wears so little clothing makes her even more vulnerable to external pathogens such as Wind or Cold. This is very much a case of the Greater Yang stage of the Cold, with clear symptoms such as floating pulse, sneezing and a runny nose accompanying the complaint.

Treatment Principle. Remove the Wind-Cold and tonify the Wei-Qi.

Cupping Application. Medium cupping on BL-12 Fengmen for 5 minutes, followed by 'A' cupping for a further 10 minutes on each visit (see Fig. 12-7).

Conclusion. The patient received eight treatments, sometimes weekly and sometimes bi-weekly, most of the time being late or missing her appointment altogether. Her cold and sneezing bouts disappeared, but the tiredness remained as part of her characteristic.

CONSTIPATION

This is one of the 'secret' complaints of Western society. In my opinion, more people are self-medicating for this complaint than for all other complaints put together. These days it is so easy and convenient to purchase one of many varieties of laxative available, some herbal and some conventional pharmaceutical products. I remember visiting a herbalist in a European country, where there was a box of herbs in the window marked 'slimming herb'. On closer inspection and a finger-taste, I discovered that it was nothing more than powdered Senna leaf. It is of some concern to consider what he might have been selling as a laxative!

Aetiology and Pathology

Constipation can be due to a Qi deficiency (seen more frequently in elderly patients); excessive consumption of food, causing 'Food blockage' (seen more in children); poor diet (although the diet factor is relatively less significant these days, owing to the much-publicized need for fibre in the diet, which has led to a general increase in fresh vegetable and fruit intake over the last 10–15 years), the consumption of raw and cold food and drink, lack of fluid intake, use of painkilling tablets, the aftermath of a febrile disease, lack of exercise (particularly walking) or emotional upsets leading to Liver-Qi stagnation.

Treatment

In general, constipation can be classified under two headings: Cold, Deficient type, the clinical manifestations of which are alternating symptoms such as diarrhoea and constipation with abdominal pain, and Hot, Excessive type, whose clinical manifestations are dry stools with constipation accompanied by thirst and a dry mouth.

Cold, Deficient-Type Constipation

TREATMENT PRINCIPLE. Warm and regulate the Stomach / Spleen-Qi, and move the bowels.

CUPPING APPLICATION

Cupping Therapy. Medium cupping on ST-25 Tianshu, Ren-12 Zhongwan, Liv-13 Zhangmen, BL-20 Pishu and BL-25 Dachangshu. For children under 7 years, massage the abdomen with olive oil using a clockwise circular motion.

Hot, Excessive-Type Constipation

TREATMENT PRINCIPLE. Remove Heat, regulate the Large Intestine and move the bowels.

CUPPING APPLICATION

Cupping Therapy. To the previous acupuncture points, add: LI-4 Hegu, LI-11 Quchi, ST-44 Neiting and Liv-2 Xingjian. Cup the same points as before, using a Stronger method when draining the Heat.

Cupping Duration. Apply 10 minutes of Moving cupping (clockwise) twice a week around the umbilicus.

CASE 12-12 **Male Patient Aged 50 (Constipation)**

Complaint. He has suffered from constipation for over 10 years. When not taking laxatives his bowel movement is once every 15 days, with great difficulty.

Present Medication. Glycerol suppositories and Senna herbal tablets.

Pulse. Rapid and strong.

Tongue. Reddish body with a thin, yellow coating.

Observation. He is a mobile mechanic by profession, which meant that he is driving long distances without much exercise or stopping for regular breaks for food or rest. His staple diet is ready-made fast food and a fizzy drink. He is of strong body build with no excess weight. He also smokes between 20 and 30 cigarettes a day while driving.

Diagnosis. Hot, Dry-type constipation with Liver-Qi stagnation – this is the result of the wrong diet and frustration brought on by driving in heavy traffic all day; he is probably also compelled to ignore 'nature's calls' as he is often on the road. Irregular, snack-type food, eating while on the move, too often having the same kind of food, lack of exercise, sitting for too long, and the fact that he does not enjoy his work have all contributed towards stagnation, leading to constipation.

Treatment Principle. Remove the Stomach Heat, assure the smooth flow of Liver-Qi, regulate and moisturize the Large Intestine.

Cupping Application. Medium cupping on Ren-12 Zhongwan, Liv-13 Zhangmen, SP-15 Daheng and BL-25 Dachangshu (Colour Plate Figure 5AB).

Conclusion. The patient was also advised to take up some form of exercise, long walks in particular, to have more regular and proper meals, and to avoid rich and greasy fast foods, drinking plenty of fresh water and eating fresh fruits rather than dried nuts. With long-term constipation sufferers, their digestive internal clock has somehow come to a stop. To restart this, a disciplined regimen of proper meals, rest and plenty of exercise is essential. Taking laxatives for a long period of time is not a sensible solution for constipation. After 3 months of weekly treatment the patient's condition has much improved and he is passing well-formed stools once every other day.

COUGH

Everyone contracts a cough at some time or another – winter or summer, the season does not seem to make much difference. Children, adults and the elderly alike are equally susceptible to coughs, and they can quite often turn into a distressing condition, especially in children or the elderly.

Aetiology and Pathology

The primary cause of cough is an attack of the external pathogen of Wind-Cold or Wind-Heat, which in both cases causes injury to the Lung-Qi. Deficient Lung-Qi fails to direct the Qi downward, causing coughing. Broadly speaking, coughs can be classified under two headings: Wind-Cold and Wind-Heat. These pathologies can also be further subdivided; however, within the context of this book only the clinical manifestations of Wind-Cold and Wind-Heat will be discussed.

Treatment

Wind-Cold

Clinical manifestations include cough with watery sputum, thin, white nasal discharge, sneezing, aversion to cold, slight or no raised temperature, body aches and a stiff neck.

TREATMENT PRINCIPLE. Expel the exterior Wind-Cold, restore the descending action of the Lung-Qi, encourage sweating and stop the coughing.

CUPPING APPLICATION

Cupping Therapy. Dingchuan Extra, GB-21 Jianjing, BL-12 Fengmen and BL-13 Feishu, or 'A' cupping (see Fig. 12-7, Fig. 12-13).

Reported Additional Cupping Points in the Treatment of Cough for Children's Respiratory Disorders (Cui & Zhang, 1989). The treatment of *whooping cough* was published in the 1960s, with cupping over Du-12 Shenzhu point only. A different practitioner used cupping over Ren-21 Xuanji and ST-14 Kufang, alternating with BL-13 Feishu and Du-14 Dazhui. For *chronic bronchitis in infants* (7 to 12 months), pricking of Du-14 Dazhui for bloodletting was followed by cupping. For *acute*

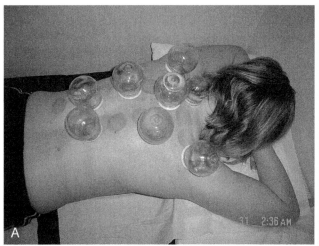
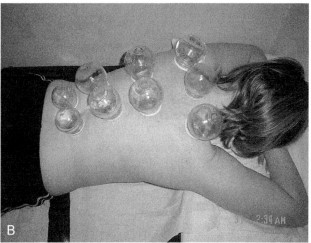
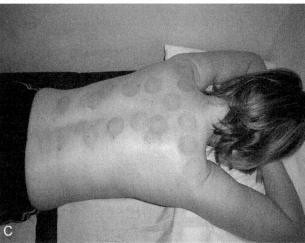

FIGURE 12-13 (A–C) Treating colds and cough.

bronchitis in children, cupping to BL-13 Feishu, K-25 Shencang and K-24 Lingxu was used bilaterally and alternately. For *phlegmy dyspnoea*, Water cupping over BL-12 Fengmen, BL-13 Feishu, BL-43 Gaohuangshu, Ren-21 Xuanji, Ren-20 Huagai and ST-15 Wuyi has been employed.

Cupping Duration
Children

- **Under 5 years:** 2–3 minutes, Empty or Weak cupping
- **5–7 years:** Up to 10 minutes, Empty or Weak cupping
- **7–14 years:** Up to 15 minutes, Weak or Medium cupping.

Adults

- **Young adults:** Strong or Moving cupping, up to 20 minutes
- **The weak and frail:** Light to Medium cupping, up to 10 minutes.

Wind-Heat

Clinical manifestations include dry cough, sore throat, sticky thick phlegm, thick nasal discharge, headache, raised temperature and some sweating.

TREATMENT PRINCIPLE. Clear the Lung Heat, restore the descending action of the Lung-Qi and stop the coughing.

CUPPING APPLICATION
Cupping Therapy. Use a stronger cupping technique to the same points as in the common cold, with the addition of LU-1 Zhongfu (see Fig. 4-2).

DYSMENORRHOEA

Dysmenorrhoea is very common complaint in modern society. The clinical manifestations include abdominal pain before, during or after the onset of menstruation, often accompanied by other symptoms such as lower backache, dizziness, nausea, restlessness, agitation, tiredness and heart palpitations. Failure to protect and nurture the body during menstruation is a key factor in dysmenorrhoea. Television advertisements often imply that a woman wearing a tampon can easily go about her daily routines, including swimming and mountain climbing! Not long ago, and in many different cultures around the world, a woman during menstruation stayed at home doing little and resting. Some cultures also have a degree of religious or superstitious belief that menstruation is 'unclean'.

Aetiology and Pathology

The pain is the result of stagnation of Qi (Liver-Qi) and Blood in the uterus, or Cold-Damp invading the uterus, Damp-Heat retention in the Liver channel and deficiency of Qi and Blood. Excessive, Full-type dysmenorrhoea is characterized by severe lower abdominal pain during the flow; Deficient, Empty-type dysmenorrhoea is characterized by a dull, lingering lower abdominal pain towards the end of the period.

Treatment

Stagnation of Liver-Qi and Blood

Clinical manifestations include breast distension, pain before or during the flow, some blood clots, agitation and restlessness.

TREATMENT PRINCIPLE. Remove the Liver-Qi stagnation, move Qi and Blood, and stop pain.

Cold-Damp Invading the Uterus

Clinical manifestations include feeling cold, especially in the lower extremities and abdomen, colicky pain before or during menstruation, lower backache, tiredness and pain relieved by hot water bottle application.

TREATMENT PRINCIPLE. Warm the lower abdomen with Moxa, remove Cold, and restore the movement of Qi and Blood (Fig. 12-14).

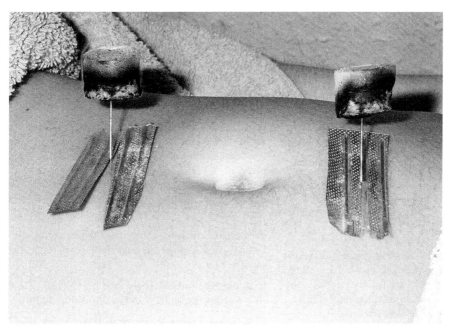

FIGURE 12-14 Moxa (Hot Needle) cupping on the points Ren-4 and Ren-12; this is excellent for tonifying the energy of the body.

Damp-Heat Retention in the Liver Channel

Clinical manifestations include distending pain in the lower abdomen, a short cycle, dark-red flow with clots, restlessness and agitation.

TREATMENT PRINCIPLE. Resolve Dampness; clear Heat and stagnation.

Deficiency of Qi and Blood

Clinical manifestations include postmenstrual pain, pain relieved by pressure, a long cycle, large amounts of menstrual flow, pale complexion, dizziness, palpitations and tiredness.

TREATMENT PRINCIPLE. Tonify Qi and Blood; remove stagnation in the uterus.

As seen in the above four differentiations, all pathological conditions cause *stagnation* of the Qi and Blood, leading to dysmenorrhoea. Therefore, *tonifying* the Empty, *draining* the Excess, *warming* the Cold and *cooling* the Heat are the treatment principles applied.

CUPPING APPLICATION

Cupping Therapy. In all four situations, various strengths of cupping are applied to the same points, depending on the energetic condition of the particular patient: Liv-13 Zhangmen, Ren-4 Guanyuan and ST-29 Guilai. In cases of back pain, use the lower back cupping points in the section on Back pain (Colour Plate Figure 13).

Reported Additional Cupping Points in the Treatment of Gynaecological Disorders (Cui & Zhang, 1989). In the last 40 years, conditions of *leukorrhoea*, *labour* and the *mammaries* have been treated by cupping therapy. *Oligomenorrhoea* and *infertility* are treated by needling BL-23 Shenshu in a downward direction, combined with Moving cupping to the same point, and *leukorrhoea* by prickly needling and cupping at Yaoyan Extra under the third lumbar vertebra and the area around Balio (BL-31 to BL-34). The treatment of 47 cases of uterine pain has been reported, by the Longyan District Hospital, by cupping to Ren-4 Guanyuan combined with needling of ST-36 Zusanli and Ren-4 Guanyuan (Cui & Zhang, 1989). For *postpartum deficiency of milk secretion*, acupuncture to BL-15 Xinshu followed by cupping to the same point has been employed.

Cupping Duration

- **Under 16 years:** Up to 10 minutes
- **Under 50 years:** Up to 20 minutes.

PRECAUTION

Do not apply Strong or Moving cupping to the abdominal points.

CASE 12-13   Female Patient Aged 26 (Dysmenorrhoea)

Complaint. Bad period pains just before the period and after onset for 2 days, then the pain subsides.

Present Medication. She is taking the contraceptive pill and co-proxamol analgesics.

Pulse. Wiry, weak at the Kidney pulse.

Tongue. Nothing of significance.

Observation. The patient is a very slender girl, studying and working at the same time. The fear of gaining weight prevents her eating proper meals, therefore she eats only once a day. With period pains she also has painful breasts and becomes moody with weepy spells. For the first 2 days of her period she stays at home because of the severity of the pain. She sleeps well and suffers no particular bowel problems.

Diagnosis. Qi and Blood deficiency with pronounced Liver-Qi stagnation. Depriving the body of proper nutrition for a long period of time has led to this deficiency. Working and studying for her accountancy course has contributed further towards her deficiency. The anxiety of having to take 2 days off work every month, coupled with the heavy mental demands of her studies, has resulted in stagnation of the Liver-Qi – hence the mood swings and the distended and painful breasts during menstruation.

Treatment Principle. Tonify the Qi and Blood, disperse the Liver-Qi and remove the stagnation, regulate the Uterus and stop the pain.

Cupping Application. Light cupping on Liv-13 Zhangmen, Ren-4 Guanyuan and ST-29 Guilai (see Fig. 12-14).

Conclusion. The weekly treatment was continued for 3 months, by which time the period pains were much reduced and the patient was able to continue with her work during the onset. She received ten further monthly booster treatments.

FEVERS

Complementary medicine practitioners, when presented with a condition that accompanies a fever, are sometimes placed in a dilemma whether to advise the use of antibiotics, or to try to manage the disease and reduce the fever using alternative remedies alone. Chinese doctors have long recognized the diseases caused by fever, and have contributed such classics as the *Treatise on Febrile Diseases caused by Cold* by Zhang Zhongjing (c. 220 AD), also known as the *Shanghan Lun*, and the diseases caused by Wind-Heat, the 'School of Warm Diseases' (Wen Bing School, late 1600s).

Aetiology and Pathology

From the Western medicine point of view, having a raised temperature or fever indicates an infection, and it is treated with antibiotics or antipyretic drugs. In general, antibiotics are prescribed for a short period of time (1 or 2 weeks). Sometimes, however, people are on low-dose antibiotics for as long as 3–4 years.

From the Chinese medicine point of view, fever is caused by the external pathogenic factors of Wind-Cold or Wind-Heat attacking the Exterior (Wei Qi). When the fever is not cleared at the Wei-Qi level, it penetrates into the deeper energetic layers (i.e. the Qi, Nutritive-Qi and the Blood levels) where it turns into a Warm disease. Conditions such as meningitis, measles, chickenpox and German measles are included in this category. The most common clinical presentations are fever and infection.

Treatment

TREATMENT PRINCIPLE. Always disperse the Heat first, before dealing with other symptoms.

CUPPING APPLICATION

Cupping Therapy. Bleeding cupping method on the Du-14 is the most effective for treating Fever attacks. Alternatively, you can use Strong cupping method on Du-14 Dazhui, Du-10 Lingtai and BL-17 Geshu. Apply Empty cupping method on the upper back if the patient is lethargic (Colour Plate Figures 14 and 15AB).

Reported Additional Cupping Points in the Treatment of Fever. Dr Wang (in Chen & Deng 1989: 22) believes that a number of diseases are the result of Blood Heat and stagnation. He used Bleeding cupping to remove Blood stagnation, activate the blood circulation, dispel the pathogenic factors and regulate the channel Qi. A patient with flu, headache and a high fever was treated with Bleeding cupping to Du-14 Dazhui, BL-13 Feishu and BL-15 Xinshu. Another patient with high fever, accompanied by abdominal pain, diarrhoea with pus and bloody stools, was treated twice with Bleeding cupping to Du-14 Dazhui, BL-20 Pishu and BL-25 Dachangshu.

In 1972, Dr Qu (Chen & Deng, 1989: 165) treated infantile toxic indigestion accompanied by dehydration and venous collapse with Moving cupping, using a medium-sized cup dipped in warm ginger water; this was used 30 times on bilateral Huatuojiaji points, followed by local cupping to Ren-12 Zhongwan, ST-25 Tianshu and Ren-4 Guanyuan 60 times in order to activate the internal organs and expel the pathogenic Heat.

Cupping Duration
Children (including infants)

- **Under 5 years:** 2–3 minutes, Empty or Weak cupping
- **5–7 years:** Up to 10 minutes, Empty or Weak cupping
- **7–14 years:** Up to 15 minutes, Weak or Medium cupping.

Adults

- **Young adults:** Bleeding cupping, Strong or Moving cupping, up to 20 minutes
- **The weak and the frail:** Light to Medium cupping, up to 10 minutes.

As always, the individual's energy level should be taken into account, and the patient treated accordingly, not overzealously. Sometimes patients with fever may look quite energetic and have abundant Yang (Fire) symptoms. This, however, can be very deceiving as the Yin (Fluids) may be depleted, resulting in dryness, tiredness and listlessness.

CAUTION

Patients arriving with a temperature above 37.8°C (100°F), particularly children, should be referred to hospital or advised to see a doctor without delay.

GROWING PAINS

Growing pains mostly occur in children between the ages of 3 and 12 years. The pain is usually concentrated in the muscles and not the joints. The thighs, calves and backs of the knees are the common pain locations. According to Julian Scott, Dampness and Phlegm in the channels are the main causes of growing pains in children (Scott & Barlow, 1999).

Aetiology and Pathology
Spleen controls the muscles. Liver-Blood nourishes the extremities. Deficient Spleen-Qi will lead to poor transformation and transportation of nutrients leading to accumulation of Damp and pain.

Treatment
TREATMENT PRINCIPLE. Tonify the Spleen and promote blood circulation to the legs.

CUPPING APPLICATION. Alternate the cupping treatment between moving the Blood and Qi and tonifying the Spleen, treating twice a week if possible. Apply a Flash or Light cupping method for between 3 and 5 minutes to each leg, concentrating on the Liver and the Gall Bladder channels. On alternate days apply Weak cupping for 3 to 5 minutes to the Liv-13 Zhangmen, Ren-10 Xiawan, Ren-6 Qihai, ST-30 Qichong, BL-20 Pishu and BL-28 Panggunagshu points (Fig. 12-15).

HYPERTENSION

Blood pressure is considered to be elevated when the systolic (upper) value is 160 mmHg or above, and the diastolic (lower) value is 90 mmHg or above. Both these values indicate the pressure of the blood on the walls of the vessels, the former being during heart contraction and the latter being the resting period between contractions. Blood pressure normally increases slightly with age, during pregnancy, and with kidney disorders and emotional circumstances such as grief, excitement or fear.

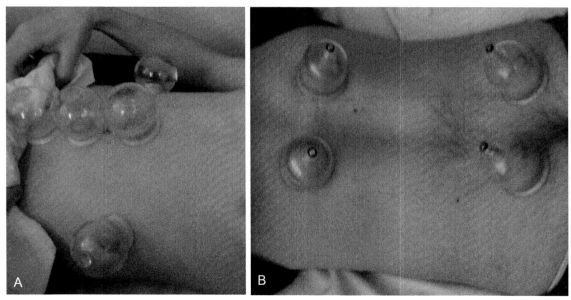

FIGURE 12-15 (A, B) Treatment of growing pain.

Aetiology and Pathology

As far as TCM is concerned, 'hypertension can be due to either Kidney-Yang or Kidney-Yin deficiency' (Maciocia, 1994). When the Kidney-Yang (Fire) is deficient the Yin (Water) accumulates, and when the Kidney-Yin (Water) is deficient the Liver-Yin is not nourished; this leads the Liver-Yang to ascend, causing elevated blood pressure. Classic symptoms of hypertension are light-headedness, occipital or vertical headache, blurred vision, tinnitus, dizziness and, in severe cases, stroke caused by a cerebral haemorrhage.

Treatment

TREATMENT PRINCIPLE. Tonify the Kidneys and subdue the Liver-Yang.

CUPPING APPLICATION

Cupping Therapy. Bleeding cupping on Du-14; up to 100 mL of blood can be extracted (Colour Plate Figure 15AB).

CASE 12-14 Male Patient Aged 37 (Hypertension)

Complaint. He had high blood pressure of 180/110 and insomnia. He was discovered to have elevated blood pressure during a routine check-up 3 years previously; he suffered no noticeable adverse effects. A civil servant by profession and a keen sportsman, running and weight-lifting are his main sporting activities. He also manages to sleep only 3 to 4 hours during the night, waking up early and failing to go back to sleep again. This pattern has not changed in the last 5 to 6 years.

Present Medication. Over the 3 years various types of vasodilators and beta blockers have been prescribed to reduce and control the hypertension. He does not take sleeping pills.

Pulse. Strong on the surface, weak at the deeper level.

Tongue. Red body with a thin, yellow coating and a pronounced red tip.

Observation. This patient entered the civil service on leaving school and worked his way up to a managerial position; he enjoys his work tremendously. He has no financial problems and

his girlfriend has just given birth to a boy. On the surface he looks and acts very happy and content. During our conversations, however, I noticed a certain degree of insecurity as far as his job was concerned, but he did not acknowledge this. Lack of sleep was also taking its toll; by most lunchtimes he would be very tired, but continued to work. He had a good appetite and ate well-balanced meals.

Diagnosis. Hypertension resulting from Liver-Yang rising. This case was a mixture of excesses and deficiencies. Work-related worry and anxiety resulted in Heart Fire (tip of the tongue red), leading to insomnia. Overwork and excessive physical activity caused Kidney-Yin and Liver-Yin deficiency, leaving the Liver-Yang to ascend.

Treatment Principle. Nourish the Liver- and Kidney-Yin, clear the Heart Fire and subdue the Liver-Yang.

Cupping Application. Bleeding cupping to Du-14 Dazhui on each visit.

LARYNGITIS

Laryngitis is inflammation of the larynx (voice box).

Aetiology and Pathology

Speaking, singing or shouting for long periods of time can damage the Qi circulation in the larynx. Symptoms include: sore throat, loss of voice, difficulty in speaking, high fever, headache and irritating cough.

Treatment

TREATMENT PRINCIPLE. Regulate the flow of Qi and clear the pathogenic Heat from the throat.

CUPPING APPLICATION. Medium cupping on BL-13 Feishu, Dingchuan, LI-11 Quishi, LI-4 Hegu and on the Du-14 Dazhui points (Bleeding cupping on Du-14 if the patient is over 14 years old) (Fig. 12-16).

MUSCULOSKELETAL PAIN ('BI' SYNDROME)

Easily the most frequently seen complaints by alternative practitioners all over the world are the musculoskeletal disorders (i.e. painful 'Bi' syndrome). In the young this could be the result of excessive physical activity or trauma, and in the elderly to lack of activity, arthritis or rheumatism.

Aetiology and Pathology

An external attack of Damp or Wind-Cold invades the channels and collaterals causing constriction of the flow of Qi and Blood. Clinical manifestations are muscular and joint pain, sometimes with numbness or swelling. The meaning of 'Bi' is obstruction of the circulation of Qi and Blood. The external pathogenic factors such as Damp or Wind-Cold can penetrate the channels easily, particularly when the body's Wei Qi is weak. There are five variations of painful 'Bi' Syndrome:

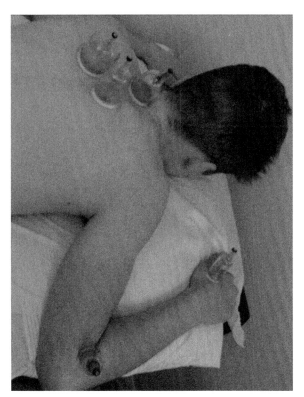

FIGURE 12-16 Treatment of laryngitis.

- Wind or wandering painful 'Bi' syndrome, characterized by wandering pain, moving between the joints or muscles
- Damp painful 'Bi' syndrome, characterized by severe fixed pain and swelling of the joints, aggravated by damp or cold weather
- Cold painful 'Bi' syndrome, characterized by severe pain in the joints, made worse by cold weather
- Febrile 'Bi' syndrome, characterized by pain with local redness and hot, swollen joints
- Bone painful 'Bi' syndrome, characterized by painful and swollen joints and bone deformities (this type of 'Bi' Syndrome cannot be treated with cupping therapy).

Treatment

TREATMENT PRINCIPLE. Nourish the Blood when treating the Wind 'Bi' syndrome, warm and tonify the Yang when treating the Cold painful 'Bi' syndrome, tonify the Spleen when treating the Damp painful 'Bi' syndrome and clear the Heat when treating the febrile 'Bi' syndrome.

CUPPING APPLICATION: UPPER BODY

Cupping Therapy. Medium, Strong, Moving, Moxa and Needle cupping methods can all be used according to differentiation on the following points: Du-14 Dazhui, GB-21 Jianjing, SI-11 Tianzong, SI-12 Bingfeng, LI-14 Binao and LI-15 Jianyu (Colour Plate Figure 16).

CUPPING APPLICATION: LOWER BODY

Cupping Therapy. Medium, Strong, Moving and Moxa cupping methods can be applied to lower back Du-3 Yaoyangguan, BL-26 Guanyuanshu and GB-30 Huantiao points (Fig. 12-17, see also Fig. 12-7). Ankle joints can be cupped if swelling is present, otherwise proper suction cannot be achieved around the ankle joint (Fig. 12-18A). When treating the knee joint, cup the area around the knee, especially ST-35 Dubi and the anterior patella (Fig. 12-18B).

Reported Additional Cupping Points in the Treatment of 'Bi' Syndrome (Cui & Zhang, 1989). For pain in the shoulder blade, cupping of SI-14 Jianwaishu and SI-11 Tianzong was reported, and, for pain in the loins, BL-23 Shenshu, BL-26 Guanyuanshu and BL-24 Qihaishu An inflamed joint was treated by Bleeding cupping to the surrounding joint to drain away congealed blood. Ninety further cases of 'Bi' syndrome were treated by plum-blossom needling followed by cupping to the local areas.

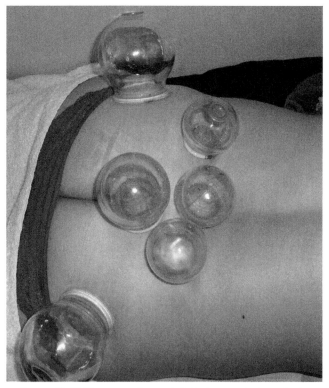

FIGURE 12-17 Treatment of musculoskeletal pain in the lower back.

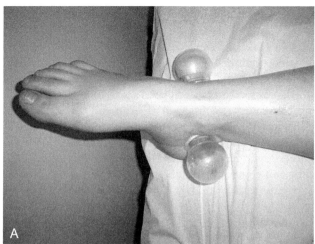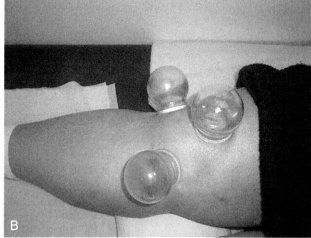

FIGURE 12-18 (A) Cupping of an ankle joint; cupping is more successful when swelling accompanies the pain. (B) Cupping a knee joint is a very common treatment method for 'Bi' syndrome of the knee.

Cupping Duration
Children

- **Under 16 years:** Light to Medium cupping, up to 15 minutes.

Adults

- **Young adults:** Medium, Strong, Moving and Moxa cupping, for up to 30 minutes
- **The weak and the frail:** Empty or Weak cupping, up to 10 minutes.

Herbal Ointment. During the treatment of the above five 'Bi' Syndromes, a herbal muscle and joint soothing 'Bi' cream, Chirali Old Remedy®1 was used extensively.[1] This particular cream contains wintergreen (*Gaultheria procumbens*), thyme (*Thymus vulgaris*), bay (*Laurus nobilis*), eucalyptus (*Eucalyptus globulus*), evening primrose (*Oenothera biennis*) and BP soft paraffin.

Action. Moves Qi and Blood, opens the channels and eliminates 'Bi'.

CASE 12-15 Male Patient Aged 50 (Muscular Pain – 'Bi' Syndrome)

Complaint. He had suffered pain around the shoulders, neck and chest, radiating to the arms, for over 5 years.

Present Medication. Co-proxamol, up to 8 tablets per day.

Pulse. Weak and slippery.

Tongue. Red body with a thick, yellowy-black coating.

Observation. This patient had in fact checked into a hospital demanding a diagnosis, after his own doctor referred him to a psychiatrist believing that his 'pain is all in your mind'. Following various neurological and blood tests and a 3-day hospital stay, he was discharged without any findings. He was quite agitated and the pain prevented him having a good night's sleep. He smoked a pack of cigarettes a day and enjoyed drinking beer. He is tall with a strong physical appearance and good body weight. On questioning he also complained of stomach acid regurgitation over a long period, and was now taking antacid tablets. He had irregular eating habits, with snack foods dominating his diet. A hot sensation in the upper back muscles and a large dark skin patch between the shoulder blades accompanied the pain.

Diagnosis. Febrile 'Bi' syndrome, with retention of Damp-Heat in the channels. The thick, yellowy-black tongue coating is a clear indication of Stomach Heat. Muscular pain with a hot sensation is a sign of obstruction in the channels caused by Damp-Heat. The dark skin patch on the back indicates Blood stasis. The Heart-Qi is also strained by the Damp-Heat, resulting in restlessness and agitation.

Treatment Principle. Clear the Heat, resolve Damp, remove the obstruction from the channels and stop the pain.

Cupping Application. Bleeding cupping on Du-14, followed by Moving cupping on both shoulders and the Bladder channel.

Herbal Prescription. Chirali Old Remedy®1 (herbal muscle and joint soothing 'Bi' cream).

Conclusion. The patient received 15 weekly treatments, sometimes twice in one week. His sleep was much improved and the pain in the chest, arms, shoulders and neck much reduced. He occasionally has setbacks, but these are not as severe as previously. He continues with the treatment, with long intermissions in between visits.

SKIN COMPLAINTS

Patients with skin conditions such as acne, rosacea, eczema and psoriasis are increasingly turning to alternative therapy for their complaints. Judging from this increase, especially in the use of Chinese medicine, it is clear that the benefits derived from the systematic use of corticosteroid creams and anti-biotics (the standard prescriptions used by orthodox medical practitioners) are short lived and far from satisfactory. The energetic properties of corticosteroids are considered as 'Cold' substances, and when applied to a warm or hot skin usually push the Heat into the inner layers of the body, thus bringing only a temporary respite and comfort to the sufferer. Because this 'cooling' effect is momentary, repeated application of the corticosteroid cream is necessary to maintain long-lasting relief. In most cases the patient is aware of the side-effects caused by corticosteroids, and therefore becomes reluctant to use such agents. Suppression of the symptoms may also lead to stronger reaction of a different nature later on, such as an asthma attack.

Aetiology and Pathology

When treating skin complaints as diverse as the above, a number of differing aetiologies are inevitable. As far as TCM is concerned, such conditions share few mutual aetiological factors, such as deficiency of the Lung- and Kidney-Qi, invasion of Wind-Heat or Damp-Heat, and deficiency of Blood (Liver). The correlation between the skin and the Lung-Qi is traditionally well documented: Lung-Qi controls the skin, and the Kidney-Qi, together with the Lung-Qi, helps nourish it. Blood (Liver) deficiency can give rise to internal Wind-Heat, which is characterized by the itching on the skin. Damp-Heat is the result of Stomach- and Spleen-Qi deficiency, resulting in the accumulation of Phlegm, and is characterized by wet, oozing fluid and itchy skin.

Treatment

Traditionally, where there is an excess pathological condition draining, and where deficiency syndrome is the predominant factor, tonifying methods are employed. In many cases of chronic skin complaints it is possible to see a deficiency syndrome and an excess condition coexisting.

TREATMENT PRINCIPLE. Nourish the Blood in order to clear the internal Wind-Heat. Tonify the Stomach/Spleen to resolve Damp-Heat. Clear Heat-poison, subdue the Wind and stop the itching.

CUPPING APPLICATION
Cupping Therapy. Strong or Bleeding cupping on Du-14 Dazhui, with Moving cupping to the Bladder channel on both sides of the spine, until red cupping marks appears on the skin surface. When applying Moving cupping, avoid skin lesions and open wounds (Colour Plate Figure 17).
Cupping Duration
Children

- **Under 5 years:** No cupping
- **5–7 years:** Up to 5 minutes, Empty cupping only
- **7–14 years:** Up to 10 minutes, Light to Medium cupping.

Adults

- **Young adults:** Bleeding or Moving cupping, up to 15 minutes
- **The weak and frail:** Light to Medium cupping, up to 10 minutes.

Herbal Remedies

- For Damp-Heat, wet skin conditions, Chirali Old Remedy®3 is used. This contains *Juniperus oxycedrus* extract. Its action is to clear Damp-Heat and nourish the skin.

PRECAUTION

Avoid direct cupping on the lesions, especially wet and oozing type skin conditions. Cups can be applied around the lesion with good effect.

CASE 12-16 Male Patient Aged 17 (Skin Complaint – Eczema)

Complaint. He has had dry and very itchy skin, mainly on the arms, neck and face, since the age of 10.

Present Medication. He has used corticosteroid creams in the past, but now uses only an aqueous moisturizing cream.

Pulse. Rapid and strong at all levels.

Tongue. Red body with a thin yellow coating.

Observation. He is a student and is preparing for his university entrance exams. He has also been involved in vigorous sporting activities from a very young age. He is the only son of the family, and is expected to do well. Restless in nature, he would rather do something physical than work in an office. On his first visit his face and the eyes were quite red and itchy; according to his mother 'he had had a few difficult days at school'.

Diagnosis. Wind-Heat, resulting from Lung- and Kidney-Qi deficiency, and Liver-Qi stagnation. Prolonged and excessive exercise have injured the Lung- and the Kidney-Qi resulting in Liver-Yin deficiency. This causes Liver-Wind, manifesting as itching on the skin. Frustration causes Liver-Qi stagnation, which further exacerbates the Liver-Blood and results in increased Heat.

Treatment Principle. Clear the Wind-Heat, soothe the Liver-Qi stagnation, tonify the Lungs and the Kidneys, nourish the skin and stop the itching.

Cupping Application. Moving cupping on the Bladder channel on each visit.

STROKE (WIND-STROKE) BELL'S PALSY – FACIAL PARALYSIS

This condition was definitely the most common disorder treated in the acupuncture departments in various Nanjing Hospitals during my studies there – so much so that quite a few of my colleagues complained of not being able to treat conditions other than facial paralysis! Electromagnetic stimulation of the acupuncture points alongside cupping was a popular treatment protocol.

Young and old are equally affected by this condition. The clinical manifestations of central and peripheral facial paralysis, as defined by Western medicine, are much the same, except that in the former the movement of the eyebrow is not impaired, whereas in the latter the movement of the eyebrow is affected, as well as other symptoms. The most common presentations are drooping of one corner of the mouth, salivation, inability to frown, inability to whistle or to close the eye fully, slurred speech, numbness of the affected side, sometimes pain in the jaw, and the lips deviating to one side.

Aetiology and Pathology

Paralysis is the invasion of facial channels by internal Wind or by external Wind-Cold causing channel distortion and deviation.

Treatment

TREATMENT PRINCIPLE. Treatment for both conditions is very similar: clear the Wind from head and face, remove the obstruction from the channels and invigorate Qi and Blood locally and throughout.

CUPPING APPLICATION

Cupping Therapy. I believe cupping to be the most effective therapy when treating facial paralysis. I often use it as the main treatment modality, supported by acupuncture and moxibustion. Apply up to ten small cups (number 2 to 3) cups to *both sides* (five on each side), daily or twice a week for better and faster results (Fig. 12-19). Also, advise the patient to blow into a balloon for exercise, to rest and to keep away from draughts.

Reported Additional Cupping Points in the Treatment of Wind-stroke. Facial paralysis was treated by acupuncture to local points, followed by cupping over Du-14 Dazhui (Cui & Zhang, 1989). Deviation of the mouth and eyes was treated by cupping over Taiyang Extra and ST-4 Dicang. A further 800 cases were treated by 'point to point acupuncture' and cupping to the affected side. Bell's palsy, with all the classic symptoms, was successfully treated by applying Empty (Flash) cupping, four sessions to the affected side of the face (Chen & Deng, 1989: 22, 165).

Cupping Duration

Children

- **Under 14 years:** Up to 10 minutes, Empty or Light cupping.

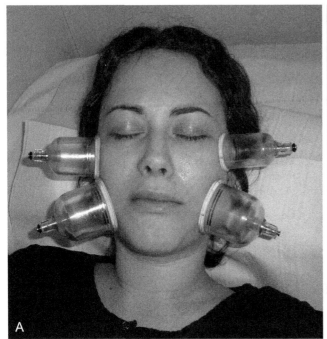 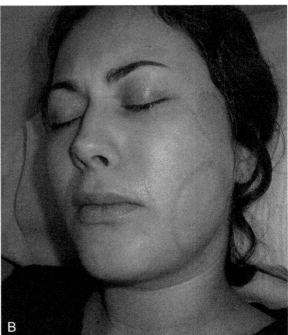

FIGURE 12-19 (A, B) Facial cupping for treating Wind-stroke.

Adults

- **Young adults:** Light to Medium cupping, up to 20 minutes
- **The weak and frail:** Empty to Medium cupping, up to 10 minutes.

PRECAUTION

> When cupping on facial points, extra care is needed in order to avoid cupping marks and blistering. The facial skin is considerably thinner than in other parts of the body, especially in the elderly. It is therefore relatively easy to cause the fine capillaries to burst under the skin, even with Light or Medium cupping. During moxibustion the practitioner should place his hand over the treatment area so that he can feel the heat derived from the moxa; do *not* rely solely on the response from the patient, as his or her sense of feeling may be impaired by the paralysis.

CASE 12-17 Male Patient Aged 52 (Facial Paralysis)

Complaint. He has had facial paralysis for 3 months. He woke up one morning with his mouth deviated to the left, feeling numb in the right cheek, and his right eye remained open with constant lacrimation. No pain was experienced at any time.

Present Medication. He was given a steroid injection to the local area at the time of onset.

Pulse. Floating and weak.

Tongue. Red body with a thin white coating.

Observation. The patient works for the Water Board, and part of his job is to inspect reservoirs in the countryside. He is of strong build and otherwise healthy. About 10 days prior to the paralysis, despite having a good night's sleep, he felt tired and sleepy during the day.

Diagnosis. Wind-Cold invading the facial channels, resulting in the stagnation of Qi and Blood, most probably caused by a draught when he left his warm, heated car and was exposed to the cold wind during the course of his work.

Treatment Principle. Expel the Wind-Cold, restore the circulation of Qi and Blood, and nourish the local muscles and tendons.

Cupping Application. Using small (number 1 to 2) cups, up to four cups were applied at Medium strength to the affected side on each visit (see Fig. 12-19; Colour Plate Figure 20AB).

Conclusion. He received a total of 15 weekly treatments, after which his condition was completely restored to normal.

CASE 12-18 Male Patient Aged 84 (Lower Limb Paralysis due to Stroke)

Complaint. Right leg paralysis due to stroke accompanied by oedema of the right foot.

Present Medication. Aspirin 75 mg, perindopril 4 mg, citalopram 20 mg, dipyridamole 200 mg and simvastatin 40 mg.

Pulse. Weak-floating (soft).

Tongue. Pale and dry with a thin body.

Observation. This patient has been visiting me for many years, firstly complaining of a 'tense neck and shoulders' and later on continuing to come once a month as a 'maintenance course'. He paints as a hobby and enjoys reading. He takes his painting quite seriously and, together with his wife and daughter, displays at various art exhibitions at least once a year. Long hours of standing or sitting and leaning over while painting aggravates the neck and shoulder pains. He responds to acupuncture well but dislikes cupping therapy as he finds it 'quite painful'. Before he suffered a stroke he had often complained of dizzy spells and felt 'unsteady' when walking.

On the day of the stroke he collapsed to the ground, knocking his head on a hard object, and lost consciousness for 2 days. Following his stroke he was kept in hospital for 6 weeks and was discharged from the hospital unable to stand or walk. A physiotherapist visited three times a week for the first 2 weeks and once a week for a further 3 weeks. At the end of 5 weeks he was told that he would not walk again and the home visits stopped. Five months after the stroke I visited the patient once a week and administered cupping therapy alongside acupuncture treatment.

Both his hands had good grip and movement, although he sometimes complained of 'pins and needles' in both hands. The right leg did not respond to any stimulation, and he complained of pain in the right inner-thigh muscle and the knee; he also felt cold in the same leg and considerable muscle wasting was observed throughout this leg. He had a good appetite but slept poorly owing to the pain in his right knee.

Diagnosis. Wind-stroke affecting the channels to the lower body (Gall Bladder, Bladder, Liver, Stomach, Spleen and Kidney channels).

Treatment Principle. Restore and regulate the normal flow of Qi and Blood to the affected meridians.

Cupping Application. Light to Medium cupping is regularly administered to the following points: GB-21 Jinanjing, BL-23 Shenshu, BL-26 Guanyuanshu, GB-30 Huantiao, GB-31 Fengshi, GB-34 Yanglingquan, ST-31 Biguan, ST-32 Futu and SP-10 Xuehai. Six cupping locations are chosen for each session lasting between 15 and 20 minutes (Colour Plate Figure 21).

Conclusion. After almost 18 months of regular weekly treatments (he is still receiving treatment at the time of writing) the patient can now voluntarily flex and extend his right leg at his own will. The flexing action, however, is much stronger than the extending action. With the help of a gutter-frame and under the watchful eye of his extremely compassionate wife, he is at present experimenting with standing and putting weight on both legs.

TIREDNESS

The single most common condition following any complaint in a patient is tiredness. From school-aged children to pensioners, this malady usually accompanies the main complaint. It is true to say that today's lifestyle does not allow enough time for rest and recuperation. Children as young as 7 are often rushed to various after-school activities, such as music classes, dancing, foreign languages or sport. I am sure that the parents are equally tired as a result of all this activity. When this routine is repeated between three and five times a week, tiredness becomes 'normal'. Only when the patient becomes ill and a visit to a practitioner is inevitable do people complain of tiredness. In other words, people seldom seek help when tiredness alone is the symptom. I frequently warn my patients that feeling tired is often the first bodily signal that all is not well in the energy department. Most of the time people continue with work as normal, drawing on and depleting their energy reserves.

Aetiology and Pathology

Tiredness is a sign of deficiency, and in very general terms it can be grouped into two categories: *deficiency of Qi* and *deficiency of Blood*. This should not be seen as a clear-cut attempt to differentiate between the two: this is not possible – one always overlaps the other. Excessive pathogenic factors such as Phlegm or Damp-Heat also cause considerable tiredness.

Clinical Manifestations

DEFICIENCY OF QI. Pale, white complexion, tiredness, breathlessness, poor appetite, muscular weakness, depression, feeling cold at the extremities and lack of sex drive. This type is more pronounced in men, and contributed to by heavy lifting, long standing, overwork or excessive sexual activity.

DEFICIENCY OF BLOOD. Extreme tiredness, palpitations especially when tired, poor memory, lack of concentration, insomnia, dizziness, depression, pale lips and complexion, and dry skin. This type is more pronounced in women, owing to monthly menstrual blood loss, miscarriage or childbirth.

EXCESSIVE PATHOGENIC FACTORS, PHLEGM OR DAMP-HEAT. Tiredness accompanied by a heavy feeling of the body, sleepiness, obesity, vaginal discharge and poor concentration.

Treatment

TREATMENT PRINCIPLE. Tonify Qi and Blood, resolve Phlegm and clear Damp-Heat.

CUPPING APPLICATION

Cupping Therapy. Because this is primarily a deficiency syndrome, a Light to Medium or an Empty cupping method is employed on both sides of the Bladder channel on the back of the body. When the tiredness is described as 'total exhaustion' by the patient, apply Empty cupping first, followed by moxibustion treatment (Colour Plate Figure 22).

Cupping Duration

Children

- **Under 7 years old:** Up to 5 minutes, Empty cupping
- **7–14 years:** Up to 10 minutes, Empty cupping.

Adults

- **Young adults:** Light, Medium or Empty cupping, up to 10 minutes
- **The weak and the frail:** Empty cupping only, up to 5 minutes.

PRECAUTION

It is very easy to be complacent and ignore the simple rule: 'don't drain when Empty, and don't tonify when Full'. Care is necessary when treating the Excess, Damp-Heat type of condition. The patient may have a deceptively strong physical appearance; pulse and tongue diagnosis should confirm otherwise: usually one notices a full and slippery pulse at the superficial level, and very faint one at the deeper level. A swollen tongue with a thick, yellowish coating is the classic appearance of Damp-Heat presence in the body.

CASE 12-19 Male Patient Aged 14 (Tiredness)

Complaint. Constantly feeling tired, lack of concentration and depression.

Present Medication. None, only multivitamin tablets.

Pulse. Noticeably faint, at all levels.

Tongue. Thin and pale.

Observation. He is the youngest child, after three girls in the family. Both his parents were in their 40s when he was born. He is pale and his handshake is very limp. His eyes are everywhere in the room, except on me, during our conversations. He is tall and with a good body weight. He is very restless, intelligent and demands attention, especially from the people around him. He is often weepy and depressed. He finds concentration very difficult and taxing, and gets into considerable mischief at school; consequently, he is often reprimanded.

Diagnosis. Inherited Qi deficiency – it is very common for the offspring of a middle-aged couple to lack the necessary strong Kidney-Qi during conception. Lack of energy results in stagnation, and stagnation impairs the movement of Qi and Blood. Concentration is difficult because the deficient Qi and Blood fail to nourish the brain. Excessive masturbation in young boys depletes the Kidney-Qi further (although he would not admit to this). Tiredness is the result of the Kidney-Qi (especially Kidney-Yang) deficiency.

Treatment Principle. Tonify Qi and Blood, and eliminate the stagnation of Qi.

Cupping Application. Empty cupping for 5 minutes on and alongside the Bladder channel was performed on each visit (see Fig. 9-9).

Conclusion. During the treatment, especially after the sixth visit, his energy level and depression improved and he was able to take part in school activities. His concentration, however, still remained poor. He was reluctant to continue with the treatment, as the only reason for coming so far was to please his parents! My opinion was that he required up to 1 year of weekly treatment, along with some counselling.

VEINS (VARICOSE/BROKEN)

This is more of a female affliction. The twisted and dilated veins are most commonly seen in the legs; gravity causes the blood to accumulate in the leg veins, where valves allow the blood to flow in one direction only (i.e. towards the heart). An increase in intra-abdominal pressure caused, for example, by pregnancy, an abdominal tumour, chronic constipation, lifting or continued coughing, increases the pressure in the leg veins. This causes the capillary blood vessels to protrude and flow into the veins, and web-like, broken, fine clusters of capillaries develop in the skin. Cupping is employed to remove the stagnant Blood from these fine capillaries. This form of cupping is classified as a *cosmetic cupping therapy*, as its purpose in the majority of cases is always the same (i.e. cosmetic).

Treatment

TREATMENT PRINCIPLE. Drain the excess and eliminate the Blood stagnation.

CUPPING APPLICATION

Cupping Therapy. Bleeding cupping is performed on each visit. When treating single capillaries, puncture the capillary from both ends, using a fine-gauge needle, and immediately apply a Strong cupping method over it. Within a few seconds blood should exude into the cup. If this fails, either the bleeding or the strength of the suction was insufficient. Repeat the procedure until blood is extracted from the capillary. When treating a cluster of broken veins, use a plum-blossom needle and tap gently over the veins until the area is bled. Select a single cup, large enough to accommodate the entire cluster, and apply over the desired position employing a Strong technique. Blood is extracted more quickly from large clusters. There is no need to be alarmed, as the blood will coagulate and stop of its own accord, usually within a minute. Avoid Strong cupping when treating facial capillaries; Medium strength or a fast, Empty method is preferred (Fig. 12.20).

Cupping Duration
Adults only

- **First visit:** Up to 5 minutes
- **Follow-up visits:** Up to 15 minutes.

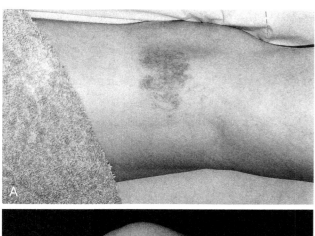
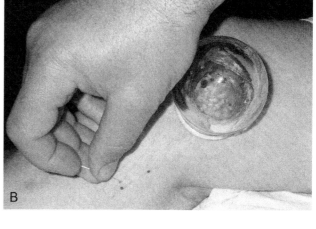
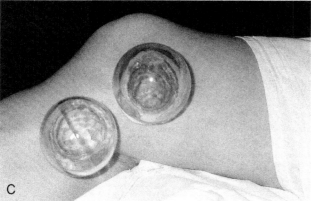

FIGURE 12-20 (A–C) Treatment of broken veins.

PRECAUTIONS

Under no circumstances should cupping be applied directly on the main varicose veins.

As dark red cupping marks following the treatment are inevitable, warn the patient in advance. This is less of a problem when the cupping marks can be covered by clothing, as it can take up to 10 days for the marks to subside.

Extra care is also required when removing the cup (see Chapter 9, Full [Bleeding/wet] cupping).

CASE 12-20 Female Patient Aged 25 (Broken Veins)

Complaint. Broken veins on the right leg.

Present Medication. She has been taking the contraceptive pill for over 15 months.

Pulse. Slippery and strong.

Tongue. Red tip, and curling up.

Observation. The patient was a shop assistant, which meant that she was on her feet all day. Since taking the pill, her weight and the broken veins have increased. The broken veins were in a single cluster, 2 cm in diameter.

Diagnosis. Stagnation of the Qi and Blood, most probably caused by the pill.

Treatment Principle. Remove the local Blood stagnation.

Cupping Application. Tapping with a plum-blossom needle, the area was bled; this was immediately followed by a Strong cupping with a large (number 4) cup. Around 30 mL of blood were exuded during the first application. With a further three applications the cluster of veins was reduced by 80%.

Conclusion. This patient was advised to see the practitioner who prescribed the pill, or to seek an alternative method of contraception. In most cases following treatment the broken veins either disappear completely or gradually become inconspicuous. With this patient, regular exercise, especially leg exercises, and a low-fat diet were also advised.

WEAK/POOR CONSTITUTION

Individuals suffering from weak constitution are prone to ongoing illnesses. They never seem to recover fully from one condition before they are down with another. Children under 7 years of age are usually born with this condition. Children between 7 and 14 years old can compromise their immune system by an unhealthy home environment, such as parents going through a divorce or straightforward bad dietary habits. In teenagers older than 14 years old adults, contributory factors include too much work and not enough play. Long-term emotional or mental stress, physical overactivity and ongoing financial worries can all lead to breakdown in the immune system, which in turn may result in a diminished immune response.

Treatment

TREATMENT PRINCIPLE. Tonify the Qi and the Blood and lift up the spirit (Shen); also concentrate on the Lungs, Spleen, Liver and the Kidney corresponding points.

CUPPING APPLICATION. To the front of the body: administer Empty cupping method to the Lung Front-Mu points (LU-1), also to Ren-15, Ren-17, the Front-Mu points of the Spleen (Liv-13) and Stomach (Ren-12), Ren-4 and Ren-6 (Fig. 12.21A, B). To the back of the body: employ Light-moving cupping over the Bladder channel, starting from the lower back (BL-52), massaging up towards the neck (BL-10) and moving towards the shoulders (GB-21) points (Fig. 12-21C). *It is important that you move the cup from the Lower to the Upper Jiao in order to 'bring the Qi up'.* This method of cupping improves the appetite and is also greatly mentally and physically uplifting as well as relaxing.

ENDNOTES

1. Chirali Old Remedy® ointments are the innovation of the author and are trademark registered in England as non-medicinal herbal skin preparations. They include: Muscle and Joint Soothing 'Bi' Cream Chirali Old Remedy®1, Dry Skin Cream Chirali Old Remedy®2 and Damp-Heat Cream Chirali Old Remedy®3. Information regarding the ointments can be obtained from the author at 163 Upton Road, Bexleyheath, Kent DA6 8LY, UK, or the website www.cuppingtherapy-hejama.com.

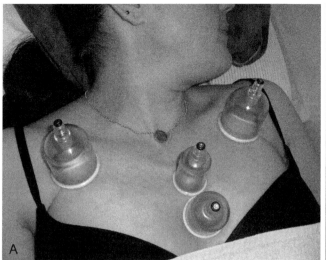

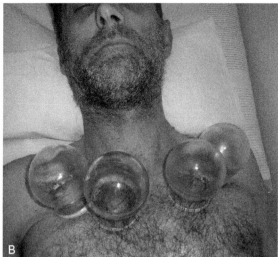

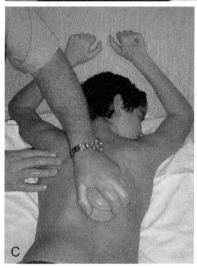

FIGURE 12-21 (A–C) Treatment of weak/poor constitution.

REFERENCES

American Psychiatric Association, 1994. Diagnostic and Statistical Manual of Mental Disorders. Fourth ed American Psychiatric Publishing, Arlington VA.

Bayfield, S., 1823. A Treatise on Practical Cupping. E. Cox & Son, London, pp. 60–62.

Bensky, D., Barolet, R., 1990. Chinese Herbal Medicine Formulas and Strategies. Eastland Press, Seattle WA.

Chen Bin, 1995. Personal Communications. China Nanjing International Acupuncture Training Centre.

Chen, J., 1982. Anatomical Atlas of Chinese Acupuncture Points. Shandong Science and Technology Press, Jinan.

Chen, Y., Deng, L., 1980. Essentials of Chinese Acupuncture. Foreign Languages Press, Beijing.

Chen, Y., Deng, L., 1989. Essentials of Contemporary Chinese Acupuncturists' Clinical Experiences. Foreign Languages Press, Beijing, pp. 22–23, 165, 166.

Cui, J., Zhang, G., 1989. A survey of thirty years' clinical application of cupping. J. Tradit. Chin. Med. 9, 151–153.

Ellis, A., Wiseman, N., Boss, K., 1989. Grasping the Wind. Paradigm Publications, Brooklyn MA.

Maciocia, G., 1989. The Foundations of Chinese Medicine. Churchill Livingstone, Edinburgh.

Maciocia, G., 1994. The Practice of Chinese Medicine. Churchill Livingstone, Edinburgh.

Scott, T., Barlow, J., 1999. Acupuncture in the Treatment of Children. Eastland Press, Seattle WA.

Sherwood, P., 1992. The Back and Beyond. Arrow Books, London.

Zhang, R.F., Wu, X.F., 1986. The Illustrated Dictionary of Chinese Acupuncture. Sheep's Publications (HK) Ltd. People's Medical Publishing House, China.

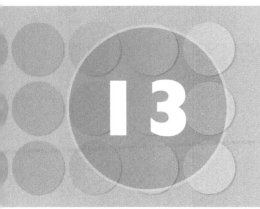

13 TREATING MISCELLANEOUS DISORDERS WITH CUPPING THERAPY

CHAPTER CONTENTS

ALLERGIC RHINITIS (HAY FEVER), 184
ANKYLOSIS SPONDYLITIS, 185
BRONCHITIS, 186
CARPAL TUNNEL SYNDROME, 186
CHRONIC FATIGUE SYNDROME (ENCEPHALOMYELITIS), 186
COLITIS, 187
DEPRESSION, 187
DIARRHOEA, 190
EYE CONDITIONS, 190
EPILEPSY, 191
FEMALE CONDITIONS, 192
FORGETFULNESS, 200
GOUT, 201
HANGOVER, 201
HEADACHE/MIGRAINE, 201

HICCUPS, 202
INSOMNIA, 202
MALE SEXUAL COMPLAINTS, 203
MUMPS, 204
NIGHT SWEATING (HYPERHIDROSIS), 206
POOR APPETITE, 206
PROLAPSE OF THE BLADDER AND THE UTERUS, 208
PSORIASIS, 208
RESTLESSNESS AND HYPERACTIVITY, 208
TRIGEMINAL NEURALGIA, 208
TOOTHACHE, 209
TORTICOLLIS (WRY NECK), 210
REFERENCES, 210
FURTHER READING, 210

This section is an addition to Chapter 12 and describes a short treatment protocol to miscellaneous children's and adults' conditions. I have put these conditions together as a result of visiting and observing various clinics around the globe. It may not necessarily present the 'whole picture' such as the full traditional Chinese medicine (TCM) differentiations of the disease. It is, however, imperative that practitioners use their particular skills to address the underlying pathological conditions before and during treatment.

ALLERGIC RHINITIS (HAY FEVER)

This is a seasonal allergy due to increased pollen count in the atmosphere. Hay fever is characterized by sneezing bouts and a blocked, itching and runny nose; many people develop the additional symptom of red and runny eyes. In TCM, hay fever is considered to be Wind-Cold invading the Lungs at its initial onset, then becoming a Wind-Heat syndrome in the later stages.

TREATMENT PRINCIPLE. Remove Wind-Cold and 'open' the chest. If not treated in time, Wind-Cold may turn into Wind-Heat with its own characteristic features (Maciocia, 1994).

CUPPING THERAPY
   Wind-Cold Stage. Medium to Strong cupping on GB-21 Jiangjing, BL-13 Feishu and Dingchuan Extra (Fig. 13-1A).

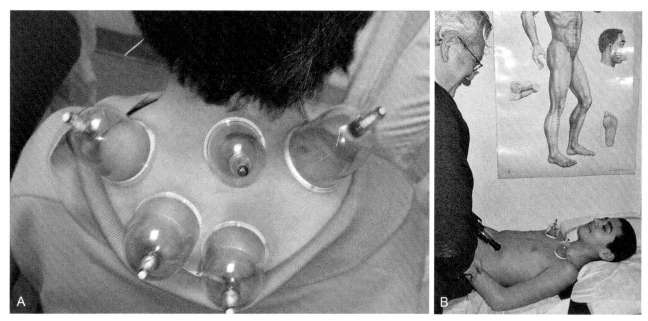

FIGURE 13-1 (A, B) Treating allergic rhinitis.

Wind-Heat Stage. In addition to the above points, also apply Light to Medium cupping on LU-1 Zhongfu and Light-moving or Moving cupping to the Upper Zone (Fig. 13-1B, see also Fig. 6-1).

ANKYLOSIS SPONDYLITIS

This is a chronic arthritis condition where the spinal joints, ligaments and the sacroiliac joints become inflamed. Bones of a joint can also fuse together. This causes pain and stiffness in the neck and back.

CUPPING THERAPY. Apply 15–20 minutes of Light to Medium cupping, to both sides of the Bladder channel, across the lower back including Du-3 Yaoyangguang, BL-26 Guanyuanshu, BL-28 Pangguangshu and GB-30 Huantiao. If the patient can tolerate it, apply a further 5 minutes of Light-moving cupping on both side of the spine Huatuo Jiaji Extra points (Fig. 13-2).

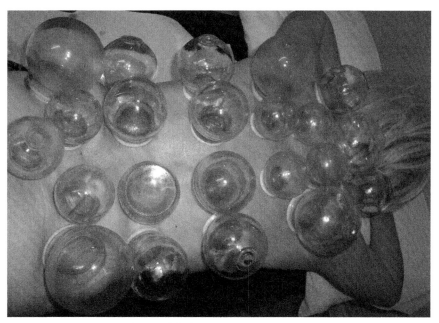

FIGURE 13-2 Treating ankylosis spondylitis.

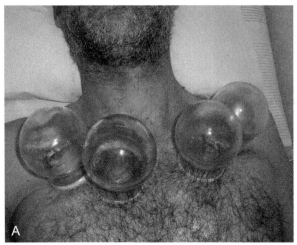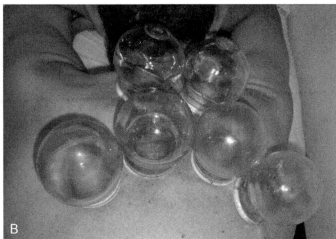

FIGURE 13-3 (A, B) Treating bronchitis.

BRONCHITIS

This condition in an inflammation of the mucous membrane of the bronchi (the main airways of the lungs). Symptoms include cough accompanying yellow/grey phlegm, sore throat, wheezing and a blocked nose.

CUPPING THERAPY. Apply Medium cupping application to LU-1 Zhongfu and Ren-17 Tanzhong; Strong cupping method to P-4 Ximen and Du-14 Dazhui; Medium cupping to BL-12 Fengmen, Dingchuan Extra point and BL-13 Feishu (Fig. 13-3).

CARPAL TUNNEL SYNDROME

This condition is an obstruction or entrapment of the median nerve at the wrist, causing paraesthesia (numbness and tingling feeling, like pins and needles) and pain in the affected wrist and fingers.

TREATMENT PRINCIPLE. Clear the obstruction in the channels and return the normal flow of Qi and Blood to the wrist and fingers.

CUPPING THERAPY. Apply four to five Medium to Strong strength cups on the inner aspect of the arm starting 1 cun above the point P-4 Ximen, and terminating at P-8 Laogong, making sure that a cup is also placed on P-7 Daling (Fig. 13-4).

CHRONIC FATIGUE SYNDROME (ENCEPHALOMYELITIS)

Chronic fatigue syndrome (CFS), or encephalomyelitis (ME), as it is also known, affects many people of all ages. Yet many conventional doctors are refusing to recognize or acknowledge this condition as a disease. It is, however, quite a debilitating condition. The manifestations are disabling fatigue after a minimum of physical effort, headaches, muscular pains, gastrointestinal complaints, poor memory and difficulty in concentration, poor sleep patterns, catching colds several times a year, reduced immune system (CFS is sometimes described as the 'immune system deficiency syndrome'), painful lymphatic glands and generally feeling unwell.

In TCM pathology, Dampness – especially the Damp-Heat type pathogen – is considered the primary cause of CFS/ME. Qi deficiency is the next major factor. Long-term Qi deficiency will almost always cause stagnation of various types, in particular Qi and Blood stagnation that may lead to physical symptoms such as pain as well as extreme tiredness. (For more detailed reading on the subject of CFS/ME, see the *Journal of Chinese Medicine* Issues 35, 40 and 44.)

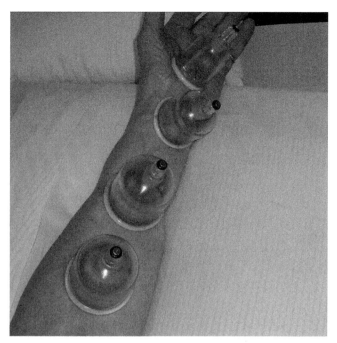

FIGURE 13-4 Treating carpal tunnel syndrome.

TREATMENT PRINCIPLE

1. Resolve phlegm and clear pathogens such as Damp and Heat
2. Tonify and move the Qi in order to resolve Qi and Blood stagnation and improve the energy level.

CUPPING THERAPY

1. Apply short (10 minutes) of Empty to Light cupping to the Middle and Upper Zones twice a week
2. Apply short (10 minutes) of Light-moving cupping to the entire back, concentrating on the Bladder channel twice a week.

If memory and poor concentration are part of the complaint, try stimulating the Du Mai (Governing Vessel) either by applying Light-moving cupping or gentle massage on the channel (Fig. 13-5).

COLITIS

Colitis is an inflammation of the colon, also called 'mucous colitis' or 'irritable bowel syndrome', where the patient suffers pain and spasm of the muscles of the colon. Symptoms are: abdominal pain, diarrhoea, cramping, urgency, weight loss, change in the bowel habits, blood in the stools, distension and fatigue.

CUPPING THERAPY. Rub the entire abdomen and the back of the body with warm olive or sesame oil. Apply Light cupping on Ren-8 Shenque, Ren-10 Xiawan, Ren-12 Zhongwan, ST-25 Tianshu, Ren-3 Guanyuan, Ren-6 Qihai, ST-37 Shangjuxu, BL-20 Pishu, BL-49 Yishe and BL-28 Pangguangshu. For children under the age of 14 years old, choose up to six treatment points per treatment, and employing Empty or Light cupping methods only (Fig. 13-6).

DEPRESSION

Emotional disturbances such as anxieties, phobias, mood swings and depression often accompany behavioural symptoms. Changes in sleep pattern, tension headaches, irritability, panic attacks, chest pains, general tiredness and altered appetite are common. Treatment depends on the particular situation. Psychotherapy or antidepressant medication, or both, are the standard treatments offered to patients within the mainstream medical system. Patients coming to complementary therapy clinics are those who are seeking a drug-free approach.

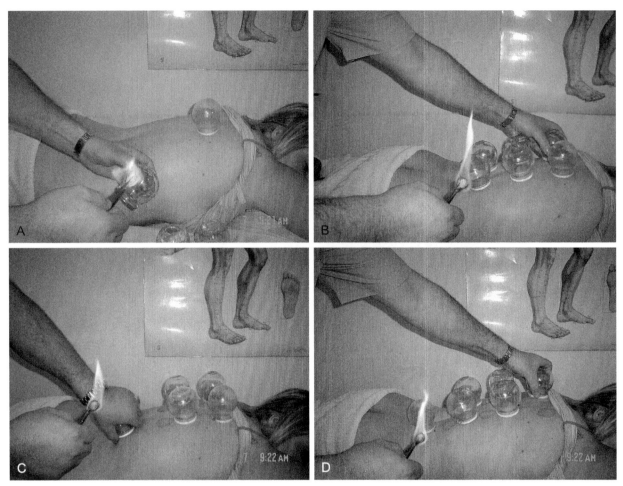

FIGURE 13-5 (A–D) Cupping therapy for chronic fatigue syndrome (encephalomyelitis).

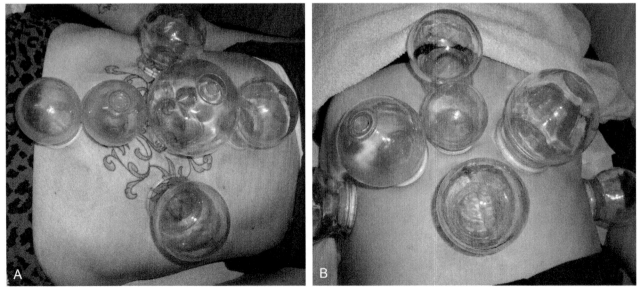

FIGURE 13-6 (A, B) Treating colitis.

As far as TCM is concerned, mental and emotional conditions are intimately linked to the Zang-Fu (Internal Organs) and reciprocally influence each other's energies. *Anger and frustration,* for instance, affect the Liver; *excessive joy* affects the Heart; excessive or *prolonged worry* affects the Lungs and the Spleen; long-term *pensiveness* affects the Spleen; long-lasting *sadness* or *grief* affects the Lungs; *fear,* even in the short term, affects the Kidneys; *shock,* again even a brief shock, can affect the Heart and the Kidneys; *love* (especially unreciprocated) affects the Heart; *hatred* affects the Heart and the Liver; continuous *craving* affects the Heart; long-term *guilt* affects the Kidneys and the Heart (Cui & Zhang, 1989). However, particular emphasis is placed upon the Liver (responsible for smooth flow of the Qi), the Heart (which houses the Shen-Spirit and the Mind) and the Spleen (responsible for Blood production). During cupping treatment, the above factors must also be taken into account.

Liver Pattern Qi Stagnation

Rebellious (i.e. flowing the wrong way) Liver-Qi and deficiency of Qi both cause Qi stagnation.

TREATMENT PRINCIPLE. In both cases the treatment should be directed towards *releasing and maintaining a smooth flow of the Qi.*

Rebellious (Excessive) Liver-Qi Causing Stagnation

Symptoms include frustration, short temper, red eyes, restlessness, depression, anger, intolerance and a feeling of fullness in the chest; they also include premenstrual tension and breast distension in women.

CUPPING THERAPY. Apply Medium to Strong Moving cupping to the Middle and Upper Zones, concentrating on the Bladder meridian.

CUPPING DURATION. Up to 15 minutes on each side.

Deficiency of Qi Causing Stagnation

Symptoms include pale appearance, depression, apathy, inward personality, lack of spirit and exhaustion.

CUPPING THERAPY. Apply Light to Medium Moving cupping to the Middle and Upper Zones, concentrating on the Bladder meridian.

CUPPING DURATION. Up to 10 minutes on each side.

Heart Patterns

Disturbed Shen-Spirit due to inability of the Heart to store the Shen. Symptoms include depression, palpitations, weepiness, restlessness (especially during the night), nightmares or unpleasant dreams, waking up and not being able to get back to sleep.

TREATMENT PRINCIPLE. Nourish the Heart, calm the Mind and restore the free flow of the Qi.

Alongside the cupping therapy, Heart-nourishing herbal prescriptions are an essential component of this pattern. Cupping strength should be determined according to the patient's energetic condition.

CUPPING THERAPY. BL-13 Feishu, BL-15 Xinshu and BL-17 Geshu should be cupped for 3–4 weeks followed by a further 3–4 weeks of Medium Moving cupping to the Upper Zone.

Spleen Patterns

Overwork, too much thinking, constitutional weaknesses, poor diet and worry all damage the Spleen's ability to transform and transport the Body Fluids, leading to accumulation of Fluids, particularly Phlegm, which 'clouds the Mind' causing diarrhoea, nausea, dizziness, confusion, relentless talking and mental confusion.

TREATMENT PRINCIPLE. Tonify the Spleen, resolve Phlegm and restore the free flow of the Qi.

CUPPING THERAPY. The strength of cupping therapy should depend on the energetic condition of the patient: BL-18 Ganshu, BL-20 Pishu and BL-23 Shenshu. This should be followed by Light to Medium Moving cupping to the Lower and Middle Zones.

CUPPING DURATION. Between 10 and 20 minutes (Colour Plate Figure 23).

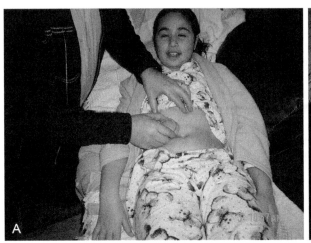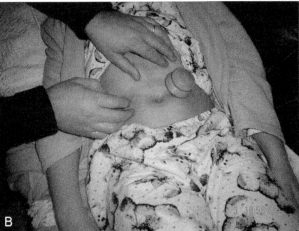

FIGURE 13-7 (A, B) Treating diarrhoea.

DIARRHOEA

Children Under 4 Years of Age

Using olive oil, *massage by hand* the entire abdomen using an anticlockwise movement around the umbilicus Ren-8 Shenque, for about 5 minutes. This exercise can be repeated several times a day.

Children Over 4 Years of Age

Oil the abdomen with olive oil and using rubber cups apply Light-moving cupping (anticlockwise) concentrating around the umbilicus for 1 minute. This treatment can be repeated two to three times per day (Fig. 13-7).

EYE CONDITIONS

Dropped Eyelid (Ptosis)

This condition is a drooping of the upper or the lower eyelid. It is caused by the weakening of the lifting muscles (levator and superiortarsal). It can affect one or both eyes and is more common in the elderly. Congenital ptosis is where a person is born with the condition.

CUPPING THERAPY. Apply Medium cupping technique to the above points starting from 2 minutes and progressively increasing to 15 minutes per application. Yintang Extra point, Taiyang Extra point, GB-14 Yangbai, GB-4 Hanyan and Moxa cupping on Ren-8 Shenque (Fig. 13-8).

Conjunctivitis

This condition is the inflammation of the conjunctiva (a transparent membrane which covers the front of the eyeball and the inside of the eyelids). This disorder is often caused by an irritation such as allergies or environmental pollution, pollen, dust and electrical flares. Symptoms are red, itchy, burning eyes with profuse lacrimation.

CUPPING THERAPY. Conjunctivitis and ophthalmitis caused by the use of electric flashes are treated by cupping to LI-4 Hegu, LI-15 Jianyu, Du-14 Dazhui and ST-12 Quepen (Cui & Zhang, 1989) (Fig. 13-9).

Lacrimation

Wind-lacrimation is treated by local acupuncture and cupping over Taiyang Extra (Cui & Zhang, 1989) (Colour Plate Figure 27).

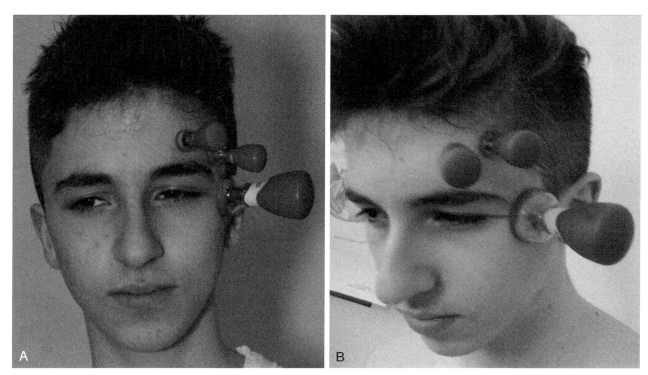

FIGURE 13-8 (A, B) Treating eyelid ptosis.

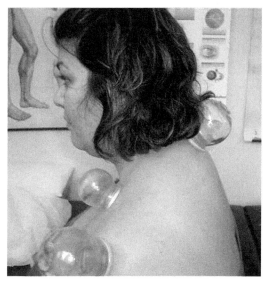

FIGURE 13-9 Treating conjunctivitis.

EPILEPSY

This is a chronic condition of the nervous system in which convulsions and loss of consciousness occur owing to chaotic brain activity. The main symptoms of epilepsy are repeated seizures, which can happen during the waking consciousness or whilst asleep.

CUPPING THERAPY. Apply Moving cupping on Ren-17 Tangzhong towards Ren-15 Jiuwei and along the Spleen channel from SP-9 Yinlingquan towards SP-8 Diji and SP-7 Lougu. Apply Bleeding cupping to Du-2 Yaoshu. Also add acupuncture to Du-1 Changqiang using perpendicular insertion to 1 cun (Fig. 13-10).

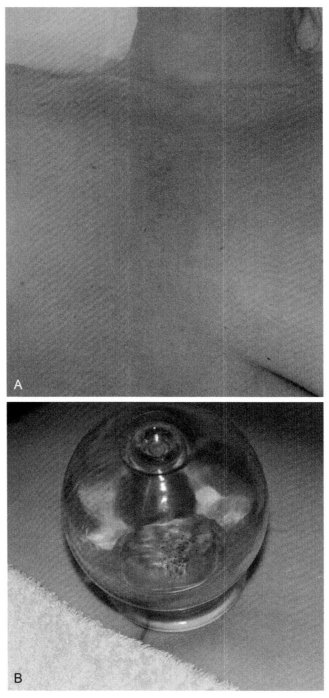

FIGURE 13-10 (A, B) Treating epilepsy.

FEMALE CONDITIONS

Amenorrhoea

This is the absence of one or more menstrual periods by 14 years of age in women and girls. Amenorrhoea is normal during pregnancy, breastfeeding, and after the menopause, but otherwise unusual in adult women.

CUPPING THERAPY. To the front of the body; apply Moving cupping from the point umbilicus Ren-8 Shenque towards Ren-2 Qugu. Also across the lower abdomen use Moving cupping on SP-12 Chongmen from Left to the Right side of the abdomen, and Medium cupping on Liv-11 Yinlian. To the back of the body, apply Moving cupping from left BL-53 Baohuang to the right Baohuang, and finally apply Medium cupping on SP-6 Sanyinjiao (Fig. 13-11).

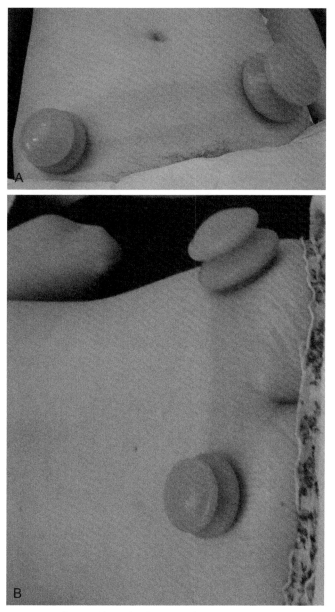

FIGURE 13-11 (A, B) Treating female conditions.

Breast Pain During Menstruation

Breast pain during the menstruating cycle is quite a common occurrence. In some women the breasts also swell and enlarge. The most common cause is believed to be an imbalance between the hormones oestrogen and progesterone.

CUPPING THERAPY. Using rubber or silicon cups, apply Light-moving cupping to the painful breast starting from under the clavicle and moving the cup following the sternum towards the ST-18 Rugen point under the breast. Apply Light-moving cupping to the Sanjiao (Triple Burner/Warmer) meridian, starting from SJ-8 Sanyangluo and moving towards SJ-5 Waiguan (Fig. 13-12). Also apply Medium cupping to SP-6 Sanyinjiao.

Female Infertility

Over the years I have employed cupping therapy in conjunction with acupuncture and moxibustion, in many cases quite successfully, to treat infertility problems. The whole experience can take an excessive toll on the patient's mental, emotional and physical states, often involving and testing the entire relationship between partners undergoing any form of assisted conception therapy. Failure to have children

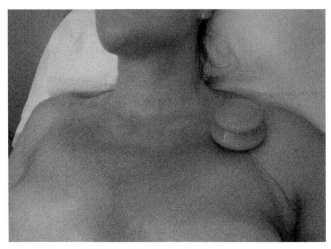

FIGURE 13-12 Treating breast pain during menstruation.

after 2–3 years of marriage, despite both partners being healthy, is sufficient to be considered infertile (Cui & Zhang, 1989).

Aetiology and Pathology

According to TCM aetiology, there are five pathological conditions that can cause infertility in women:

- Kidney deficiency
- Liver-Qi stagnation
- Phlegm-Dampness
- Blood stagnation
- Cold uterus.

Kidney Deficiency

KIDNEY-YANG DEFICIENCY. Clinical manifestations include infertility, feeling tired (especially as the day progresses), long-term back pain, a prolonged menstrual cycle with scanty periods with a light-coloured discharge or amenorrhoea, dizziness, weakness of the legs, lack of sexual desire, loose stools, a pale tongue with a white coating, a general feeling of cold and colourless facial features. However, not all the symptoms are expected to be present at the same time.

KIDNEY-YIN DEFICIENCY. Clinical manifestations include infertility, a short menstrual cycle with scanty, clear-red flow, dizziness, palpitations, insomnia, irritability, dry mouth or vagina, heat sensation in the palms, soles and chest, and a red tongue with little coating.

Liver-Qi Stagnation

Clinical manifestations include infertility, mental depression, aggression or short temper, early or late (irregular) periods, dark-coloured scanty periods (usually with clots), dysmenorrhoea, sighing, premenstrual distension and tender breasts, a normal or dark-red tongue body with a thin, white coating.

Phlegm-Dampness

Clinical manifestations include infertility, obese constitution, long history of Phlegm condition, feelings of tiredness with heaviness, prolonged menstrual cycle, sticky vaginal discharge, pale complexion, dizziness, nausea, and a pale/white tongue body with a sticky coating.

Blood Stagnation

Symptoms include infertility, dysmenorrhoea accompanied by cramps, prolonged bleeding with scanty and dark flow with clots, and a dark-purplish tongue body, sometimes accompanied by dark-red spots.

Cold Uterus

Symptoms include infertility, scanty periods with prolonged discharge and dark clots, cold lower abdomen with pain that is relieved by hot-water bottle application, and a pale/white tongue body with no coating.

TREATMENT PRINCIPLE. As well as addressing the above differentiations, one must not underestimate and overlook the importance of the *Ren Mai (Conception Vessel)* and *Chong Mai (Directing Vessel)*, the two extraordinary channels responsible for the health of the uterus, which may affect the outcome of the treatment (Low, 1983). Together with Kidney-Qi, the Ren Mai and Chong Mai are responsible for nourishing the Uterus and assisting the fertility treatment by harmonizing both channels, as illustrated below.

Treatment

Kidney Deficiency

TREATMENT PRINCIPLE. Tonify the Kidney-Qi and regulate the Ren Mai and Chong Mai.

CUPPING THERAPY. Ren-4 Guanyuan, Ren-6 Qihai, K-11 Henggu, ST-30 Qichong, GB-26 Daimai, BL-23 Shenshu and BL-52 Zhishi (Fig. 13-13).

Liver-Qi Stagnation

TREATMENT PRINCIPLE. Disperse Liver-Qi Stagnation, tonify the Kidney-Qi and regulate the Ren and Chong channels.

CUPPING THERAPY. Liv-13 Zhangmen, Liv-9 Yinbao or SP-6 Sanyinjiao, ST-30 Qichong, Ren-4 Guanyuan, Ren-6 Qihai, BL-23 Shenshu and BL-52 Zhishi.

Phlegm-Damp

TREATMENT PRINCIPLE. Remove Phlegm-Damp, tonify the Kidney-Qi and regulate the Ren and Chong Mai.

CUPPING THERAPY. Ren-12 Zhongwan, SP-6 Sanyinjiao or SP-9 Yinlingquan, ST-30 Qichong, Ren-4 Guanyuan, BL-20 Pishu, BL-23 Shenshu and BL-52 Zhishi (see Fig. 13-13C).

Blood Stagnation

TREATMENT PRINCIPLE. Remove Blood Stagnation, tonify the Kidney-Qi and regulate the Ren Mai and Chong Mai.

CUPPING THERAPY. ST-30 Qichong, Ren-4 Guanyuan, K-11 Henggu, SP-10 Xuehai, BL-17 Geshu, BL-23 Shenshu and BL-52 Zhishi (see Fig. 13-13D).

Cold Uterus

TREATMENT PRINCIPLE. Warm the uterus, tonify the Kidney-Qi and regulate the Ren Mai and Chong Mai.

CUPPING THERAPY. Hot Needle cupping technique on Ren-12 Zhongwan, Ren-4 Guanyuan, Ren-6 Qihai, K-11 Henggu, ST-30 Qichong, BL-23 Shenshu and BL-52 Zhishi (see Fig. 13-12E).

COMMENT

Moxibustion application with a moxa stick or a moxa box is extremely effective and beneficial when dealing with any form of Cold pathological condition. I would therefore urge practitioners not to overlook the importance of the warming and healing properties of moxibustion treatment.

Heavy Periods (Menorrhagia)

This is excessive bleeding during the menstrual period, which can be emotionally and physically very distressing. Some of the symptoms are: extreme tiredness, shortness of breath, palpitations and headache.

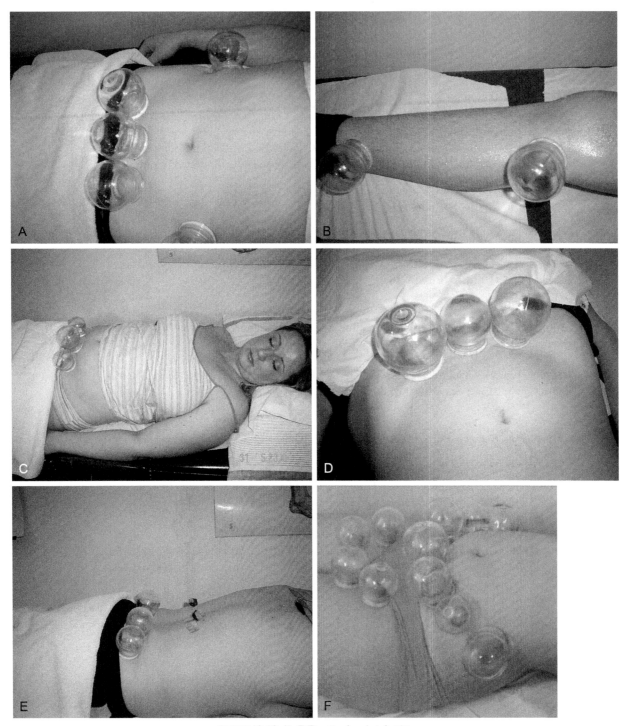

FIGURE 13-13 (A–F) Treating female infertility.

CUPPING THERAPY. Using small cups (no. 1 or 2), apply Strong cupping on SP-3 Taibai or SP-4 Gongsun, and Medium cupping on Ren-6 Qihai, SP-10 Xuehai, Liv-8 Quguan, BL-18 Ganshu and BL-23 Shenshu (Fig. 13-14).

Female Sexual Frigidity

Sexual frigidity is described as the inability to experience orgasm or sexual pleasure, or the absence of sexual desire. Causative factors can vary from the emotional to the physical. In TCM, however, frigidity in women is often differentiated into two major pathologies:

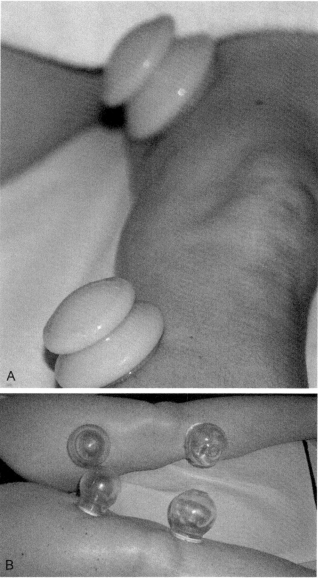

Figure 13-14 (A, B) Treating heavy periods (menorrhagia).

1. **Cold-type frigidity (Kidney-Yang deficiency):** Clinical manifestations include frigidity, tiredness, feeling of cold in the lower abdomen or in the vagina, low libido and a pale tongue with a thin coating
2. **Hot-type frigidity (Liver-Qi stagnation):** Clinical manifestations include frigidity, painful coitus, feeling of heat or itching in the vaginal region, restless with a short temper and a red to purple tongue body without coating.

Both pathological factors have a profound effect on the pelvic organs and associated energies that control sexual desire.

Kidney-Yang Deficiency

TREATMENT PRINCIPLE. Regulate the Ren Mai and Chong Mai and tonify the Kidney-Yang by warming the Lower Jiao.

CUPPING THERAPY. Apply Hot Needle cupping method on the lower abdomen and the lower back of the body, concentrating particularly on Ren-4 Guanyuan, Ren-6 Qihai, ST-30 Qichong, GB-25 Jingmen, BL-23 Shenshu and BL-20 Pishu. Treatment should be carried out two or three times a week for 5 weeks, subsequently reducing to once a week for a further 5 weeks.

MOXIBUSTION. Moxibustion should also be employed quite frequently during the treatment, in particular to the lower abdominal points as well as the lower back points with the addition of Du-4 Mingmen (Fig. 13-15A).

Liver-Qi Stagnation

TREATMENT PRINCIPLE. Dissipate Liver-Qi stagnation, harmonize the Ren Mai and Chong Mai and calm the Mind.

CUPPING THERAPY. Apply Light to Medium cupping method on Liv-5 Ligou, Liv-13 Zhangmen, GB-25 Jingmen, Ren-4 Guanyuan, Ren-6 Qihai and ST-30 Qichong. To the back of the body apply bilateral Moving cupping method to the Bladder channel, starting from BL-15 Xinshu and ending level with BL-28 Pangguangshu. Treatment should be given twice a week for 5 weeks, then reducing the frequency to once a week for a further 5 weeks (see Fig. 13-15B).

Mastitis

Mastitis is inflammation of and pain in the breast. This condition is most common in breastfeeding women. However, some women who are not breastfeeding can also develop it.

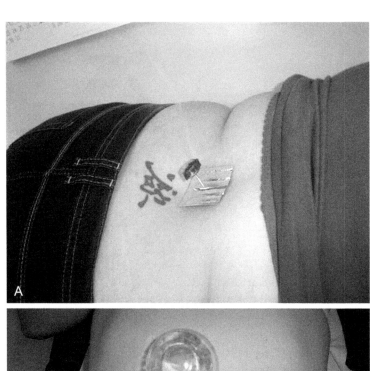
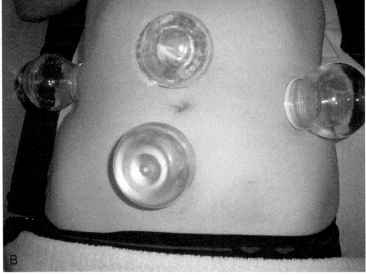

FIGURE 13-15 (A, B) Treating sexual frigidity.

CUPPING THERAPY. Apply Medium cupping to GB-21 Jianjing, and Medium strength Moving cupping to the outer Bladder channel between the points BL-44 Shentang, BL-45 Yixi and BL-46 Geguan. Finally, apply Bleeding cupping on LI-11 Quchi (Fig. 13-16).

Pelvic Inflammation

Pelvic inflammation disease (PID) is a general term to describe an infection that passes from the vagina through the neck of the cervix to the uterus and to the fallopian tubes and/or ovaries. This condition can lead to infertility in women.

CUPPING THERAPY. Apply Medium cupping to ST-30 Qichong, Liv-11 Yinlian and SP-10 Xuehai. Apply Medium to Strong cupping to Du-2 Yaoshu and Du-3 Yaoyangguan. Apply Moving cupping to the Ciliao points from BL-31 Shangliao to BL-35 Huiyang (Fig. 13-17).

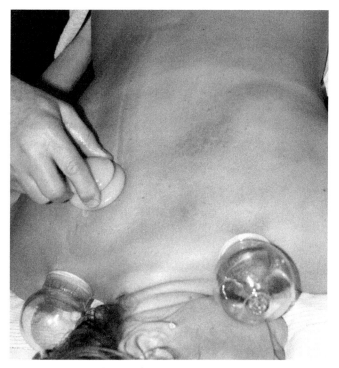

FIGURE 13-16 Treating mastitis.

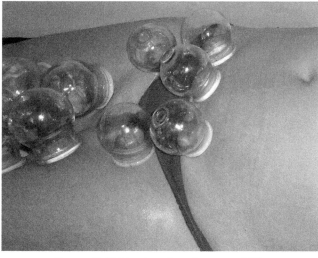

FIGURE 13-17 Treating pelvic inflammation (PID).

Vulvitis

Vulvitis is an inflammation of the vulva, which includes the external female organs such as the labia, clitoris and entrance to the vagina. Vulvitis produces intense local irritation. Apply four cups using Medium cupping method from Liv-11 Yinlian to Liv-8 Quguan, Medium cupping on SP-6 Sanyinjiao and finally Bleeding cupping to LI-11 Quchi and Liv-3 Taichong (Fig. 13-18).

FORGETFULNESS

Forgetfulness, also called amnesia, is a recurrent failure to remember events and information that people are normally able to recall. It is a normal part of ageing, but can be distressing for both the patient and the immediate family.

CUPPING THERAPY. Start the treatment with a moxibustion treatment to Du-20 Baihui. If there is no hair on the scalp, continue the treatment with Strong cupping on the same point. Apply Moving cupping to both inner and outer Bladder channels on the back (Fig. 13-19). Finally, apply Strong cupping on K-3 Taixi.

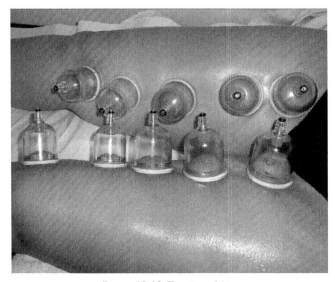

FIGURE 13-18 Treating vulvitis.

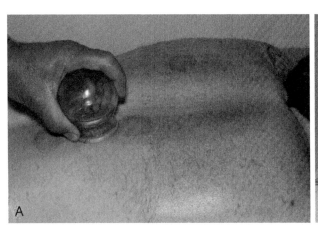
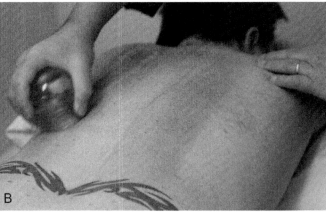

FIGURE 13-19 (A, B) Treating forgetfulness.

GOUT

Gout is considered to be a disorder of the metabolism, in which there is an excessive build-up of uric acid in the blood. Symptoms are a sudden and intense pain in one or more joints, typically the big toe.

CUPPING THERAPY. Apply Moving cupping to the Bladder channel on the back of the body. Apply Bleeding cupping to the affected joint. Avoid foods that are high in purines and drink plenty of water (2–3 litres per day) (Fig. 13-20).

HANGOVER

Overindulgence in alcohol consumption completely disrupts the entire Qi mechanism, including the direction of Qi movement. It causes dehydration, which in turn leads to Yin deficiency such as Liver- and Kidney-Yin vacuity and Empty Heat. Also the Spleen-Qi is destroyed owing to improper diet and eating habits, which is reflected in the skin texture and the overall complexion. As a result, the Qi becomes inadequate as well as rebellious (i.e. moving in the wrong direction) and restless. This complete confusion of the Qi system is the main cause of the 'sick' feeling described as a 'hangover' the next day. The symptoms of hangover can vary enormously from person to person. Some people may display more physical than psychological symptoms, and vice versa.

TREATMENT PRINCIPLE. The overall priority is to restore and regulate the smooth flow of the Qi of the Zang-Fu before dealing with other symptoms such as Empty Heat and Yin or Yang deficiency of various Zang-Fu organs.

CUPPING THERAPY. Apply Light-moving cupping for 10 minutes to the Ren Mai starting from Ren-3 Zhongji and finishing at Ren-15 Jiuwei. Apply Gua Sha technique (or massage) to Ren-17 Shanzhong for a further 5 minutes, moving towards the mouth. To the back of the body, apply a further 15 minutes of Moving cupping technique to both Bladder channels and the Du Mai if possible. Repeat this treatment up to three times a day if the symptoms persist (Colour Plate Figure 24).

HEADACHE/MIGRAINE

Headaches are probably the most common of all complaints seen in the clinic; between 6 and 12% of adults experience a headache at least once a week. The pain experienced can vary in intensity from

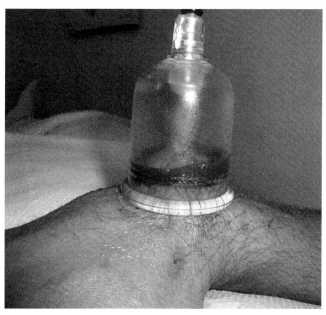

FIGURE 13-20 Treating gout.

person to person, from 'mild' headache to a 'severe' debilitating type. The causes of headaches can be emotional as well as physical. Identifying the underlying cause will help determine the treatment modality and the medication. In children, headaches that occur alongside a fever should be taken more seriously as this could be an indication of meningitis (inflammation of the meninges), which can have serious consequences. The majority of adult headaches are harmless and of very little significance.

The most common factors that bring on headaches are worry in various forms (in particular over finances), tension, tiredness and emotional upset. Less commonly, a headache may accompany an infection, such as of the teeth or sinuses. Some eye conditions can also precipitate headaches. *Migraine* is a special type of severe headache that usually affects only one side of the head and is frequently accompanied by other symptoms, such as nausea, vomiting and vision disturbance.

In this section the most commonly seen headache patterns are shown in the cupping therapy protocol. The differentiations of headache will not be discussed, however, as this is a vast subject and beyond the scope of this book.

CUPPING THERAPY. For frontal headaches, treatment by cupping of Taiyang Extra and Yintang Extra (acupuncture) is administered. For migraine, cupping on Taiyang Extra and Du-14 Dazhui is administered (Cui & Zhang, 1989) (Fig. 13-21).

HICCUPS

This condition is considered as rebellious Stomach-Qi rising upwards (whereas Stomach-Qi normally travels downwards).

Treatment

ACUPUNCTURE. A reducing method of acupuncture is applied to regulate, pacify and direct the Stomach-Qi downward: Ren-12 Zhongwan, P-6 Neiguan, ST-36 Zusanli, Ren-17 Shanzhong and BL-17 Geshu (Chen & Deng, 1989).

CUPPING THERAPY. After removing the needles, Medium to Strong cupping is applied to Liv-13 Zhangmen, Ren-12, Ren-17 and BL-17. The hiccups have reportedly stopped completely after 30 minutes (Fig. 13-22; see also Colour Plate Figure 25).

INSOMNIA

An inability to sleep, or regularly waking up after going to sleep, waking up tired and disturbed sleep patterns are all indications of insomnia. In TCM, the relationship between the Body and Mind is very intimate. For instance, Blood deficiency or Fire (especially Heart Fire) will have a profound effect on

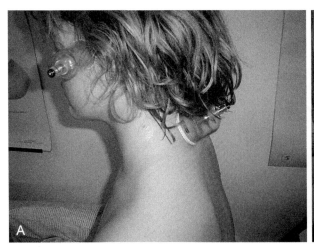 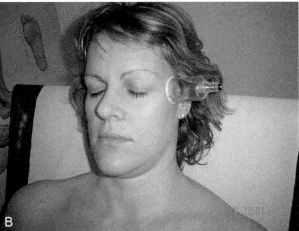

FIGURE 13-21 (A,B) Treating headache.

the Mind. Anger or frustration will affect the Liver's energies, leading to restlessness and agitation. Therefore, when treating insomnia, the underlying cause should be investigated and treated accordingly.

CUPPING THERAPY. Insomnia is treated by cupping in conjunction with massage to the same points: BL-15 Xinshu, BL-17 Geshu and BL-23 Shenshu (Colour Plate Figure 26).

MALE SEXUAL COMPLAINTS

Erectile Dysfunction

Erectile dysfunction is the inability to get and maintain an erection to achieve a satisfactory penetration during intercourse.

CUPPING THERAPY. Apply Medium to Strong cupping methods on BL-17 Geshu, BL-20 Pishu, BL-23 Shenshu, Du-2 Yaoshu, Du-3 Yaoyangguan and Du-4 Mingmen. Apply Weak or Medium cupping to Ren-3 Zhongji, Ren-4 Guanyuan and Ren-6 Qihai. Apply Light-moving cupping to the Liver meridian starting from Liv-13 Zhangmen and working towards the Liv-12 Jimai point (Fig. 13-23).

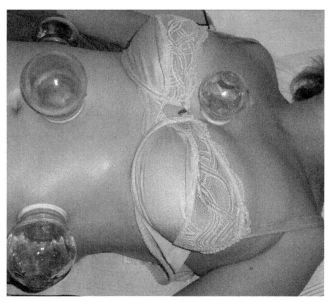

FIGURE 13-22 Treating hiccups.

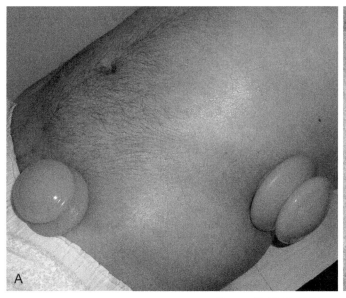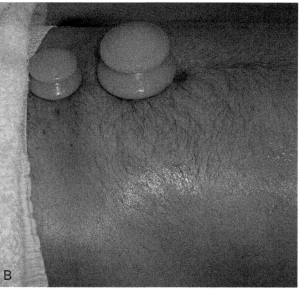

FIGURE 13-23 (A, B) Treating erectile dysfunction.

Male Infertility

Male infertility is considered when a couple cannot conceive after 1 year of regular intercourse without any form of protection.

CUPPING THERAPY. Apply Moving cupping to the five Ciliao points from BL-31 Shangliao to BL-35 Huiyang and the outer Bladder channel between the points of BL-52 Zhisi and BL-41 Fufen. Apply Moxa cupping to BL-23 Shenshu and Du-4 Mingmen, and Medium cupping to Ren-2 Qugu, Ren-3 Zhongji, Ren-4 Guanyuan and Ren-6 Qihai. Apply Moxa cupping to the same points if a Cold pattern exists (Fig. 13-24).

Prostatitis

Prostatitis is a general term to describe inflammation or infection of the prostate gland.

Symptoms can vary from individual to individual including: pain in the pelvis, lower back, or when passing urine, frequent urination (day and night), difficulty in urinating, and pain when ejaculating and high temperature (above 38°C).

CUPPING THERAPY. Apply Strong cupping to LI-4 Hegu and LI-11 Quchi, Medium cupping to Liv-8 Quguan, and Moving cupping between the points SP-7 Lougu and SP-6 Sanyinjiao (Fig. 13-25).

MUMPS

Mumps – also known as *infectious parotitis* – is mostly seen in children with fever and swelling in the salivary glands. This highly infectious viral illness characteristically begins with painful swelling of the parotid salivary glands. Following a 2–3-week incubation period there may be low fever, muscular pain and headaches. In TCM, mumps is described as 'rising of Wind-Damp infection' (Scott, 1991).

CUPPING THERAPY. Mumps is treated by applying Water cupping over the swollen glands, with good results (Fig. 13-26).

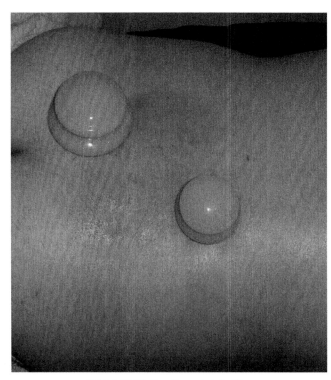

FIGURE 13-24 Treating male infertility.

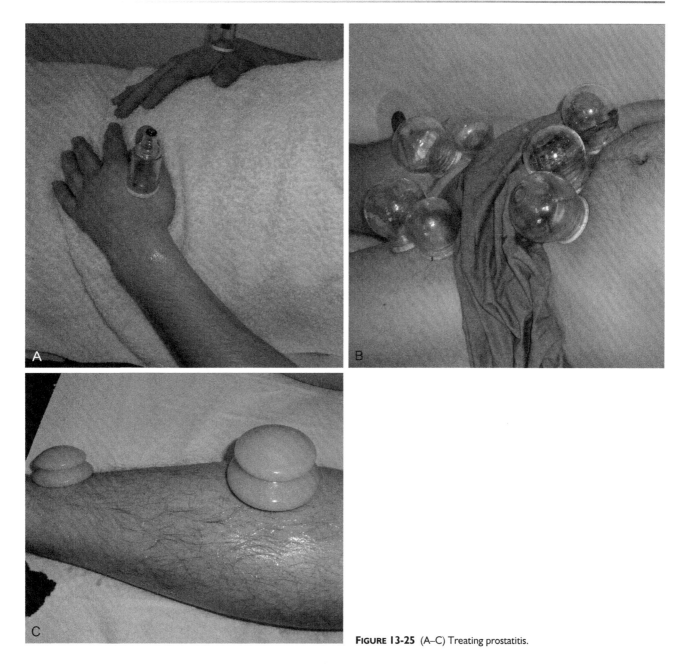

FIGURE 13-25 (A–C) Treating prostatitis.

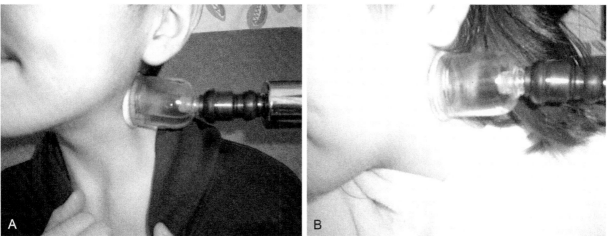

FIGURE 13-26 (A, B) Treating mumps.

NIGHT SWEATING (HYPERHIDROSIS)

Hyperhidrosis is a common condition where a person sweats excessively even when the room isn't excessively hot.

CUPPING THERAPY. Apply 'A' cupping to the upper back (see Fig. 12-7), Strong cupping to Du-14 Dazhui and BL-15 Xinshu, and Moving cupping to the Pericardium channel between the points P-7 Dailing and P-4 Ximen. Finally apply Moxa cupping on Ren-8 Shenque (Fig. 13-27).

POOR APPETITE

Adults

A decrease in appetite could be the result or a sign of emotional or physical condition; explore and if possible treat that first.

CUPPING THERAPY. Apply Moxa cupping on Ren-8 Shenque, and Medium cupping to Ren-12 Zhongwan, Ren-6 Qihai, Liv-13 Zhangmen and Liv-14 Qimen. Apply Light-moving cupping to the entire Bladder channel on the back of the body (Fig. 13-28).

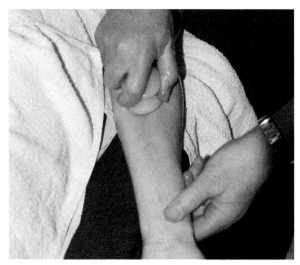

FIGURE 13-27 Treating night sweating (hyperhidrosis).

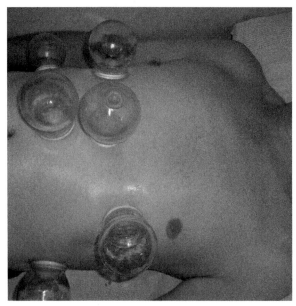

FIGURE 13-28 Treating poor appetite (adults).

Children

Short-term loss of appetite in children should present no health problem. However, sometimes parents – particularly those from Far Eastern, Middle Eastern and the Mediterranean countries – react dramatically to the problem far too early, acting as if the child has an ongoing appetite problem. In fact in most cases there is no cause for alarm. Children, like adults, lose their normal appetite from time to time and take less interest in food. A sudden loss of appetite in the very young (0–2 years old) should be taken more seriously, however, especially when accompanied by a simultaneous lack of bowel movement.

CUPPING THERAPY

Under 4 years old. Massage the chest and the entire abdominal region of the child using a *clockwise* movement. Using the entire Bladder channel on the back of the body, apply massage oil and massage gently with a minimum of pressure on the Bladder channel for 2–3 minutes, using the index and the middle fingers (Fig. 13-29).

Over 4 years and under 7 years old. Apply olive oil to the back of the body and administer Light-moving cupping on the Bladder channel for 2 minutes, preferably using silicon or rubber cupping apparatus (Fig. 13-30).

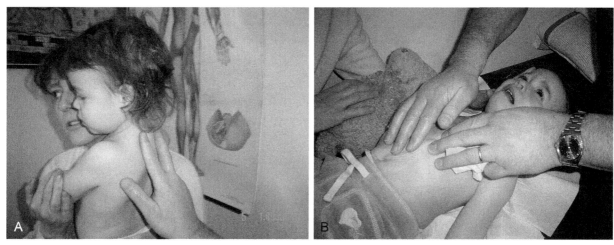

FIGURE 13-29 (A, B) Treating poor appetite (under 4 years old).

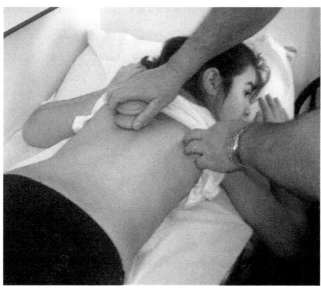

FIGURE 13-30 Rubber cupping apparatus.

PROLAPSE OF THE BLADDER AND THE UTERUS

Bladder Prolapse

Both the bladder and the uterus are held in place by muscular layers and ligaments much like a 'hammock'; this is called the 'pelvic floor'. When the pelvic floor is damaged and becomes weak it fails to hold the organs in place, causing prolapse. The most common contributory factors are heavy lifting, pregnancy, obesity, surgical interventions to the pelvic organs (e.g. hysterectomy) and age (with age all muscles and ligaments become weaker). Symptoms include pain in the lower back, heaviness with a pulling sensation in the vaginal area, incontinence with lifting or coughing, the need to urinate frequently, exertion during a bowel movement and pain during sexual intercourse.

As far as TCM is concerned, all prolapses (including those of the vagina and rectum) are due to Kidney-Yang deficiency (i.e. failure of Kidney-Yang to 'lift and hold upright' the urogenital organs). Therefore, alongside cupping therapy, Kidney-Yang tonifying herbs and acupuncture should also be applied as part of the treatment.

CUPPING THERAPY. Apply Medium to Strong cupping to Ren-3 Zhongji, ST-30 Qichong, BL-26 Guanyuanshu and BL-28 Pangguangshu (Colour Plate Figure 28).

Prolapse of the Uterus

CUPPING THERAPY. Apply Medium to Strong cupping to Ren-6 Qihai, K-12 Dahe, ST-29 Guilai, Du-3 Yaoyangguan and BL-26 Guanyuanshu (Colour Plate Figure 29).

PSORIASIS

Psoriasis is a common skin condition that can occur at any age. The lesions are bright red in colour, have clearly defined edges and a silvery scale. Typically the lesions are symmetrical, but any part of the body can be involved.

TREATMENT PRINCIPLE. Disperse and clear the Damp/Heat from the lesions as well as the body.

CUPPING THERAPY. Apply Bleeding cupping method to one lesion at a time. Using a plum-blossom needle, bleed the borders and the middle of a lesion and apply Strong cupping on the bled location. Allow some blood to exude from the location before terminating the cupping. Reapply the same cupping protocol on each visit until very little or no blood is exuding from the lesion. This mode of treatment helps to remove and disperse the Damp-Heat and the Heat-poison from the location, allowing a normal skin to grow back (see also Chapter 12, Skin Complaints) (Fig. 13-31).

RESTLESSNESS AND HYPERACTIVITY

Under 4 years old

Massage the chest and the abdominal region of the child with olive oil. Turn the child over and oil the entire back, again using olive oil. Concentrating on the Bladder channel, massage the back applying gentle pressure on this channel. This action 'opens and regulates' the Bladder channel, resulting in relaxation and removal of Heat pathogen from the body. This action can be repeated up to three or four times a day.

Over 4 and under 7 years old

Apply Light-moving cupping (preferably using rubber cups) for not more than 1 minute to the back of the body on the Bladder channel (bilaterally) (Fig. 13-32).

TRIGEMINAL NEURALGIA

Trigeminal neuralgia, also known as tic douloureux and facial neuralgia, is pain in the trigeminal nerve, which sends a stabbing and severe pain shooting across the face.

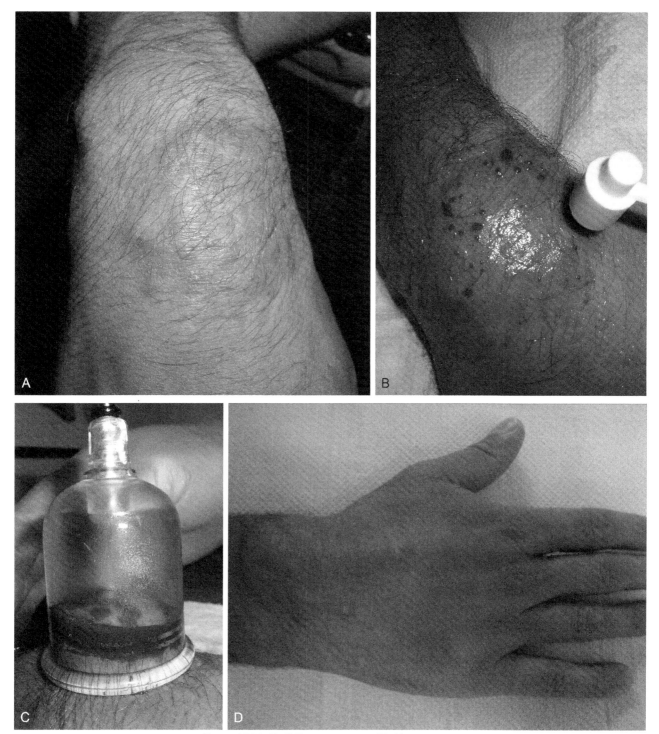

FIGURE 13-31 (A–C) Treating psoriasis: (D) After treatment.

CUPPING THERAPY. Apply Strong cupping to LI-4 Hegu and SJ-17 Yifeng. Apply Light or Medium cupping to GB-2 Tinghui, ST-6 Jiache and ST-7 Xiaguan.

TOOTHACHE

Toothache is treated by cupping over Du-11 Dashu, ST-6 Jiache and ST-7 Xiaguan, massage over SJ-17 Yifeng and acupuncture to LI-4 Hegu (Cui & Zhang, 1989) (Colour Plate Figure 31).

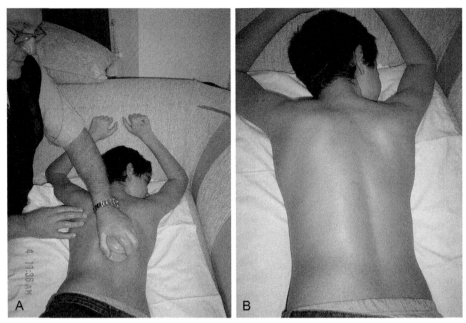

FIGURE 13-32 (A,B) Treating restlessness.

TORTICOLLIS (WRY NECK)

Torticollis (also known as wry neck) is due to the involuntary contractions of neck muscles, where the head is twisted to one side by tightening of the sternocleidomastoid muscle. Head deviation to one side, shaky head, neck pain and abnormal posture are among the symptoms. In TCM, torticollis is considered as Wind attack that injures the channels.

CUPPING THERAPY. Treatment is aimed at removing the Wind factor from the channel involved by using acupuncture, moxibustion and cupping therapy.

Torticollis is treated by applying acupuncture to GB-39 Xuanzhong in an upward direction, followed by cupping therapy to the affected site (Cui & Zhang, 1989) (Colour Plate Figure 32).

REFERENCES

Chen, Y., Deng, L., 1989. Essentials of Contemporary Chinese Acupuncturists' Clinical Experiences. Foreign Languages Press, Beijing, p. 231.
Cui, J., Zhang, G., 1989. A survey of thirty years' clinical application of cupping. J. Tradit. Chin. Med. 9, 152–153.
Low, R.H., 1983. The Secondary Vessels of Acupuncture. Thorsons, Wellingborough.
Maciocia, G., 1994. The Practice of Chinese Medicine. Churchill Livingstone, Edinburgh.
Scott, J., 1991. Acupuncture in the Treatment of Children. Eastland Press, Seattle.

FURTHER READING

Schnyer, R., Allen, J., 2001. Acupuncture in the Treatment of Depression. Churchill Livingstone, Edinburgh.

SPORTS INJURIES

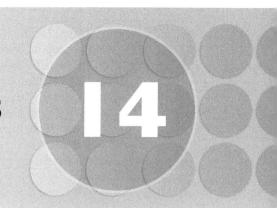

14

CHAPTER CONTENTS

INTRODUCTION, 211

WHY CUPPING THERAPY?, 212

LIGAMENT AND TENDON INJURIES, 212

SKIN INJURIES, 213

MUSCLE INJURIES, 214

BONE INJURIES, 214

CONTRAINDICATIONS WHEN DEALING
WITH SPORTS INJURIES, 215

TREATMENT: LOWER LIMBS, 215

TREATMENT: UPPER LIMBS, 225

UNDERPERFORMANCE SYNDROME, 227

BLOOD INJURY, 229

REFERENCES, 229

INTRODUCTION

Sports injuries are quite common, especially for people who tend to be active or exercise a lot. Over the years I have treated numerous sportsmen/women, applying cupping therapy in conjunction with acupuncture and many times on its own with numerous benefits to the athlete. Although many sportsmen/women come seeking help as a result of an injury, I have also treated many, and in particular long-distance (endurance) runners, *before* the event took place. Without any overstatement, I can testify that almost all athletes reported some form of improvement to their overall health, including feeling 'refreshed', 'light' and 'more flexible', and having 'less pain' and 'more energy'. For the reasons I have listed below, I believe cupping therapy can be employed quite successfully during the management phase of many injuries as well as before the sporting activity, in order to help the athlete deliver their maximum performance.

PRECAUTION

Cupping therapy immediately following sports injury should not be attempted at the site of the injury until the practitioner is absolutely certain that the bleeding into the injured tissues has completely stopped. It is of paramount importance that this safety measure is adhered to, in order to avoid further damage to the tissues involved.

In the acute stages of sports injuries the normally acceptable treatment is to apply an ice pack to minimize swelling and bleeding into the muscle. After the initial treatment has been undertaken, rest, physiotherapy or, if necessary in the case of extreme injuries, surgical intervention might be the next course of action. Cupping therapy is most effective in the subsequent stages of the injury (usually around 24 hours later) and is certainly not suggested as an immediate treatment directly following an injury.

This is because the instant physiological reaction to injury is a rush of synovial fluid and blood into the injury site in order to 'protect' the injured area (hence the swelling of the injured site). If the injury is severe, blood also escapes into the tissues, resulting in a black and blue swelling. At this stage, cupping therapy is not an appropriate form of treatment, as the condition could worsen owing to the power of suction that is created inside the cup. From the TCM energetic point of view, we can safely conclude that all forms of injury, anywhere on the body, cause local stasis and stagnation of Qi, Blood and Fluids.

The purpose of cupping therapy, therefore, is to remove and eliminate this adverse stagnation of Qi, Blood and Fluids by dispersing the stasis and harmonizing their smooth flow. Consequently, the best time to administer cupping therapy is when the practitioner is quite satisfied that the bleeding has completely stopped, which in most cases will be the next day. The cupping application forces the stagnant Blood, Fluid and Qi into movement towards the cup. When this treatment is administered by means of the Bleeding cupping technique, some blood and fluid will also be removed from the swollen site into the cup. This action will have the immediate effect of decreasing the localized pressure and reducing both swelling and pain. Consequently, it offers welcome relief and benefit to the patient.

With regard to the question 'Should cupping therapy be administered to an open wound?', the answer is, most definitely not! Wound healing takes time and depends on several factors. Local tissue oxygenation, infection, patient-related factors such as diabetes, nutritional deficiencies, smoking and medication are amongst the important healing factors (Scuderi & McCann, 2005: 103). Once again, to reiterate the point I have made above, cupping therapy is not the appropriate choice of treatment in the acute stages, but is most effective in the healing and recovery phases of the injury.

WHY CUPPING THERAPY?

One of the most authoritative books available on sports medicine is *Sports Medicine: A Comprehensive Approach* (Scuderi & McCann, 2005). In Chapter 10, entitled *Wound Healing* (contributed by Dr Susan Craig Scott), a very clear account of the healing process is described:

Factors that affect wound healing: Local tissue oxygenation (pO_2, tissue partial pressure of oxygen) is the single most important factor in wound healing. It is poor local pO_2 that ultimately accounts for healing problems in irradiated tissue or in a patient with diabetes mellitus, peripheral vascular disease, chronic infection, and pressure sores. Interestingly, the fibroblast, which lays down the collagen for wound healing, is oxygen sensitive. Collagen synthesis requires a pO_2 in the range of 90 to 95 mmHg; in patients on a normal diet with adequate vitamin C, the availability of O_2 to the fibroblast is the rate-limiting factor for collagen production. Adequate local pO_2 depends on several factors. There must be adequate inspired O_2 and haemoglobin must be adequate in level and normal in structure to allow the transfer of O_2 on demand by local tissue.

Let us take a pause for a moment and remind ourselves of the reasoning as well as the purpose of the cupping application itself. Cupping suction is due to the negative pressure created inside the cup either by introducing a fire into the cup or by manual/mechanical influences over the cup. This negative pressure forces the oxygen-rich blood to move towards the cup, thus saturating the damaged tissues with such blood and consequently precipitating the healing process. This is precisely why cupping therapy has an advantage over all other forms of healing systems, and one that is considered the most fundamental requirement in the healing process, according to Scuderi & McCann.

As far as cupping therapy is concerned, we can further group the injuries into two categories: *overuse injuries* and *on-field trauma injuries*. Overuse injuries are the result of repetitive, cumulative mini-injuries to the same part of the body. They do not appear as a sudden-onset complaint but rather as a slow-onset aggravation that gets worse with each activity or exercise. Consequently, when the complaint becomes sufficiently intolerable for the athlete to seek help, the injury has penetrated into the deeper energetic layers of body tissue, resulting in the need for much more extensive treatment. However, when on-field trauma injuries are involved, after waiting for the initial acute stage of the injury to settle, the management of the injury is more rapidly responsive. This will therefore reflect favourably on the long-term outcome of the treatment.

LIGAMENT AND TENDON INJURIES

Tendons and ligaments are both potentially vulnerable to many incapacitating sports injuries. Together they bind, support and give stability, flexibility and strength to the entire musculoskeletal system as well as being responsible for the stretching and movement of the joints. I would like to take a brief look at the structure and functions of both ligaments and tendons.

Ligaments

A ligament is a short, tough band of white, fibrous, elastic connective tissue that binds nerves and muscles together and retains tendons in place. Ligaments connect individual bones to others to form a joint. Some ligaments limit the mobility of articulations, or prevent certain movements altogether (Wikipedia, n.d.). Capsular ligaments are part of the articular capsule that surrounds synovial joints. Extracapsular ligaments unite bones together and provide joint stability (Wikipedia, n.d.). Ligaments also help support many internal organs, such as the bladder, uterus, liver and diaphragm. Ligaments are composed of 60–70% water and long, stringy collagen fibres.

Ligament injuries vary from mild injuries involving the tearing of only a few fibres to complete tears of the ligament, which may lead to instability of the joint. Ligament injuries are divided into three grades:

⊙ A grade I sprain represents some stretched fibres but clinical testing reveals a normal range of motion on stressing the ligament (Brukner & Khan, 2001: 9-18). Cupping therapy is applicable to a grade I injury.
⊙ A grade II sprain involves a considerable quantity of fibres and, therefore, stretching of the joint and stressing the ligament show increased laxity but a definite end point (Brukner & Khan, 2001: 9-18). Cupping therapy is also applicable to grade II sprains.
⊙ A grade III sprain is a complete tear of the ligament with extreme joint laxity and no firm end point. Although they are often painful conditions, grade III sprains can also be pain free as sensory fibres are completely divided in the injury (Brukner & Khan, 2001: 9-18). Cupping therapy in grade III sprains is contraindicated until after the necessary intervention (i.e. after surgery), and well into the healing and building phase of the injured tissue.

Tendons

Tendons connect or attach muscles to bones; they provide the 'pulling' action on the bones. Tendons comprise tough and flexible bands of fibrous tissue that transmit power from muscle to bone and also act as shock absorbers. Tendons often become inflamed – a condition known as tendonitis. Rupture of a tendon, especially the Achilles tendon, is a common complaint amongst sportsmen and women. The composition of a tendon is similar to that of ligament: mainly water, fibrous and collagenous fibres. Both tendons and ligaments lack blood vessels (hence the familiar grey or white colouring in anatomical charts).

In the event of an injury, both of these tissue forms are deprived of the oxygen necessary for repair work. The application of cupping therapy, either directly or proximally on the tendons and ligaments, will facilitate blood flow via the method described above, thus providing more evidence to support the opinion that cupping therapy is an effective treatment for muscular as well as tendon and ligament injuries.

Tendon rupture comes in two forms: partial and complete. The two most commonly ruptured tendons are the Achilles tendon and the supraspinatus tendon of the shoulder (Brukner & Khan, 2001: 9-18).

SKIN INJURIES

Injury to skin tissue during sporting activities is quite common, particularly in athletes involved in contact sports. The underlying structural damage to the bones, blood vessels, muscles and ligaments should always be taken into consideration. Damage to the skin resulting in an open wound should be managed appropriately:

There are three principles of treatment of all open wounds. The first is to stop any associated bleeding. The second principle of open wound treatment is to prevent infection by removing all dirt and contamination. The third principle is that, if the wound is over a constantly moving part, the area should be immobilised to encourage healing.

(Brukner & Khan, 2001: 9-18)

Cupping therapy in all three circumstances is therefore contraindicated.

MUSCLE INJURIES

Muscle Strain and Muscle Tear

Muscle tissues are strained or torn when some or all of the fibres fail to cope with the burden placed upon them. Muscle strains are among the most common sporting injuries. Common muscles affected are the hamstrings, quadriceps and gastrocnemius – all muscles that are biarthrodial (cross two joints) and are thus more vulnerable to injury. A muscle is most likely to tear during sudden acceleration or deceleration.

Muscle strains are classified into three grades:

- A grade I strain involves a small number of muscle fibres and causes localized pain but no loss of strength.
- A grade II strain is a tear of a significant number of muscle fibres with associated pain and swelling (Brukner & Khan, 2001: 9-18). In both types of strain, cupping therapy during the first 1–3 weeks should be avoided until the bleeding, swelling or inflammation is adequately managed.
- A grade III strain is a complete tear of the muscle. This is seen most commonly at the musculotendinous junction (Brukner & Khan, 2001: 9-18). Cupping therapy is once again contraindicated during the first 5–6 weeks of injury in grade III strains. However, when the underlying bleeding, swelling or inflammation is properly managed, cupping therapy can safely be administered in order to promote healing and to encourage the muscle building and strengthening process.

BONE INJURIES

Bone Fractures

Bone fractures are common sporting injuries amongst athletes. This may be the result of direct on-field trauma such as a blow or a fall. Fractures are categorized as transverse, oblique, spiral or comminuted (where the bone is broken in several places). Another type of fracture seen in athletes, particularly children, is the avulsion fracture, where a piece of bone attached to a tendon or ligament is torn away.

The clinical characteristics of a fracture are pain, tenderness, localized bruising, swelling and, in some cases, deformity and restriction of movement (Brukner & Khan, 2001: 9-18). Cupping therapy is totally contraindicated until symptoms such as bruising, swelling and deformity have disappeared or completely resolved.

Stress Fractures

Stress fractures are also a common injury amongst athletes, especially those that are engaged in running, jumping or repetitive stress. A stress fracture is a micro-fracture (tiny cracks) appearing in bones as a result of muscles becoming overtired and no longer able to absorb the shock of repeated force:

Overload stress can be applied to bone through two mechanisms: 1. The redistribution of impact forces resulting in increased stress at focal points in bone. 2. The action of muscle pull across bone. Histological changes resulting from bone stress occur along a continuum beginning with vascular congestion and thrombosis. This is followed by osteoclastic and osteoblastic activity leading to rarefaction, weakened trabeculae and micro-fracture and ending in complete fracture. Stress fractures may occur in virtually any bone in the body. The most commonly affected bones are the tibia, metatarsals, fibula, tarsal navicular, femur and pelvis. Patients with stress fractures usually complain of localised pain and tenderness over the fracture site.

(Brukner & Khan, 2001: 9-18)

A clear and definite diagnosis is difficult to reach using ordinary X-ray investigation. Magnetic resonance imaging (MRI) scan or a radioisotopic bone scan (scintigraphy) is more revealing. Traditionally, rest and avoidance of the precipitating activity are advised. Most stress fractures heal with 6 to 8 weeks of total rest. Once the injured limb is pain free and fully mobile, cupping therapy is of great value, particularly when a Light-moving cupping technique is employed and is accompanied by acupuncture.

CONTRAINDICATIONS WHEN DEALING WITH SPORTS INJURIES

Cupping therapy is contraindicated in all the following conditions: to an open wound, to inflamed or infected tissue, to a bleeding injury (external as well as internal), over a fracture and to a grade III muscle or ligament sprain, as well as in complete tendon rupture.

The *Sports Injury Bulletin* (UK), *Sports Medicine for Specific Ages and Abilities* (Maffulli et al, 2001), MedicineNet.com, *Sports Medicine: A Comprehensive Approach* (Scuderi & McCann, 2005) and *Clinical Sports Medicine* (Brukner & Khan, 2001) were the main sources of sports injuries mentioned in this chapter.

TREATMENT: LOWER LIMBS

Ankle Injuries

Sprains

Ankle sprains are one of the most common ankle injuries a healthcare practitioner will see. These injuries can comprise as much as 10% of all A&E visits (Scuderi & McCann, 2005: 407-409). Sprains can be very painful and can cause restrictions in the movement of the joint. Swelling and bruising or both can also result from sprains.

SPORTING ACTIVITIES THAT CAUSE MOST ANKLE INJURIES. Participants in Australian football, football (soccer), skiing, snowboarding, surfing, karate, Tae Kwon Do, triathlon, running, rugby, cricket, squash and netball are amongst the sufferers.

CUPPING THERAPY. Using a no. 1 or 2 glass cup, apply Medium cupping, increasing to Strong method on SP-5 Shangqiu, ST-41 Jiexi (when swelling is present), BL-62 Shenmai, BL-60 Kunlun, K-3 Taixi and K-8 Jiaoxin. Apply Bleeding cupping on ST-41 Jiexi and BL-62 Shenmai when persistent bruising or swelling occurs. Moxibustion is also applicable to ankle injuries (Fig. 14-1).

Achilles Tendon Injuries

Achilles Tendonitis and Achilles Tendon Rupture

The Achilles tendon attaches the calf muscle (gastrocnemius) to the heel bone (calcaneus) and connects the leg muscles to the foot. It facilitates walking, puts a spring in our step and helps us stand on tiptoe. The Achilles tendon is the largest and strongest tendon in the body; in mature adults it measures between 10 and 15 cm in length (Scuderi & McCann, 2005: 407-409). It lies just under the skin, has no protective covering and is therefore vulnerable to injury and inflammation.

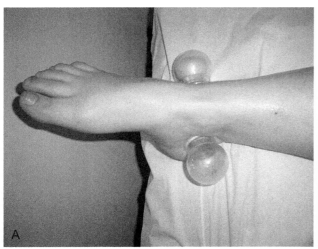 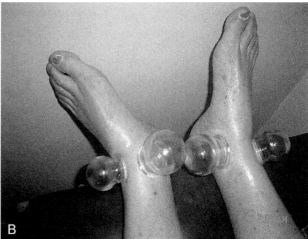

FIGURE 14-1 (A, B) Treating ankle injuries.

Achilles tendonitis is a painful and incapacitating inflammation of the Achilles tendon. It often originates from overuse or micro-injuries that go untreated and cause the tendon to become painful, less flexible and swollen. Known causes of acute Achilles tendonitis include inflexibility of the Achilles tendon, insufficient gastrocnemius strength or flexibility, functional overpronation producing a whipping action on the Achilles tendon on heel strike as the heel goes from varus (bending towards the centre of the body) to valgus (bending away from the body) in mid stance, number of years running, training pace, stretching habits, recent change in footwear and poor running shoes, recent increase in training (especially if it includes hill running), eccentric loading of a fatigued muscle–tendon unit from overtraining and running on uneven terrain (*Sports Injury Bulletin*, 2002).

Achilles tendon rupture is a complete disturbance of the Achilles tendon, usually occurring at 2–6 cm above the heel bone (calcaneus). Achilles tendon rupture is characterized by sudden-onset pain with local swelling and bruising. Patients often describe the feeling as been kicked in the back of the leg. Achilles tendon complaints may account for 5–10% of all athletic injuries (*Sports Injury Bulletin*, 2002). The blood supply to the Achilles tendon is also quite deprived; therefore, in order to help reverse this condition, cupping therapy is particularly appropriate.

SPORTS ACTIVITIES MOST AFFECTED BY ACHILLES TENDON INJURIES. Achilles tendonitis is seen in runners, jumpers, rugby players, gymnasts, cyclists and participants in football (soccer), volleyball, tennis and all other forms of racquet sports. Achilles tendon rupture is more often seen in tennis players and the incidence seems to be rising because of an increasing number of older athletes. It is also common in sports such as basketball, squash, triathlon, diving, dancing, cricket and rugby.

CUPPING THERAPY. Using a no. 1 or 2 glass cup, apply Moving cupping directly on the Achilles tendon, starting from point BL-57 Chengjin and moving the cup in the direction of the calcaneus. Continue to apply Moving cupping to the inner and outer aspects of the Achilles tendon.

MOXIBUSTION. Moxibustion therapy is of immense benefit when treating Achilles tendon rupture injuries. A burning moxa stick is held directly over the swollen tendon for between 5 and 15 minutes, following the cupping treatment (Fig. 14-2).

Calf Muscle (Gastrocnemius) Injuries

Calf muscles are amongst the strongest in the body and are designed to absorb the shock as we walk or run. The gastrocnemius is the powerful muscle that runs down the back of the calf and terminates in the Achilles tendon (*Sports Injury Bulletin*, 2002). Medial gastrocnemius muscle tear usually happens at a time of utmost force during running, jumping or change of direction. The gastrocnemius muscle has been described as a 'short-action' muscle, making it vulnerable to overstretching and rupture (Scuderi & McCann, 2005: 398). Athletes describe a sudden-onset, crippling pain in the calf. Pain, swelling and bruising are the main symptoms.

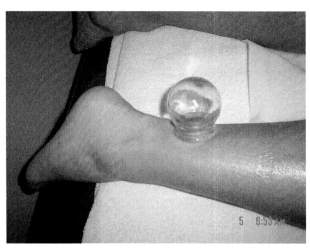

FIGURE 14-2 Treating Achilles tendon injuries.

SPORTING ACTIVITIES THAT CAUSE MOST GASTROCNEMIUS MUSCLE INJURIES. Runners (20% of all injuries) (*Sports Injury Bulletin*, 2003), high jump, rugby (40% of all injuries) (*Sports Injury Bulletin*, 2003), Australian football and football (soccer).

CUPPING THERAPY. Depending on the size of the calf muscle, use a no. 2 or 3 glass cup to apply Moving cupping on the middle of the gastrocnemius, starting from the back of the knee (BL-40 Weizhong) and moving the cup towards the heel alongside the Achilles tendon. Starting from GB-34 Yanglingquan, apply Moving cupping alongside the Gall Bladder channel, terminating at GB-37 Guangming. Finally, apply Moving cupping to the inner aspect of the gastrocnemius, starting from SP-9 Yinlingquan and following alongside the Spleen channel, terminating at SP-6 Sanyinjiao. Apply between 10 and 20 movements to all three sides of the muscle. This treatment can be repeated up to twice a day for the first 3 days, reducing to once a day for a further 3 days. Cupping therapy to the gastrocnemius is particularly effective when muscle tightness or cramp occurs (Fig. 14-3).

Medial Tibial Stress Syndrome

Medial tibial stress syndrome (shin splints, MTSS) is defined as injuries to the front of the outer leg. While the exact injury is not known, shin splints appear to result from inflammation from injury to the tendon (posterior peroneal tendon) and adjacent tissues in the front of the outer leg. Shin splints represent one member of a group of injuries called 'overuse injuries'. Shin splints occur most commonly in runners or aggressive walkers, causing pain in the front of the outer leg below the knee. The pain of shin splints is characteristically located on the outer edge of the mid region of the leg next to the shin bone (tibia). Shin splint discomfort is often described as dull at the outset. However, with continuing trauma, the pain can become so extreme as to cause the athlete to stop workouts altogether (Shiel, n.d.). The definitive location of injury in the shin area can be muscle, tendon, bone or the connective tissue wrappings that surround the muscle and tendon (*Sports Injury Bulletin*, 2000).

SPORTING ACTIVITIES THAT CAUSE MOST SHIN SPLINT INJURIES. All athletes concerned in sports that involve running and jumping are at higher risk of shin splint injuries. It is considered an overuse injury. Sportsmen/women taking part in endurance running, sprinting, triathlon, football (soccer), squash, tennis, gymnastics, handball, basketball, rugby, cricket and volleyball are amongst the high-risk athletes.

DIAGNOSIS. A correct diagnosis of MTSS is crucial during the cupping treatment as it can easily be confused with stress fracture injuries, where cupping is contraindicated. Rest diminishes the symptom in the early stages of the injury but the pain changes progressively from a 'dull ache' to more severe pain. The pain is not well localized but expands over approximately one-third of the length of the posteromedial tibia. This finding is important in distinguishing stress fractures, which are characterized by localized point tenderness. Negligible swelling may be present, but no specific mass is seen (Scuderi & McCann, 2005).

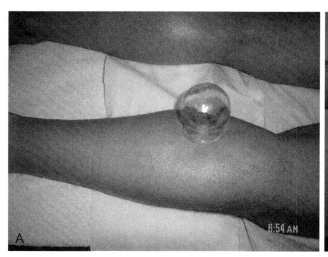
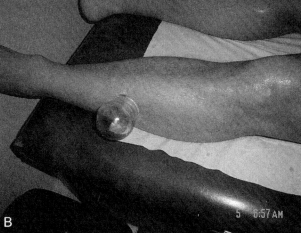

FIGURE 14-3 (A, B) Treating calf muscle injuries.

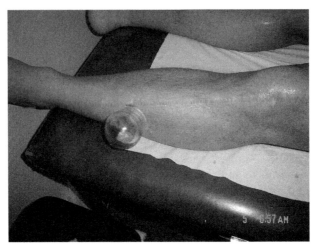

FIGURE 14-4 Treating medial tibial stress syndrome injuries.

CUPPING THERAPY. Using a no. 2 or 3 glass cup, apply Moving cupping to the outer aspect of the tibia. The cupping direction should follow the posterior tibial line, starting from ST-36 Zusanli and ending just below ST-39 Xiajuxu. A maximum of 15 minutes of daily treatment is recommended for the first 2 weeks, thereafter reducing the frequency to twice a week (Fig. 14-4).

Knee Injuries

The knee is the body's biggest, and heaviest, joint. It is enclosed in a protective, fluid-filled sac called the synovial capsule. The medial collateral ligament (MCL) and the lateral collateral ligament (LCL) connect the upper leg to the lower leg along the sides of the knee. Together they stabilize and prevent sideways movement of the knee joint. The parts of the joint are lashed together with tendons and ligaments and it is protected by a solid bony shield: the kneecap (patella). The thighbone is protected from contact with the lower leg bones by shock-absorbing cartilage. Despite all this protection, the knee is injured more often than any other joint (Scuderi & McCann, 2005). Both overuse and on-field trauma are very common knee injuries because of the demand that sportsmen/women place on the legs during strenuous sporting activities.

SPORTING ACTIVITIES THAT CAUSE MOST KNEE INJURIES. Runners (25–30% of all injuries to endurance runners) (*Sports Injury Bulletin*, 2000), basketball, volleyball, football, skiing, water skiing, snowboarding, rugby, netball, high jump, swimming, cycling, golf, cricket, and martial arts including Tae Kwon Do athletes are all prone to knee injuries.

CUPPING THERAPY. Using a no. 2, 3 or 4 size cup, apply Medium strength cupping to ST-35 Dubi, ST-34 Liangqiu, GB-34 Yanglingquan, Heiding Extra and Liv-8 Quguan. Apply Bleeding cupping to persistent swellings and bruises (Fig. 14-5).

Iliotibial Band Syndrome

Iliotibial band syndrome (ITBS) is a pain or aching on the lateral (outside) side of the knee or the hip. It is caused by friction between the iliotibial band and the knee or hip bone. The pain is often described as sharp with a burning sensation. Pain may also be present below the knee where the iliotibial band attaches to the tibia; accompanying pain may also occur much higher up – in the tensor fascia lata itself or in its tendinous connection to the hip (*Sports Injury Bulletin*, 2000).

SPORTING ACTIVITIES THAT CAUSE MOST ILIOTIBIAL BAND INJURIES. Running (12% of all running-related overuse injuries) (Fredericson et al, 2000), cycling, football, tennis, squash, weightlifting and handball.

CUPPING THERAPY. Using a no. 1 or 2 glass cup, apply Medium to Strong cupping method on the lateral side of the painful knee. Moxibustion application is also quite beneficial (before the cupping treatment). If the pain is higher up, in the tensor fascia, perform Moving cupping with a no. 3 or 4 cup,

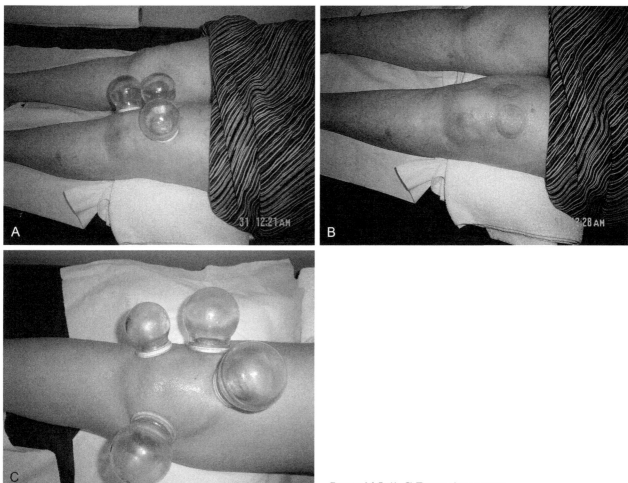

FIGURE 14-5 (A–C) Treating knee injuries.

directly on the tensor fascia. Should the pain be in the hip, Medium to Strong cupping with a no. 4 or 5 cup is applied to GB-30 Huantiao, followed by Moving cupping on the tensor fascia (Fig. 14-6).

Hamstring Injuries

The hamstring muscles are a group of muscles at the back of the thigh that flex the knee and extend the gluteus maximus (the largest of the three muscles in the buttock). The hamstring tendon is a group of tendons behind the knee that link the thigh muscles to the bones in the lower leg.

Injuries to the hamstring group of muscles can vary from a minor strain to a major rupture. Minor strains are classified as grade I tears, whereas complete ruptures are classified as grade III tears. Grade II tears are incomplete ruptures. Given the function of these muscles, it should not be surprising that grade III injuries most frequently occur in the athletically strenuous and demanding sports. Grade I injuries tend to be mild in that they usually heal fully with only minor aggravation to the injured, especially in the sedentary individual. On the other hand, in power athletes, hamstring injuries can be severe and debilitating. Hamstring injuries usually occur after sudden lunging, running or jumping (Wikipedia, n.d.). An inconsistent amount of pain is experienced. The athlete is usually unable to continue and cannot even stand.

Hamstring complaints vary from strains to 'pulls', tendonitis and tightness. Unfortunately, hamstring injuries are rather slow to heal, and athletes often spend several weeks resting or carrying out alternative activities before they are able to train without much pain (*Sports Injury Bulletin*, n.d.).

SPORTING ACTIVITIES THAT CAUSE MOST HAMSTRING INJURIES. Hamstring injuries are particularly common in sports that require short bursts of power, acceleration and deceleration, such as football (a two-season study of English football league clubs confirmed that hamstring strains are the most

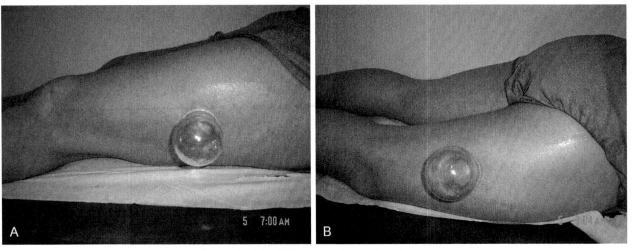

FIGURE 14-6 (A, B) Treating iliotibial band syndrome.

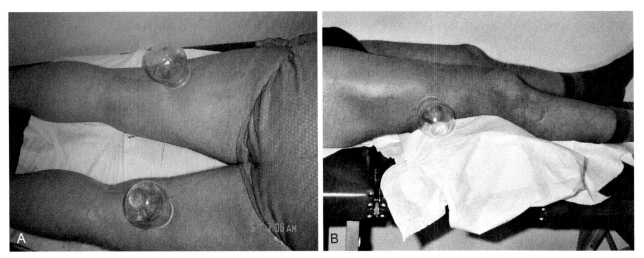

FIGURE 14-7 (A, B) Treating hamstring injuries.

common injuries in football, accounting for an average of 90 days and 15 matches misses per club per season, with a significant recurrence rate of 12%) (*Peak Performance*, 2004), rugby, cricket and American and Australian rules football (*SportEx*, 2002). Long-distance runners and in particular sprinters are well known for their hamstring injuries.

The hamstrings consist of three muscles covering the posterior thigh; the biceps femoris is the most lateral with the semitendinosus and semimembranosus making up the medial side (Scuderi & McCann, 2005: 324). The hamstring muscles are the most commonly involved muscle injury of the pelvis, hip and thigh. The injuries often occur at the musculotendinous junction, with forced flexion of the hip with a fully extended knee, or when the hamstrings are maximally stretched. The symptoms are posterior thigh pain, possibly with a 'pop' being felt, and difficulty in walking (*Sports Injury Bulletin*, 2003). Hamstring pain is sometimes described as a 'referred pain' originating from lumbar spine injuries.

CUPPING THERAPY. In order to determine the exact site of injury during the treatment phase, always refer to the hamstrings muscle group as indicated above. When treating lateral muscle injuries (biceps femoris), the cupping application should start from GB-30 Huantiao region, directing the cupping movement towards GB-32 Zhongdu (Fig. 14-7A). When treating medial muscle injuries (semitendinosus and semimembranosus), the cupping application should start from BL-36 Chengfu, moving towards BL-40 Weizhong (Fig. 14-7B).

All cupping applications relating to hamstring injuries should be a Moving cupping technique. The strength of the suction can vary from Medium suction to Light-moving method. If the hamstring pain is a 'referred pain' originating from the lumbar spine, add Du-3 Yaoyangguan, BL-26 Guanyuanshu and BL-28 Pangguangshu.

Quadriceps Femoris Injuries

The quadriceps femoris, or 'quads' for short, is the large four-part extensor muscle at the front of the thigh (rectus femoris, vastus intermedius, vastus lateralis and vastus medialis). The muscle, the tendons and their attached bones include contraction parts that stabilize the hip and knee and allow their motion:

They cross both the knee and hip joints and consequently produce flexion at the hip, moving the thigh towards the chest, and extension or straightening at the knee. Vastus medialis is particularly important for the stability of the patella during activity. The oblique pull of the quadriceps muscle is counteracted by vastus medialis and weakness can cause the knee to give way.

(University of Bristol, 2005)

An injury takes place at the weakest part of the unit. Quadriceps strains are of three types:

1. A mild (grade I) strain, which is a slightly pulled muscle without tearing of muscle or tendon fibres. There is no loss of strength.
2. A moderate (grade II) strain, which is a tearing of fibres in a muscle or tendon or at the attachment to the bone. Strength is diminished.
3. A severe (grade III) strain, which is a rupture of the muscle–tendon–bone attachment, with separation of fibres. A severe strain may require surgical repair.

Chronic strains are caused by overuse; acute strains are caused by direct injury or overstress (The BodyGuard, n.d.). Symptoms include pain when stretching or flexing the thigh, swelling of the injured muscle and weakness of the knee and the leg.

SPORTING ACTIVITIES THAT CAUSE MOST QUADRICEPS FEMORIS INJURIES. Athletes involved in contact sports such as football, Australian football and rugby, as well as cricket and all sports that require a quick start such as running, sprinting and track events are amongst the higher-end sufferers from quads injuries.

CUPPING THERAPY. Apart from a direct blow to the external muscle (vastus lateralis) and to the front muscle (rectus femoris), the inner muscle (vastus medialis) is the most treated muscle at the clinic. The majority of complaints are weakness of the leg and knee, together with pain, especially in women suffering from osteoporosis. Cupping application should always start with Light to Medium cupping technique as the vastus medialis muscle can be very sensitive to the pulling action of the cup. Moving cupping technique can be employed when treating external (vastus lateralis) and front (rectus femoris) muscles (Fig. 14-8).

Hip Injuries and Groin Pain

All complaints about hip and/or groin pain should be taken seriously and examined thoroughly, since this region accommodates a complex array of vital organs, such as the reproductive organs, as well as the ligaments, tendons, arteries, veins, nerves and bony structures of the hip and corresponding attachments. This is also an area that deals with a constant and demanding burden during sporting activities as well as while carrying out our daily chores.

The hip is a ball-and-socket joint where the head of the femur attaches itself to the pelvis. Walking, running and jumping all affect the hip. Weakness of the lower back muscles as well as inappropriate footwear can contribute to hip pain. Most hip pain is due to a hip sprain caused by trauma during a contact sport: contusions, fractures, dislocations, ligament or tendon injuries, muscle contraction and overuse injuries.

The groin is a junction at each side of the body where the lower abdomen joins the top of the thigh. Groin pain can be triggered by a variety of factors including groin strain, or stretch and tear or rupture of the adductor longus muscle.

SPORTING ACTIVITIES THAT CAUSE MOST HIP INJURIES AND GROIN PAIN. Athletes involved in running and twisting sports such as football, Australian football, rugby, golf and basketball are all susceptible to hip and groin injuries.

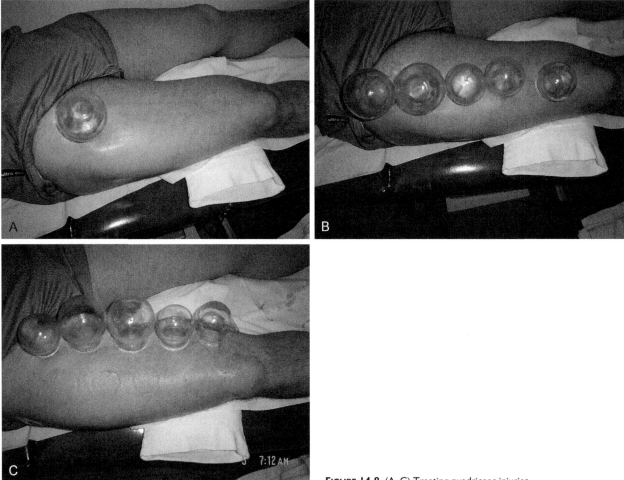

FIGURE 14-8 (A–C) Treating quadriceps injuries.

CUPPING THERAPY. As well as dealing with pain, back strengthening should also be part of the treatment when addressing hip and groin injuries. Starting with a Medium cupping method and increasing to a Strong cupping method, apply cups on the lower back points BL-28 Pangguangshu, BL-53 Baohuang, EM-Yaoyan (extra point, also known as Guihai) and GB-30 Huantiao. When treating groin pain, apply Moving cupping, starting from BL-28 Pangguangshu and moving the cup towards GB-28 Weidao (this helps to relax the adductor longus muscle as well as strengthening the back muscles). Moxibustion with moxa box should also be included as part of the treatment if pathogens such as Cold or Wind-Cold are present. Treatment should consist of at least one course of therapy, twice weekly for the first 3–4 weeks then reducing the frequency to once a week for a further 6 weeks (Fig. 14-9).

Buttock Pain

Buttock pain is most frequently seen in athletes involved in kicking or sprinting sports. It can occur in isolation or may be associated with low back or posterior thigh pain. The diagnosis of buttock pain can be difficult as pain may arise from a number of local structures in the buttock or can be referred from the lumbar spine or sacroiliac joint (Brukner & Khan, 2001). The most common causes of buttock pain are referred lower back problems including the lumbar spine, the sacroiliac joint and the hamstring attachments on the ischial tuberosities (bony parts of the buttock). There are, however, some more serious conditions that can also be the cause of buttock pain, including spondyloarthropathies, ankylosing spondylitis, Reiter's syndrome (reactive arthritis), psoriatic arthritis, arthritis associated with inflammatory bowel disease, malignancy and bone and joint infections (Brukner & Khan, 2001).

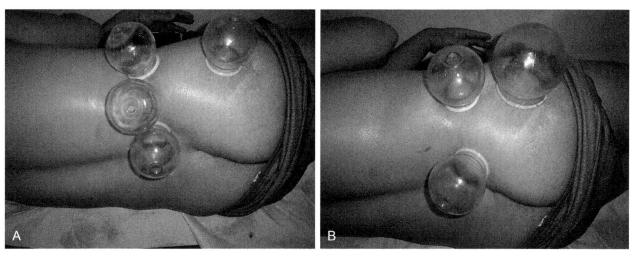

FIGURE 14-9 (A, B) Treating hip injuries.

SPORTING ACTIVITIES THAT CAUSE MOST BUTTOCK PAIN. Athletes involved in kicking and sprinting sports, cyclist and runners are amongst the sufferers from buttock pain. Female athletes are more susceptible to it (Brukner & Khan, 2001).

CUPPING THERAPY. Correct diagnosis and elimination of more serious conditions such as bowel disease, malignancy or bone infection are essential before any form of cupping treatment is administered:

⊙ **For localized buttock pain:** Apply Medium to Strong cupping method to GB-30 Huantiao, BL-28 Pangguangshu, BL-54 Zhibian and Extra point EM-Yaoyan (see Plate 36 in the colour plate section).
⊙ **For a spreading buttock pain:** As well as the above applications, add Moving cupping therapy using a medium-sized cup (no. 3 or 4), following the path of the gluteus maximus muscle.

Lower Back Injuries

Without any doubt, lower back pain is the single most common complaint amongst the general population – and athletes are no exception! The most common back complaints in sportsmen/women are due to tightness or strain of the lower back muscles. When a muscle is strained or tightened it goes into spasm; this in turn results in constrained blood supply to the muscle tissue, which leads to even more muscular tension, pain and restricted movement. On-field injury, overuse or inflammation of the lumbar spine also results in lower back pain. In the case of overuse, repeated rotational movements of the spine such as the swinging motions required for baseball, cricket, tennis, squash, handball, racquetball or golf may eventually lead to injury or inflammation of the vertebrae, spinal discs, ligaments of the spine or the spinal muscles themselves, mainly in individuals whose lower back muscles are functionally weak (*Sports Injury Bulletin*, 2000).

Spinal stress fractures resulting from a serious blow to the lower back during contact sports can also leave the athlete in constant pain and out of action for a considerable length of time. It is also worth reminding the practitioner that if there is any doubt about a potential spinal injury, such as fractures, then treatment with cupping therapy should not be attempted.

The majority of injuries to the lower back are soft tissue injuries. Most of these injuries are contusions, musculotendinous strains and ligament sprains. Contusions result from blunt trauma sustained by a direct blow. Often the athlete is able to remember an incident responsible for the injury. On physical examination, a contusion will present as a relatively separate area of point tenderness with the occasional overlying bruise (Scuderi & McCann, 2005: 217).

SPORTING ACTIVITIES THAT CAUSE MOST LOWER BACK INJURIES. Most running athletes and those taking part in sports that require a back-twisting action are susceptible to lower back injuries. Golfers, especially amateur golfers, are more prone to lower back injuries (*SportEx*, 2004); four out of five

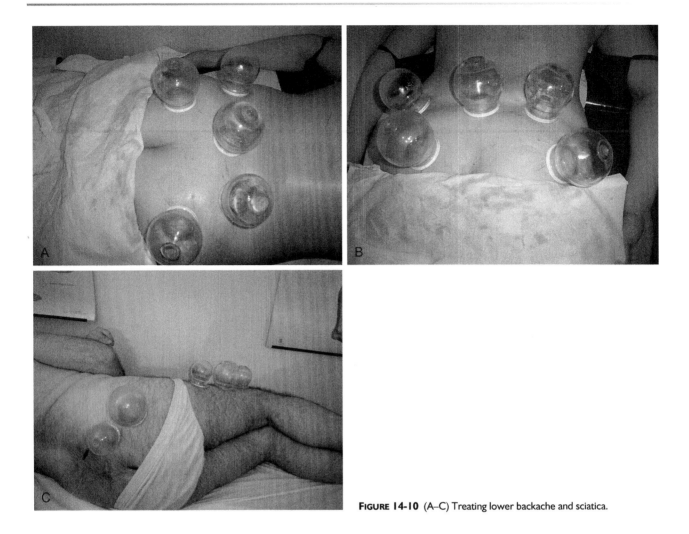

FIGURE 14-10 (A–C) Treating lower backache and sciatica.

golfers, at all levels, will suffer low back pain at some time during their pursuit (*Sports Injury Bulletin*, 2004). Cricket bowlers are reported to suffer as much as 20% from low back injuries (*Sports Injury Bulletin*, 2004) and female players' bowling-related back injuries were reported to be as high as 60% (*Sports Injury Bulletin*, 2004). Rugby, baseball, tennis, squash, handball, racquetball and weight-lifting athletes are amongst the highest on the list of sufferers.

CUPPING THERAPY. For lower back injury pain, the following point combinations are most effective:

- If the pain is across the lower back, apply cupping treatment to Du-3 Yaoyangguan, BL-26 Guanyuanshu and BL-28 Pangguangshu.
- If the pain is still in the lower back but is radiating towards the buttocks, the cupping application should be modified as follows: Du-3 Yaoyangguan, BL-53 Baohuang and BL-54 Zhibian point combinations (Fig. 14-10).

In the acute stage of pain, always start the treatment by applying Light to Medium cupping methods for around 15 minutes at a time. The strength of the cupping application can be increased to a Strong method after the third or fourth visit; as above, retain the cup in position for at least 15 minutes at each session. Conversely, when dealing with long-term or chronic lower back injury pain, the cupping application should commence by applying Medium or even Strong method, and similarly retaining the cup in position for between 10 and 20 minutes.

Moving cupping is also a suitable method when dealing with 'tense/stiff-back' or 'moving pain' syndromes. However, as far as the direction of the cupping movement is concerned, in order for the damaged muscular structures to benefit it is important to follow the correct procedure. For example, when treating the erector spinae muscle, the cupping movement should follow the path of the muscle (i.e. in a vertical motion rather than a horizontal motion). The extent of the treatment can vary between 10 and 20 visits, depending on the severity of the injury and the time factor between injury and commencement of the treatment. Typically, the longer the duration of the injury, the more likely it is that longer treatment will be required.

TREATMENT: UPPER LIMBS

Shoulder Injuries

Shoulder injuries are amongst the most frequent sports-related complaints presented at the clinic, following back injuries. Shoulder injuries are also amongst the most challenging regions to treat, requiring time and patience, since the shoulder is a complex joint that is kept in place with an array of small, strap-like muscles and strong ligaments called the 'rotator cuff'. In fact, the shoulder joint is made up of three bones – the scapula, the humerus and the clavicle – and four joints – the glenohumeral (GH) joint (the 'ball and-socket' joint between the upper arm, or humerus, and the shoulder blade, or scapula), the acromioclavicular (AC) joint (the joint between the collarbone, or clavicle, and the highest point on the shoulder, called the acromion, which is part of the scapula), the sternoclavicular (SC) joint (the joint between the sternum and the clavicle) and the scapulothoracic (ST) joint (the 'false joint' between the scapula and the rib cage). Furthermore, there is more movement possible at the shoulder joint than at any other joint in the body. Over 1600 positions in three-dimensional space can be assumed by the shoulder (*Sports Injury Bulletin*, 2004). The soft protective cushion, called the 'bursa', which is located between the shoulder joint and the rotator cuff, is a fluid-filled sac that prevents the rotator cuff from rubbing against the shoulder.

COMMON SHOULDER INJURIES AND CUPPING THERAPY. All collision and throwing sports players and 'overhead athletes', such as Australian football, volleyball, tennis, hockey, rugby, and baseball players and cricket bowlers, golfers, freestyle and butterfly swimmers, cyclists, javelin throwers, shotputters, weightlifters, and gymnasts who perform on the rings or horizontal, parallel and uneven bars, are highly susceptible to various degrees of shoulder injury, either during training or throughout their performance. AC joint injuries are amongst the highest in shoulder-related injuries; they account for 3% of all shoulder injuries and 40% of shoulder sports injuries (*Sports Injury Bulletin*, 2003). The most common cause of an AC joint injury is a fall directly onto the adducted shoulder. The force of the fall dictates the severity of injury to the AC joint: in grade I and grade II shoulder injuries the prognosis is good; however, grade III injuries may require surgical intervention (Brukner & Khan, 2001: 240-256). Depending on the force of the fall, symptoms may vary accordingly; severe pain, a bump on the shoulder, painful restricted movement (particularly horizontal flexion), considerable local swelling and bruising are common. Stress is also a known contributory factor to shoulder tension, spasm and pain.

Acromioclavicular (AC) Joint Arthrosis (Degeneration)

Excessive use of the shoulder or a direct blow resulting in AC joint separation may contribute to the development of acromioclavicular arthrosis. Symptoms and signs of AC joint degeneration are pain and discomfort to the front of the shoulder joint. Pain may radiate towards the neck, arm or chest, getting worse when the arm is brought forward across the chest.

Adhesive Capsulitis (Frozen Shoulder)

Adhesive capsulitis or 'frozen shoulder' is rarely seen in active and healthy athletes. Conversely, it is a commoner occurrence in the older athlete. Adhesive capsulitis, a painful condition that causes severe loss of movement in the shoulder, is not generally connected with any particular sport. It may precede an injury to the shoulder, or may appear as gradual onset without any warning or injury. This condition occurs as a result of inflammation of the GH joint and its surrounding capsule; other associated factors include diabetes, trauma, breast surgery and hypothyroidism (Brukner & Khan, 2001: 240-256).

Dislocated Shoulder

The shoulder joint is the body's most mobile joint; it turns in many directions, and is secured to the scapular cavity (glenoid) by the rotator cuff muscle, tendons and ligaments. This advantage in terms of mobility, however, also makes the shoulder more susceptible to dislocation. Shoulder dislocation occurs as a result of the humeral head popping out of its socket caused by a fall onto an extended arm, accident or traumatic sporting injury. Symptoms include numbness, local swelling, weakness in the arm and the hand, and bruising. On examination, the dislocated shoulder has a characteristic appearance with a prominent humeral head and a hollow below the acromion (Brukner & Khan, 2001: 240-256).

Cupping treatment is more suitable during the rehabilitation period, rather than in the earlier, acute stage of the injury. It is aimed at strengthening the muscular structure as well as eliminating the local stagnation from the shoulder joint. Moving cupping is contraindicated when dealing with dislocated shoulder injuries.

Rotator Cuff Injuries

The rotator cuff muscles are the small but strong muscles around the shoulder; they comprise the supraspinatus, infraspinatus, teres minor and subscapularis. The subscapularis is an internal rotator of the GH joint, whereas the infraspinatus and teres minor muscles are external rotators. The rotator cuff as a whole functions to centre the humeral head in the glenoid for stability and to allow utmost pull during shoulder movements. As the arm is abducted away from the body or flexed, 'impingement' or squeezing of the rotator cuff between the head of the humerus below and the coracoacromial arch above can occur. Any overhead activity that involves the arm being taken often enough from below shoulder level to above shoulder level has the capacity to damage the rotator cuff. With repeated impingement, a poorly trained and conditioned cuff can become damaged, and a cycle of cuff damage, impaired function, further impingement and worsening cuff damage is initiated (*Sports Injury Bulletin*, n.d.).

CUPPING THERAPY. Administering up to four cups by means of number 2 or number 3 small size jars, apply Medium to Strong cupping starting with 10 minutes and increasing to up to 30 minutes at each visit, close to the shoulder joint, and concentrating on LU-2 Yunmen, SP-20 Zhourong, SI-9 Jianzhen, SI-10 Naoshu, SI-11 Tianzhong, LI-16 Jugu and SJ-14 Jianliao. If pain is radiating to the arm, add LI-15 Jianyu, LI-14 Binao and SJ-13 Naohui. If pain is radiating towards the neck, add SI-12 Bingfeng and SJ-15 Tianliao. With the exception of dislocated shoulder injuries, Moving cupping is also applicable in all shoulder conditions, following the path of the muscle when moving the cup. If the shoulder tension or pain is due to stress, apply Empty cupping to both shoulders and the upper back for 10 minutes at each visit (Fig. 14-11).

Note: In all types of shoulder injury complaints, external pathogens such as Cold and Wind-Cold are considered extremely harmful factors that need to be addressed. Subsequently, when these external pathogens are presented, local application of Moxa (Hot Needle) cupping or direct moxibustion (rotation or spreading technique) becomes an indispensable tool. The duration of moxibustion therapy may vary between 5 and 15 minutes at each visit.

Elbow and Forearm Injuries

Elbow and forearm injuries are quite common amongst athletes participating in racquet and throwing sports. The majority of injuries to the arm and the elbow are the overuse injuries and may affect the bony parts, joints, muscles, ligaments, tendons or nerves. Acute elbow or forearm injuries are most often collision-related on-field injuries that normally require treatment in the Accident and Emergency Department. Lateral epicondylitis ('tennis elbow') is the single most common elbow injury reported by active athletes:

This inflammatory condition, often accompanied by stiffness, soreness, and outright pain, affects up to 45% of regular racket sports participants. Basically, tennis elbow is an overuse injury caused by repeated contractions of muscles connected to the elbow joint of the arm used to hit the ball.

(Peak Performance, 2002)

Cupping therapy is mostly administered in the overuse type of injury. It should also be noted that it is contraindicated in the acute stages of injury to the elbow and forearm.

SPORTING ACTIVITIES THAT CAUSE MOST ELBOW AND FOREARM INJURIES. Tennis and all other forms of racquet sports, golf, swimming, javelin, cricket, baseball, basketball, waterskiing, bowling, volleyball, football, gymnastics, weightlifting, shotput, canoeing, kayaking, archery and rock climbing are amongst the highest contributors (Brukner & Khan, 2001: 251).

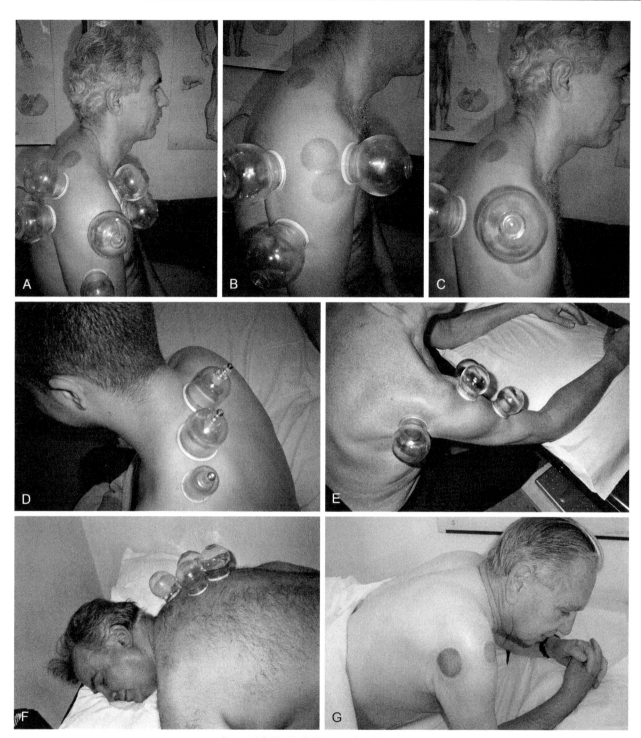

FIGURE 14-11 (A–G) Treating shoulder injuries.

CUPPING THERAPY. A combination of static and Moving cupping is employed during the rehabilitation period of elbow and forearm injuries. The main purpose of the cupping treatment is to help strengthen the forearm muscles and remove stagnation from the elbow joint (Fig. 14-12).

UNDERPERFORMANCE SYNDROME

Athletes, like the rest of us, can suffer from occasional loss of performance and energy. However, they usually recover fairly quickly and return to original form. Regrettably, however, some are very slow to

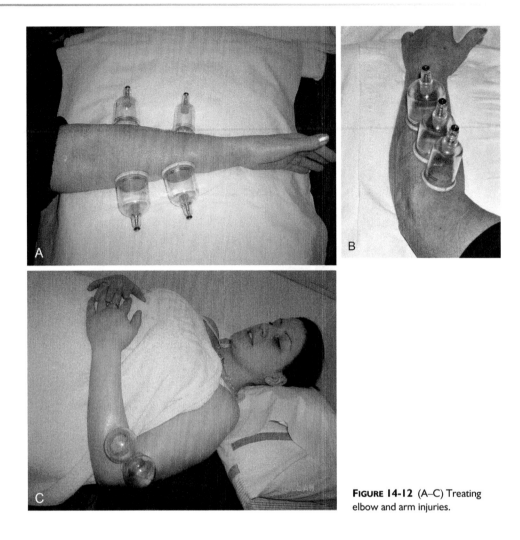

FIGURE 14-12 (A–C) Treating elbow and arm injuries.

recover or fail to do so, even after considerable rest. This is how the highly respected sports journal *Sports Injury Bulletin* (2002) describes this debilitating condition:

The 'unexplained underperformance syndrome' (UUPS) is defined as a history of objective loss of performance, without a medical cause and despite two weeks of rest. This definition was arrived at by a group of experts in Oxford in 1999. UUPS is almost exclusively a condition of endurance athletes, commonly occurring after a period of heavy training and competition. There is often a history of frequent minor infections. Anecdotally it is thought that between 2% and 10% of elite endurance athletes suffer significant episodes of UUPS during their sporting careers.

(Sports Injury Bulletin, 2002)

Fatigue is the key presenting symptom. This fatigue persists despite rest and leads to underperformance. The athlete may lose motivation and often complains of sore muscles and poor sleep. Sometimes they may experience a loss of libido and appetite. They also often become depressed. Less common symptoms of UUPS include: frequent minor infections, stiff or sore muscles, nocturnal hot sweats, minor changes in bowel habit, an elevated heart rate at a given intensity of training, an elevated resting heart rate, an inability to alter pace at the end of a race, mood disturbance and profound loss of motivation.

(Sports Injury Bulletin, 2004)

Unfortunately, we are living in a highly competitive sporting world and, when the trainer or the coach is faced with an underperforming athlete, the universal approach is to increase the training load in order to improve performance and 'get more' from the athlete, hence temporarily solving the problem. However, when this cycle is frequently repeated it actually leads to more tiredness, reduced productive activity and worsening underperformance. I believe that the TCM diagnostic technique of pulse and tongue diagnosis is a superior method of correctly diagnosing the underlying factor(s) in the unexplained underperformance syndrome.

BLOOD INJURY

How the Blood is 'Injured' and What This Means

As discussed in Chapter 1, Blood is described as a kind of material transformed from the essence of Food produced through functional activity of Qi, which circulates through the blood vessels and nourishes the body tissue. Blood has a different role to play in traditional Chinese medicine from that of Western medicine. One of the most important characteristics of the Blood in TCM is that it contains Qi (energy). Qi is considered to be the locomotive of Blood. Where Qi moves, Blood also moves, and vice versa: where Blood moves, Qi follows.

There is a very intimate relationship between Qi and Blood. Blood injury occurs through poor diet and excessive demands on the body, such as overwork without having adequate rest or sleep in between, long-lasting bleeding, excessive sexual activity and a demanding exercise regimen despite poor, ineffective recovery from a previous activity or physical injury. All the above activities, when practised in excess, will result in depletion of Qi, which is literally the 'driving force' of Blood. 'Blood injury', therefore, is a unique TCM terminology that describes irreversible damage to the Blood's functional properties.

There is, however, a distinction between depletion of Qi and an injury to Blood. Chronic Qi depletion or deficiency may present itself as a feeling of lethargy, breathlessness, profuse sweating, loss of appetite and, most of all, lack of both motivation and a desire to move. Blood injury symptoms may include all the above as well as the additional symptoms of pale and colourless facial features, dizziness, palpitations, insomnia and, most importantly, aching bones, muscles and tendons.

CUPPING THERAPY. In both scenarios the aim is to stimulate Blood and Qi into motion in order to reverse the current 'stale' situation and promote a healthy and smooth flow of Qi and Blood throughout the body. In doing so, fresh and oxygen-rich blood and the dormant Qi are both forced into action to eliminate stagnation or stasis, at the same time helping to bring about a lasting recovery from past injuries and a quick return to form.

As described in Chapter 9, apply Empty cupping treatment to the front of the chest for 15 minutes every day for 10 days, concentrating on LU-1 Zhongfu and LU-2 Yunmen and the entire back (torso) of the body (see also Fig. 13-5).

Where muscular pains are present, apply Light-moving cupping every day for 10 days on the painful areas of the body. Every application should be performed for only 5 minutes on each painful area.

Repeat the treatment procedure for several weeks after giving the patient a week's rest in between 10 sessions. During the entire period of the treatment, it is equally important for the athlete to refrain from intense training and to pursue a more gentle exercise regimen.

REFERENCES

Brukner, P., Khan, K., 2001. Clinical Sports Medicine, second ed. McGraw Hill, Sydney, pp. 9–18, 240–256.

Fredericson, M., Guillet, M., DeBenedictis, L., 2000. Quick solutions for iliotibial band syndrome. Phys. Sportsmed. 28 (2), 53–68. Online. Available: www.physsportsmed.com.

Maffulli, N., Chan, K.M., Macdonald, R., et al., 2001. Sports Medicine for Specific Ages and Abilities. Churchill Livingstone, Edinburgh.

Peak Performance, 2002. (168). Online. Available: http://www.pponline.co.uk/encyc.

Peak Performance, 2004. (196). Online. Available: http://www.pponline.co.uk/encyc.

Quads, 2005. Information Leaflet. University of Bristol.

Quadriceps injuries. The BodyGuard. Online. Available: www.antibodywear.com/articles/quadricep-injuries-symptoms-treatment.asp.

Scuderi, G.R., McCann, P.D., 2005. Sports Medicine: A Comprehensive Approach, second ed. Mosby, St Louis, p. 103, 217, 324, 398, 407–409.

Shiel Jr., W.C., Shin splints. Online. Available: www.medicinenet.com/shin_splints/article.htm.

SportEx, 2002. (13). Online. Available: http://www.sportex.net.

SportEx, 2004. (21). Online. Available: http://www.sportex.net.

Sports Injury Bulletin, 2000. 1, 7, 9. Online. Available: http://www.sportsinjurybulletin.com.
Sports Injury Bulletin, 2002. (24), 19, 21. Online. Available: http://www.sportsinjurybulletin.com.
Sports Injury Bulletin, 2003 (26), 33. Online. Available: http://www.sportsinjurybulletin.com.
Sports Injury Bulletin, 2004. (36, 38, 39). Online. Available: http://www.sportsinjurybulletin.com.
Sports Injury Bulletin. (109). Online. Available: http://www.sportsinjurybulletin.com.
Wikipedia: the free Encyclopaedia. Ligament. Online. Available: http://en.wikipedia.org/wiki/ligament.
Wikipedia: the free Encyclopaedia. Pulled hamstring. Online. Available: http://en.wikipedia.org/wiki/Hamstring.

MYOFASCIAL TRIGGER POINTS CUPPING THERAPY

15

CHAPTER CONTENTS

BACKGROUND, 231
THE PRACTICAL APPLICATION OF
CUPPING THERAPY ON MYOFASCIAL
TRIGGER POINTS, 232

CUPPING APPLICATION ON
MYOFASCIAL TRIGGER POINTS, 232
REFERENCES, 246

BACKGROUND

Musculoskeletal tender points and their therapeutic values were first identified by Froriep in 1843, in the publication *Muskel Schweile*; trigger points (TrPs) were described as 'extremely tender, palpable hardenings in muscles that, when treated, afforded the patient much pain relief' (Simons et al, 1999). Between 1843 and 1997, numerous results and scientific papers were additionally published. The most notable and the one widely accepted as the most authoritative publication on trigger points is *Myofascial Pain and Dysfunction: The Trigger Point Manual* by Simons and colleagues, who describe the myofascial trigger point as 'a hyper-irritable spot in skeletal muscle that is associated with a hypersensitive palpable nodule in a taut band. The spot is painful on compression and can give rise to characteristic referred pain, referred tenderness, motor dysfunction, and autonomic phenomena. Types of myofascial trigger points include: active, associated, attachment, central, key, latent, primary, and satellite' (Simons et al, 1999).

From the traditional Chinese medicine perspective, trigger points are similar to *ashi* points (also known as *pressure points*) as described in TCM pathology. These are sensitive spots that cause pain when pressed upon. However, a subtle difference remains – that when pressure is applied on trigger points *the sensation generated is often radiated or is referred to a predictable course*. These referred sensations can include pain, numbness, a tingling sensation, muscle stiffness and muscle weakness. Trigger points represent stagnation of Blood or Qi at a deeper musculoskeletal level. These points are usually located in the centre of a muscular structure (Baldry, 2005). Apart from being 'sensitive' when gently stroked or pressed, trigger points can also be felt as a tight band or a 'lump', not under the superficial layers of the skin, but in the deeper layers within the muscular structure and sometimes close to the bone.

What Causes Trigger Points?

Generally speaking, any action or movement that puts extra load on the musculoskeletal system can be the culprit. Persistent wrong posture while sitting or walking, carrying or lifting heavy loads, accidents, strains, falls, overwork, overuse of a particular muscle group and a stressful lifestyle can all contribute to trigger point formation.

Treatment Methods

According to Simons et al (1999) any physical intervention will influence a trigger point release (deactivation). Methods discussed in *The Trigger Point Manual* include acupuncture, spray and stretch, injecting trigger points with local anaesthetic such as procaine (the most-used method), trigger point pressure release, deep stroking (and other) massage, application of heat, posture correction, exercise, transcutaneous electrical nerve stimulation (TENS) and therapeutic ultrasound techniques – all described in detail.

THE PRACTICAL APPLICATION OF CUPPING THERAPY ON MYOFASCIAL TRIGGER POINTS

During the cupping application a strong, *negative pressure* is created over the trigger point. This in turn will result in the stimulation of the stagnant Blood or Qi into movement towards the direction of the cup. The negative pressure will also force oxygen-rich blood to flow into the trigger point, releasing the muscular knot/lump. Sometimes trigger points are difficult to obliterate completely, especially when dealing with long-established trigger points. These may require more frequent cupping application, which can be as often as three times per week.

Because trigger points are located at the deeper layers of the muscle tissues, a Strong cupping method is often required to be effectual. As recommended earlier in this book, the treatment should begin by administering a Medium cupping method, at least for the first two visits, and subsequently gradually increasing the strength of the cupping to a Strong cupping method. Typically a single cup is applied to the trigger point, with several additional cups to the borders of the muscular structure or the path of pain. Not all trigger points are suitable for cupping therapy, owing to their anatomical location. In these cases other methods of trigger point release should be employed.

One of the most suitable and effective types of apparatus for conducting trigger point cupping is the pistol-handle cupping set. As well as giving the practitioner total control over the strength of the suction, the small cups in the set also make it an ideal tool when treating points on the neck and face.

How to Locate an Active Trigger Point

Here is how Simons et al (1999) describe active and the latent trigger points:

- **Active myofascial trigger point**: A myofascial trigger point that causes a clinical pain complaint. It is always tender, prevents full lengthening of the muscle, weakens the muscle, refers a patient-recognized pain on direct compression, mediates a local twitch response of muscle fibres when adequately stimulated and, when compressed within the patient's pain tolerance, produces referred motor phenomena and often autonomic phenomena, generally in its pain reference zone, and causes tenderness in the pain reference zone.
- **Latent myofascial trigger point**: A myofascial trigger point that is clinically quiescent (dormant) with respect to spontaneous pain; it is painful only when palpated. A latent trigger point may have all the other clinical characteristics of an active trigger point and always has a taut band that increases muscle tension and restricts range of motion.

Both types of trigger point share similar physical characteristics: well-defined, tense, palpable myofascial tightness, with a distinct painful nodule when pressed. An experienced tactile therapy practitioner has no difficulty in identifying these tight nodules: as well as feeling taut or tense, the patient will always respond and react (sometimes with an extreme wrench) to the stimulation of trigger points.

CUPPING APPLICATION ON MYOFASCIAL TRIGGER POINTS

To be absolutely certain that the correct trigger points are selected, Simons et al (1999) insist that four conditions must be met: 'the detection of spot tenderness, palpation of a taut band, the presence of referred pain, and reproduction of the subject's symptomatic pain'. In the following section on treatment protocol (see Figs 15.1–15.31), I have indicated the trigger points' cupping locations (○) as the 'most likely' locations, because these myofascial trigger points are not predetermined fixed points, but rather ones that can be discovered by the practitioner only after carefully palpating the myofascial structure. To demonstrate the pain pattern of trigger points, the main pain reference zone of the trigger points is indicated in these figures in dark grey and the overflow zone in lighter grey.

Head, Neck and Shoulder Pain

Masseter Muscle (Fig. 15-1)

SYMPTOMS. Restricted jaw opening, and pain during biting and chewing; masseter muscle TrPs may also refer pain toward the eyebrow, in front of the face and under the eyes, the ear and the upper or lower molar teeth (Simons et al, 1999).

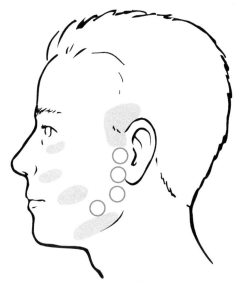

FIGURE 15-1 Masseter muscle trigger points.

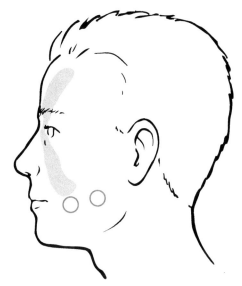

FIGURE 15-2 Cutaneous facial muscle trigger points, left zygomatic major muscle.

Cutaneous Facial Muscle: Zygomatic Major Muscle (Fig. 15-2)

SYMPTOMS. Zygomatic major muscle TrPs refer pain to the front of the face over the bridge of the nose and reaching to the middle of the forehead (Simons et al, 1999).

Semispinalis Capitis (Fig. 15-3)

SYMPTOMS. Semispinalis capitis TrPs refer pain to the back of the skull and reaching to the temple and forehead (Simons et al, 1999).

Splenius Capitis and Splenius Cervicis Muscles (Fig. 15-4)

SYMPTOMS. Splenius capitis TrPs refer pain to the vertex of the head. The upper splenius cervicis muscle TrPs refer pain to the occiput – 'ache inside the skull'. The lower splenius cervicis muscle TrPs refer pain down to the shoulder girdle and to the angle of the neck (Simons et al, 1999).

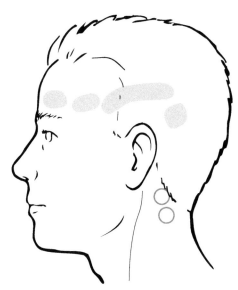

FIGURE 15-3 Semispinalis capitis trigger points.

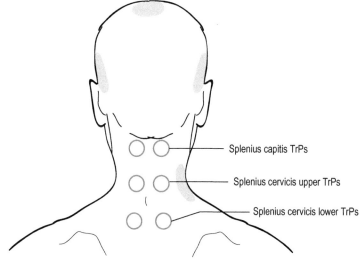

Splenius capitis TrPs

Splenius cervicis upper TrPs

Splenius cervicis lower TrPs

FIGURE 15-4 Splenius capitis trigger points, splenius cervicis upper trigger points and splenius cervicis lower trigger points.

Trapezius Muscle (Fig. 15-5)

SYMPTOMS. The trapezius muscle consists of three sections: the upper, the middle and the lower. The TrPs in the upper trapezius muscle refer pain towards the neck, behind the ear and to the temple. The TrPs in the middle trapezius muscle refer pain towards the vertebrae and to the interscapular region. The TrPs in the lower trapezius muscle refer pain in the upper part of the trapezius muscle towards the posterior neck and the mastoid area (Simons et al, 1999).

Levator Scapulae Muscle (Fig. 15-6)

SYMPTOMS. Limited neck rotation and 'stiff neck' syndrome (Simons et al, 1999).

Supraspinatus Muscle (Fig. 15-7)

SYMPTOMS. Supraspinatus muscle TrPs refer deep pain in the shoulder region, often extending down to the arm and forearm, concentrating over the lateral epicondyle of the elbow (Simons et al, 1999).

Infraspinatus Muscle (Fig. 15-8)

SYMPTOMS. Infraspinatus muscle TrPs refer pain to the front of the shoulder, radiating down the anterolateral aspect of the arm (Simons et al, 1999).

Teres Minor Muscle (Fig. 15-9)

SYMPTOMS. Teres minor muscle TrPs refer deep and sharp pain below the subacromial bursa, imitating bursitis (Simons et al, 1999).

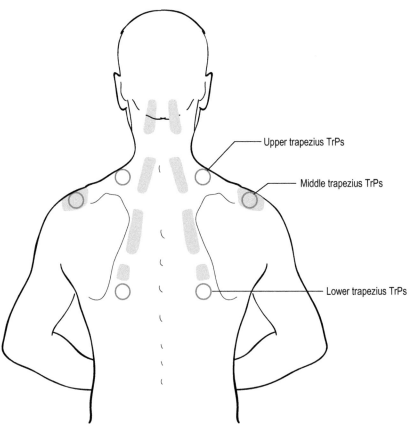

FIGURE 15-5 Trapezius muscle trigger points (upper trapezius muscle, middle trapezius muscle and lower trapezius muscle).

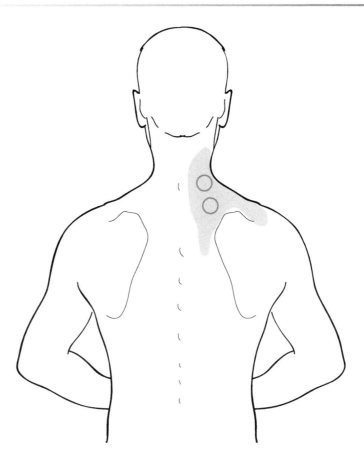

FIGURE 15-6 Levator scapulae muscle trigger points.

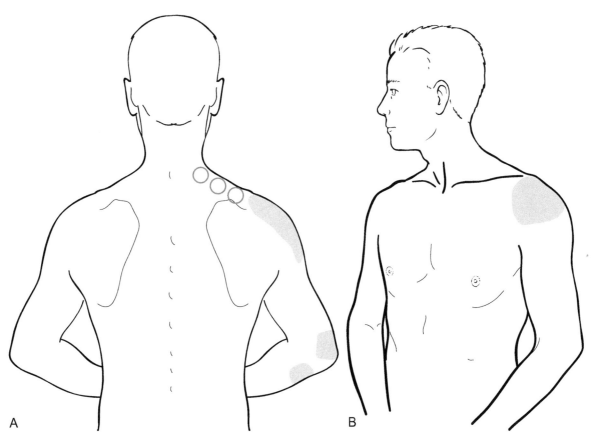

A

B

FIGURE 15-7 (A) Supraspinatus muscle trigger points (B) Supraspinatus muscle trigger points.

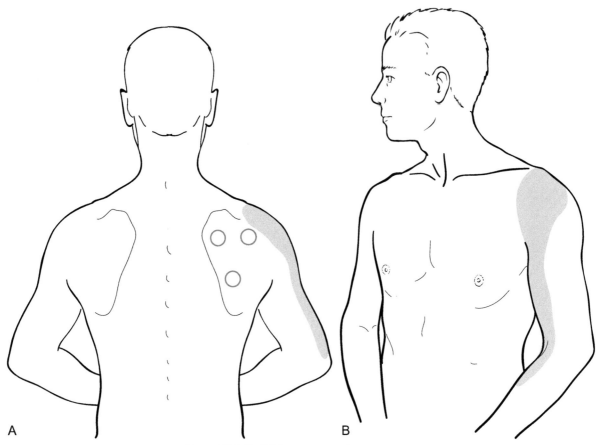

A   B

FIGURE 15-8 (A, B) Infraspinatus muscle trigger points.

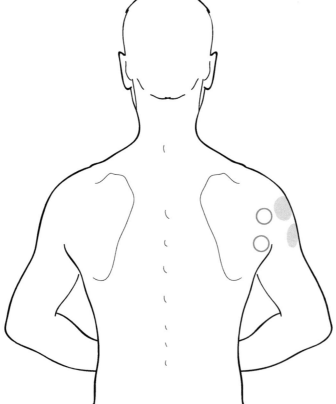

FIGURE 15-9 Teres minor muscle trigger points.

Latissimus Dorsi Muscle (Fig. 15-10)

SYMPTOMS. Latissimus dorsi muscle TrPs refer pain to the lower scapula and to the mid-thoracic region of the back (Simons et al, 1999).

Rhomboid Major and Minor Muscles (Fig. 15-11)

SYMPTOMS. Rhomboid major and minor muscles TrPs refer pain along the medial vertebral border of the scapula (Simons et al, 1999).

Deltoid Muscle (Fig. 15-12)

SYMPTOMS. Deltoid muscle Local TrPs refer pain to the anterior, middle or posterior part of the muscle (Simons et al, 1999).

Coracobrachialis Muscle (Fig. 15-13)

SYMPTOMS. Coracobrachialis muscle TrPs refer pain over the anterior aspect of the proximal humerus; pain also extends to the back of the arm and to the back of the hand (Simons et al, 1999).

Biceps Brachii Muscle (Fig. 15-14)

SYMPTOMS. Biceps brachii muscle TrPs mainly refer pain upwards over the muscle to the front of the shoulder, which may also cause restriction in arm motion (Simons et al, 1999).

Triceps Brachii Muscle (Fig. 15-15)

SYMPTOMS. Triceps brachii muscle TrPs refer pain mostly up and down the posterior aspect of the arm and to the lateral epicondyle. Pain may also radiate towards the upper part of the suprascapular region (Simons et al, 1999).

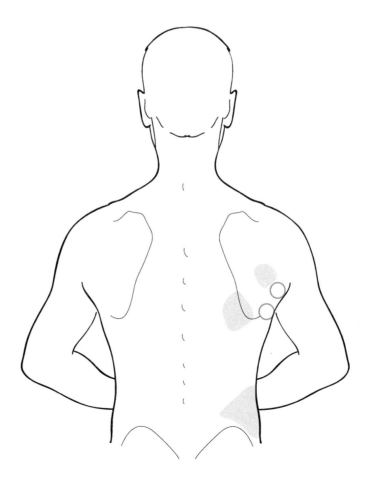

FIGURE 15-10 Latissimus dorsi muscle trigger points.

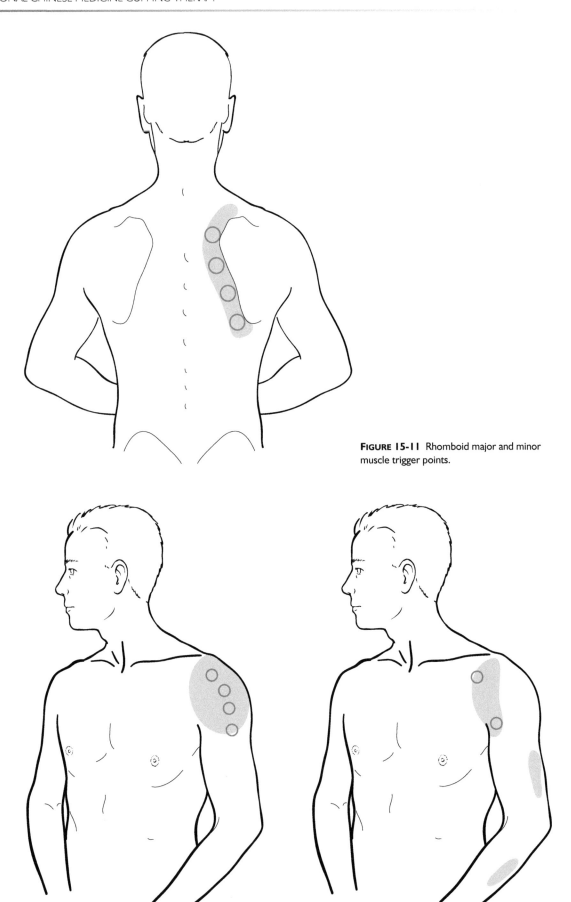

FIGURE 15-11 Rhomboid major and minor muscle trigger points.

FIGURE 15-12 Deltoid muscle trigger points.

FIGURE 15-13 Coracobrachialis muscle trigger points.

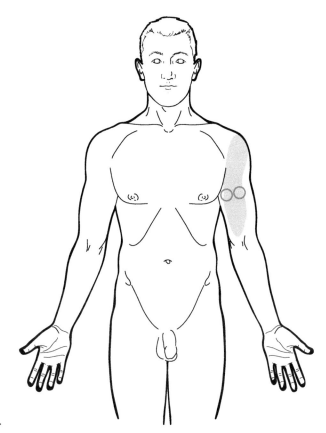

FIGURE 15-14 Biceps brachii muscle trigger points.

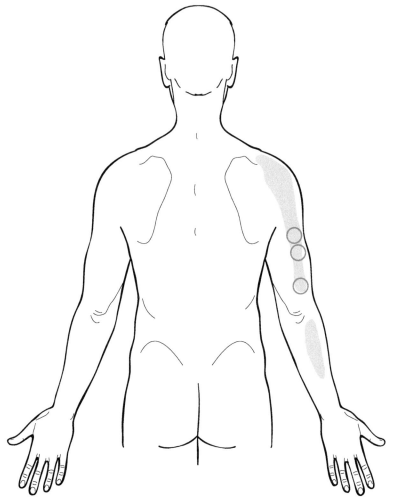

FIGURE 15-15 Triceps brachii muscle trigger points.

Forearm and Hand Pain (Extensors and Flexors)

Extensor Carpi Ulnaris, Extensor Carpi Radialis Brevis and Extensor Carpi Radialis Longus Muscles (Fig. 15-16)

SYMPTOMS. Pain originating from TrPs in the extensors carpi radialis longus and brevis appears over the lateral epicondyle, over the back aspect of the forearm, and reaches the back of the hand. The extensor carpi ulnaris TrPs radiate pain to the back of the ulnar side of the wrist (Simons et al, 1999).

Palmaris Longus Muscle (Fig. 15-17)

SYMPTOMS. The palmaris longus muscle TrP refers needle-like, prickling pain in the palm (Simons et al, 1999).

Flexor Carpi Radialis and Flexor Carpi Ulnaris Muscles (Fig. 15-18)

SYMPTOMS. The flexor carpi radialis muscle TrP refers pain towards the centre of the wrist and into the palm. The flexor carpi ulnaris muscle TrP refers pain to the ulnar side of the wrist and into the palm (Simons et al, 1999).

Adductor Pollicis Muscle (Fig. 15-19)

SYMPTOMS. The adductor pollicis muscle TrP refers aching pain along the outside of the thumb and hand at the base of the thumb distal to the wrist crease (Simons et al, 1999).

Upper Chest Pain

Pectoralis Major Muscle (Fig. 15-20)

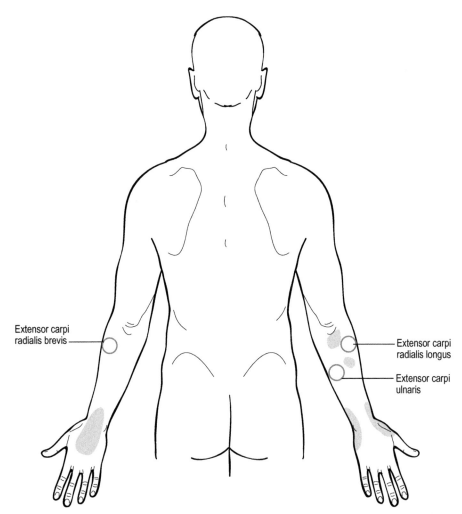

FIGURE 15-16 Hand extensor muscle trigger points (extensor carpi radialis longus, extensor carpi ulnaris and extensor carpi radialis brevis).

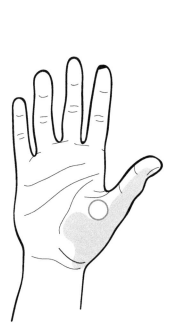

FIGURE 15-17 Palmaris longus muscle trigger point.

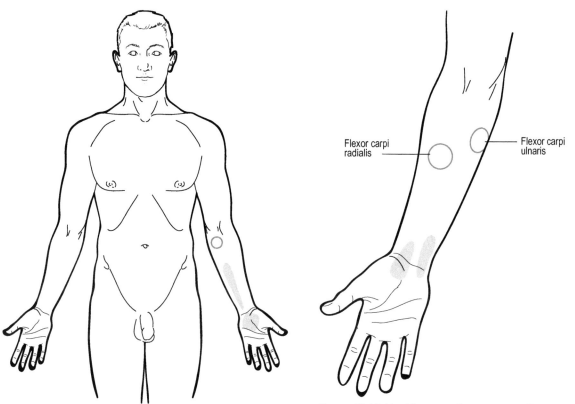

FIGURE 15-18 Hand flexor muscle trigger points (flexor carpi radialis and flexor carpi ulnaris).

Flexor carpi radialis

Flexor carpi ulnaris

FIGURE 15-19 Adductor pollicis muscle trigger point.

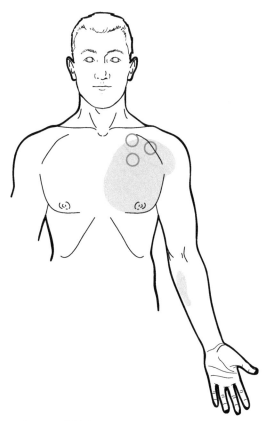

FIGURE 15-20 Pectoralis major muscle trigger points.

SYMPTOMS. Pectoralis major muscle TrPs refer pain into the breast as well as to the chest region, which imitates the pain of cardiac deficiency in persons with no previous history of cardiac disease (Simons et al, 1999). Pain may also extend towards the ulnar aspect of the arm. It is also common to have several TrPs on this muscle.

Lower Back, Lumbar and Buttock Pain

Serratus Posterior Inferior Muscle (Fig. 15-21)

SYMPTOMS. Serratus posterior inferior muscle pain is at a local point close to the TrP. The pain usually radiates over and around the serratus posterior inferior muscle (Simons et al, 1999).

Iliocostalis Lumborum Muscle (Fig. 15-22)

SYMPTOMS. The iliocostalis lumborum muscle TrP refers pain to the mid-buttock (Simons et al, 1999).

Longissimus Thoracis Muscle (Fig. 15-23)

SYMPTOMS. The longissimus thoracis muscle TrP refers pain to the sacroiliac region and the buttock (Simons et al, 1999).

Quadratus Lumborum Muscle (Fig. 15-24)

SYMPTOMS. Quadratus lumborum muscle TrPs refer pain down to the outer side of the iliac crest and over the greater trochanter, and sometimes into the groin (Baldry, 2005).

Lower Leg Pain

Piriformis Muscle (Fig. 15-25)

SYMPTOMS. The piriformis muscle TrP refers pain in the buttock to the hip, extending down the back of the leg in parallel with the sciatic nerve (Baldry, 2005).

Vastus Lateralis Muscle (Fig. 15-26)

SYMPTOMS. The vastus lateralis muscle TrP refers pain up the side of the thigh; pain may also extend into the greater trochanter (Baldry, 2005).

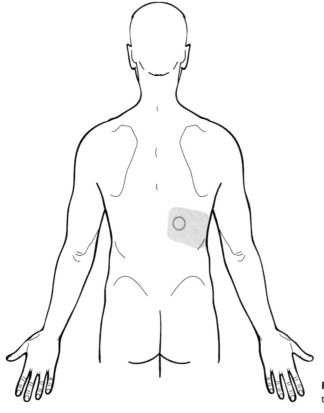

FIGURE 15-21 Serratus posterior inferior muscle trigger point.

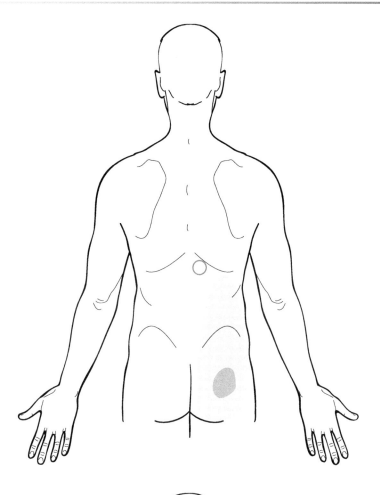

FIGURE 15-22 Iliocostalis lumborum muscle trigger point.

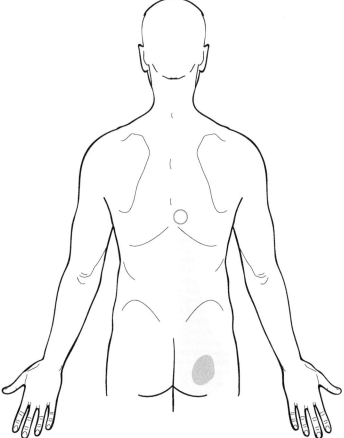

FIGURE 15-23 Longissimus thoracis muscle trigger point.

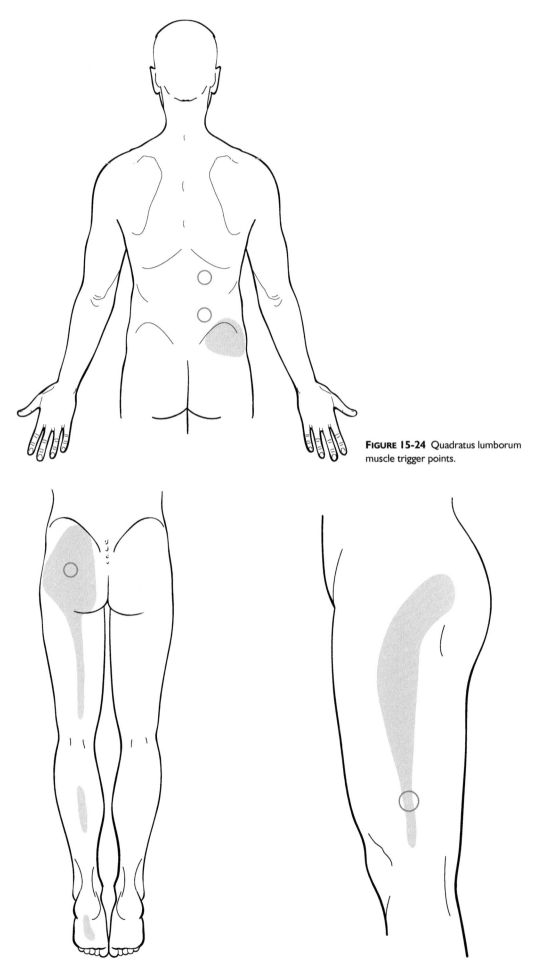

FIGURE 15-24 Quadratus lumborum muscle trigger points.

FIGURE 15-25 Piriformis muscle trigger point.

FIGURE 15-26 Vastus lateralis muscle trigger point.

Vastus Medialis Muscle (Fig. 15-27)

SYMPTOMS. The vastus medialis muscle TrP refers pain to the inner side of the knee (Baldry, 2005).

Tibialis Anterior Muscle (Fig. 15-28)

SYMPTOMS. The tibialis anterior muscle TrP refers pain down the front of the tibia, the inner side of the ankle and the foot (Baldry, 2005).

Gastrocnemius Muscle (Fig. 15-29)

SYMPTOMS. The gastrocnemius muscle TrP refers pain down the calf; pain may sometimes extend to the sole of the foot (Baldry, 2005).

Soleus Muscle (Fig. 15-30)

SYMPTOMS. The soleus muscle TrP refers pain along the Achilles tendon; pain may also extend to the heel (Baldry, 2005).

Peroneal Longus and Brevis Muscles (Fig. 15-31)

SYMPTOMS. TrPs on the peroneal longus and brevis muscles refer pain to the outer side of the leg and foot, concentrating on the outer side of the ankle (Baldry, 2005).

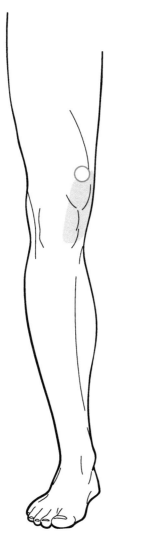

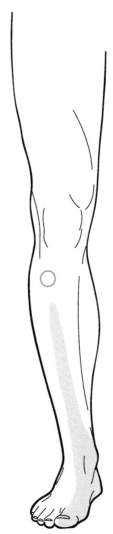

FIGURE 15-27 Vastus medialis muscle trigger point.

FIGURE 15-28 Tibialis anterior muscle trigger point.

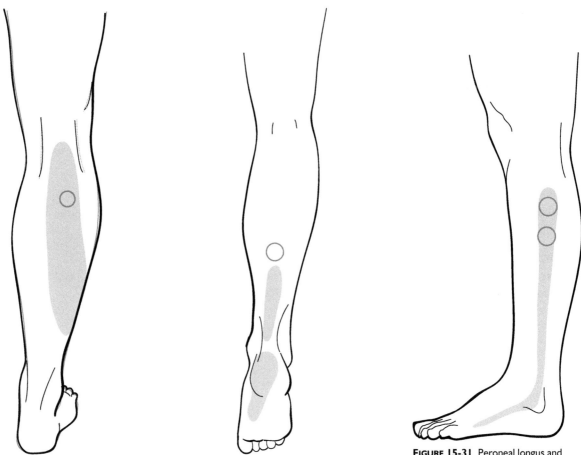

FIGURE 15-29 Gastrocnemius muscle trigger point.

FIGURE 15-30 Soleus muscle trigger point.

FIGURE 15-31 Peroneal longus and brevis muscle trigger points.

Abdominal Muscles

I have deliberately omitted abdominal muscle trigger points cupping therapy, as it is difficult to differentiate pain associated with internal organs such as the Heart, Liver, Kidney, and digestive, urinary or gynaecological origin complaints. Furthermore, abdominal trigger points can cause both internal and external abdominal pain, and misdiagnosis is common (Davis, 2004).

REFERENCES

Baldry, P., 2005. Acupuncture, Trigger Points and Musculoskeletal Pain, third ed Churchill Livingstone, Edinburgh, pp. 302–344.

Davis, C., 2004. The Trigger Point Therapy Workbook. New Harbinger Publications, Oakland, Canada, pp. 146–148.

Simons, D., Travell, J., Simons, L., 1999. Myofascial Pain and Dysfunction: The Trigger Point Manual, second ed. Williams & Wilkins, Philadelphia, pp. 14–913.

CUPPING THERAPY EVIDENCE-BASED RESEARCH

CHAPTER CONTENTS

INTRODUCTION, 247
Research Study 1: Effects of Cupping Therapy on Various Haematological Parameters, 248
INTRODUCTION, 248
METHODS, 248
RESULTS AND DISCUSSION, 248
CASE STUDIES, 250
Research Study 2: The Effects of Cupping Therapy on the Plasma Concentration of Inflammatory Mediators (Unpublished Research Findings), 251
ABSTRACT, 251
INTRODUCTION, 252
METHODS, 255
RESULTS, 255
DISCUSSION AND CONCLUSION, 255
Research Study 3: Cupping and Myofascial Pain Syndrome, 256
ABSTRACT, 256

INTRODUCTION: EXAMINING THE EFFECT OF CUPPING ON THE MANAGEMENT OF MYOFASCIAL PAIN SYNDROME, 257
METHODS, 257
RESULTS, 263
DISCUSSION, 263
CONCLUSION, 276
Research Study 4: A Systematic Literature Review of Clinical Evidence-Based Research, 277
ABSTRACT, 277
INTRODUCTION, 277
METHODS, 278
RESULTS, 279
DISCUSSION, 286
CONCLUSION, 287
APPENDIX, 288
ENDNOTES, 304
REFERENCES, 304
FURTHER READING, 309

INTRODUCTION

Although cupping therapy has been practised for more than five thousand years – first by various folklore and traditional medicine practitioners (cupping was systematically used by the Ancient Egyptians 3150 BC) and later on by a diversity of contemporary CAM practitioners in different parts of the world – scientific research material has been in short supply, particularly during the early 1990s when the first edition of this book was being prepared. I am glad to report that this situation is now rapidly changing, however, and as far as research into cupping therapy is concerned we are entering an incredibly stimulating period. This chapter brings together such existing cupping research studies as myself and the contributing authors of this edition have managed to assemble, and we hope that this will both provide readers with much-needed and so far missing research material, and also prompt future cupping studies.

Research Study 1   Effects of Cupping Therapy on Various Haematological Parameters

Ilkay Zihni Chirali

INTRODUCTION

For many years I have searched for academic papers that will demonstrate 'scientific proof' of cupping therapy and its effect upon Blood and Body Fluids. At the time of writing the first edition of this book in 1996, no such work had been published, although its efficacy was apparent through the work of many practitioners. In consequence, in 1996 I decided to undertake a limited trial myself (with 6 patients over a 14-day period). This involved patients with various complaints/conditions and analysis by a biochemist with modern laboratory facilities. Once I had raised the necessary funding (through friends and relatives) I undertook this trial with an unbiased 'open mind' approach. The biochemist, Metin Erduran, enquired, 'what kind of changes do you expect or are looking for?' My reply was quite unscientific: 'I do not know. You have to let me know of any abnormalities, if any, when your results are ready!'

METHODS

Treatment protocol: Cupping therapy
Duration of the trial: 15 days (every other day, except weekends)
Patients: Six (5 female and 1 male)
Age group: 26–69 years
Place: North Cyprus
Date: First test 3 January 2004; final test 16 January 2004
Biochemist: Mr Metin Erduran (Biochemist specialist), Erduran Laboratory Girne, North Cyprus

Inclusion Criteria

1. To have received no acupuncture or cupping treatment within the last 6 months
2. If on medication, this should be 'stable' and patients were to continue taking the medication as normal.

Treatment Protocol

Cupping therapy was given every other day. Blood analysis from specimens was taken on three occasions: before the cupping treatment commenced, after 7 days (halfway through the treatment) and finally on the 15th day of the trial following the last cupping treatment. Because of limited funds and my timescale on the island where the research was done (North Cyprus), I could not embark on a trial that would last many months and involve large numbers of people. I therefore decided to commence and complete the trial within a 2-week period, involving only six patients with various disorders. Some of the patients were referred to me by the biochemist with existing (known to him) pathological conditions; some were relatives or friends complaining of various ailments.

At the end of each full blood analysis, 22 different values were recorded, but only 7 of these were monitored as the rest were considered irrelevant to our trial or did not show any changes at all. The seven values were: uric acid, erythrocyte sedimentation rate (ESR), pH, rheumatoid factor (RF), white blood count (WBC), red blood count (RBC) and haemoglobin (Hgb).

RESULTS AND DISCUSSION

Table 16-1 details the blood test results for these six patients before, during and at the end of cupping. For almost all the patients involved in this trial, there were small fluctuations in the WBC, RBC, uric acid, RF, pH and Hgb values. There was, however, in almost every case, one major change: a reduction in the ESR levels, which was by far the most significant outcome of this trial. The biochemist, Metin Erduran (with 15 years of experience) commented he had 'never witnessed such a drastic reduction in

TABLE 16-1	Blood Screening Test Results Before, During and at the End of Cupping Therapy					
Name	Test	Normal Values	Pre-Treatment	7 days	14 days	−% Results
O.G.	Uric acid	2.5–6.00	2.8 mg/dL	2.8 mg/dL		
42 yrs old	ESR 1h	4.00–11.00	11 mm/h	8 mm/h		−37
Female	ESR 2h	6.00–20.00	28 mm/h	16 mm/h		−75
	WBC	4.5–10.5	7.8	8.5		+8.2
	RBC	4.00–5.550	5.11	5.35		+4.5
	Hgb	12.0–16.0	11.2	11.2		
	RF (latex)	<8 U/L	Negative	Negative		
	pH	Acid	7.5	7.4		
M.B.	Uric acid	2.5–7.00	4.3 mg/dL	4.7 mg/dL	4.7 mg/dL	
54 yrs old	ESR 1h	4.00–11.00	8 mm/h	4 mm/h	5 mm/h	−60
Male	ESR 2h	6.00–20.00	22 mm/h	10 mm/h	11 mm/h	−100
	WBC	4.5–10.5	6.4	?	5	
	RBC	4.00–5.550	5.63	?	5.69	
	Hgb	12.0–16.0	14.3	15.3	14.6	
	RF (latex)	<8 U/L	128 U/L	128 U/L	128 U/L	
	pH	Acid	7.4	7.4	7.5	
P.Y.	Uric acid	2.5–6.00	4.5 mg/dL	4.4 mg/dL	3.9 mg/dL	−15
69 yrs old	ESR 1h	4.00–11.00	22 mm/h	11 mm/h	11 mm/h	−100
Female	ESR 2h	6.00–20.00	45 mm/h	24 mm/h	21 mm/h	−114
	WBC	4.5–10.5	4.3	3.8	3.7	−16
	RBC	4.00–5.550	4.33	4.17	3.97	
	Hgb	12.0–16.0	13.8	12.9	12.1	−14
	RF (latex)	<8 U/L	Negative	Negative	Negative	
	pH	Acid	7.45	7.5	7.5	
C.Y.	Uric acid	2.5–6.00	6 mg/dL	5.9 mg/dL	5.9 mg/dL	
59 yrs old	ESR 1h	4.00–11.00	16 mm/h	8 mm/h	8 mm/h	−100
Female	ESR 2h	6.00–20.00	44 mm/h	19 mm/h	16 mm/h	−175
	WBC	4.5–10.5	6.5	6.5	6.6	
	RBC	4.00–5.550	5.95	5.95	5.82	
	Hgb	12.0–16.0	11.5	11.4	10.8	
	RF (latex)	<8 U/L	Negative	Negative	Negative	
	pH	Acid	7.45	7.5	7.5	
A.Y.	Uric acid	2.5–6.00	3 mg/dL	3 mg/dL	3 mg/dL	
56 yrs old	ESR 1h	4.00–11.00	15 mm/h	14 mm/h	13 mm/h	−15
Female	ESR 2h	6.00–20.00	38 mm/h	31 mm/h	28 mm/h	−35
	WBC	4.5–10.5	6.5	7.3	5.8	
	RBC	4.00–5.550	5.39	5.6	5.75	
	Hgb	12.0–16.0	11.2	11.4	11.2	
	RF (latex)	<8 U/L	Negative	Negative	Negative	
	pH	Acid	7.4	7.5	7.45	
S.A.	Uric acid	2.50–6.00	4.2 mg/dL	4.2 mg/dL	4 mg/dL	
26 yrs old	ESR 1h	4.00–11.00	16 mm/h	16 mm/h	14 mm/h	−14
Female*	ESR 2h	6.00–20.00	33 mm/h	33 mm/h	19 mm/h	−73
	WBC	4.5–10.5	5.1	5.1	3.7	−37
	RBC	4.00–5.550	4.95	4.95	4.83	
	Hgb	12.0–16.0	11	11	10.9	
	RF (latex)	<8 U/L	Negative	Negative	Negative	
	pH	Acid	7.4	7.4	7.4	

ESR, erythrocyte sedimentation rate; Hgb, haemoglobin; RBC, red blood count; RF, rheumatoid factor; WBC, white blood count.
* This patient started treatment a week late, hence the pre-treatment and 7-day values are identical.

such a short time, even with patients on strong medications'. During this trial, the highest drop in ESR level recorded was 64%; the lowest drop recorded was 15%.

What is the Erythrocyte Sedimentation Rate?

The ESR blood test is an easy, inexpensive, non-specific test that has been used for many years to help diagnose conditions associated with acute and chronic inflammations, including infection, cancer and autoimmune disease. ESR is said to be non-specific because increases do not tell the doctor exactly where the inflammation is in your body or what is causing it; therefore it is often used in conjunction with other tests. The ESR test is helpful in diagnosing two specific inflammatory diseases: temporal arteritis and polymyalgia rheumatica, where a high ESR is one of the main test results used to confirm the diagnosis. It is also used to monitor disease activity and response to therapy in both these diseases. A moderately elevated ESR occurs with inflammation, but also with anaemia, infection, pregnancy and advanced age. A rising ESR can mean an increase in inflammation or poor response to a therapy, whereas a decreasing ESR can mean a good therapeutic response (source: Lab Tests Online, a public resource on clinical laboratory testing).

According to the above, a drop in the ESR level is indicative of a *positive* response to therapy and the opposite is true when the ESR level is on the increase. Although my study shows a clear picture of *reduction* in ESR levels (see Table 16-1), it is by far too small a trial to claim a major result. I therefore urge my TCM colleagues and doctors, in particular, immunologists, to undertake further investigation on this subject.

CASE STUDIES

CASE Female Patient Aged 42 (O.G.)

Complaints/Symptoms. Tennis elbow (pain and restricted movement of the arm for 2 years). No medication.

Pulse. No significant signs.

Tongue. Normal appearance.

Treatment Protocol. Medium to Strong cupping on the local points; Moving cupping on the inside and outside of the arm.

Prognosis. 50% pain reduction with 80% more movement was reported by the patient.

- ESR 1h: from 11 mm/h to 8 mm/h. Reduction of 37%
- ESR 2h: from 28 mm/h to 16 mm/h. Reduction of 75%

CASE Male Patient Aged 54 (M.B.)

Complaints/Symptoms. He has been suffering from constant upper back and chest (ribs) pain. Ten years ago he was diagnosed with rheumatoid arthritis. He is on maximum pain tablets.

Pulse. Liver pulse, strong and slippery.

Tongue. Purple-red body and slightly swollen.

TCM Diagnosis. Blood and Liver-Qi stagnation.

Treatment Protocol. Medium to Strong cupping on BL-11 and BL-17. Light to Medium cupping on the local chest points.

Prognosis. At the end of the course he noticed considerable pain reduction in the mornings, but still had pain towards the end of the day.

- ESR 1h: from 8 mm/h to 5 mm/h. Reduction of 60%
- ESR 2h: from 22 mm/h to 11 mm/h. Reduction of 100%

CASE Female Patient Aged 69 (P.Y.)

Complaints/Symptoms. Right knee pain for 4 years, slightly swollen, pain worse when walking.

Pulse. Very fine and thready.

Tongue. Dry with red body.

TCM Diagnosis. Yin Xu (deficiency) with Hot Bi syndrome.

Treatment Protocol. Medium to Strong cupping.

Prognosis. Patient reported 50% reduction of her symptoms.

- ESR 1h: from 22 mm/h to 11 mm/h. Reduction of 100%
- ESR 2h: from 45 mm/h to 21 mm/h. Reduction of 114%

CASE Female Patient Aged 59 (C.Y.)

Complaints/Symptoms. Gets tired and out of breath on effort. Upper back and shoulder pain for 6 years.

Medical History. She had had an angioplasty due to an arterial blockage.

Medication. Aspirin, atenolol and simvastatin.

Treatment Protocol. Light to Medium cupping on LI-15, GB-21, BL-11, BL-15 and BL-17.

Prognosis. Patient reported 60% reduction in her symptoms.

- ESR 1h: from 16 mm/h to 8 mm/h. Reduction of 100%
- ESR 2h: from 44 mm/h to 16 mm/h. Reduction of 175%

CASE 16-5 Female Patient Aged 56 (A.Y.)

Complaints/Symptoms. She has been complaining of left shoulder and left shoulder blade pain for 14 months. She describes the pain as 'moving pain'.

Pulse. Rapid and faint at all levels.

Tongue. Pale, slightly swollen.

TCM Diagnosis. Cold-Damp Bi syndrome

Treatment Protocol. Total of six treatments (every other day). Medium cupping method on LI-14, LI-15, SI-10, SI-11 and on the ashi points.

Treatment Time. Starting from 10 minutes (first visit) and increasing to 20 minutes (last visit).

Prognosis. Patient reported 40% reduction in her symptoms.

- ESR 1 h: from 15 mm/h to 13 mm/h. Reduction of 15%
- ESR 2 h: from 38 mm/h to 28 mm/h. Reduction of 35%

CASE 16-6 Female Patient Aged 26 (S.A.)

Complaints/Symptoms. Pain in the knees, shoulders and neck; also feeling tired most of the time. Symptoms have become worse in the last 6 months.

Medical History. She is diagnosed as anaemic. She has a 'normal periods, but very painful the second day'. Her appetite is good. Her facial appearance is quite pale.

Medication. She has been taking low-dose steroid tablets together with painkillers.

TCM Diagnosis. Severe Blood and Qi Xu leading to exhaustion and pain.

Treatment Protocol. Empty (flash) cupping on the entire back for 5 minutes only.

Prognosis. Patient reported 30% reduction in her symptoms.

- ESR 1 h: from 16 mm/h to 14 mm/h. Reduction of 14%
- ESR 2 h: from 33 mm/h to 19 mm/h. Reduction of 73%

Research Study 2   The Effects of Cupping Therapy on the Plasma Concentration of Inflammatory Mediators (Unpublished Research Findings)

Ilkay Zihni Chirali / Roslyn Gibbs / Mark Bovey

(This paper was accepted for a 'poster presentation' at the Society for Acupuncture Research 2007 Conference in Baltimore, MD, USA.)

ABSTRACT

Methods. 14 individuals presenting with a range of chronic musculoskeletal complaints were recruited into the study. Full informed consent was obtained from each subject. A traditional diagnosis (TD) was then performed on each subject by Ilkay Chirali and the cupping treatment strategy was determined accordingly (Light, Medium, Strong, Needle). Each patient then received six cupping treatments at weekly intervals. Prior to the first treatment, and thereafter at weekly intervals, subjects completed a MYMOP (Measure Yourself Medical Outcome Profile) questionnaire in order to assess clinical outcome. Venous blood samples were also obtained before treatment, after three treatments, after six treatments and 6 weeks post treatment. The following analyses were performed on blood samples: full blood count, haemoglobin concentration, erythrocyte sedimentation rate (ESR), serum concentration of fibrinogen, C-reactive protein (CRP), immunoglobulin G (IgG) and ferritin. Serum samples were also analysed for the concentration of inflammatory cytokines (interleukins [IL-1β, IL-6, IL-10] and tumour necrosis factor alpha [TNF-α]). Data obtained were analysed by one-way ANOVA with matched values and Dunnett's Multiple Comparisons Test using Instat2 software.

Results and conclusion. Nine females (aged 23–52 years) and five males (aged 37–62 years) were recruited into the study. One female participant subsequently withdrew from the study at week 3. The TDs performed indicated that patients presented with either Empty, Mixed or Full conditions.

The MYMOP questionnaires, completed by subjects at weekly intervals, indicated that 95% of the subjects reported improvements in their symptoms as a result of treatment and, overall, this improvement was found to be significant.

Complete data sets from blood and serum analysis (before, during and after treatment) were obtained for 11 subjects. The 6-week post-treatment follow-up was 54%. Analysis of data revealed statistically significant increases in the platelet count ($p = 0.0373$) and lymphocyte count ($p = 0.0001$), and decreases in the serum concentration of fibrinogen ($p = 0.0008$) and ferritin ($p = 0.0024$). Ferritin and fibrinogen are inflammatory markers and their reduction during cupping therapy is concomitant with a reduction in the inflammatory status of the patient. Platelets and lymphocytes may increase as a result of local vascular damage from the cupping therapy itself or from a reduction in the adherence of these cells to areas of activated endothelium, associated with inflammation. No changes were measured in the serum concentration of pro-inflammatory cytokines, with the exception of one patient where slight increases above normal levels were seen in TNF-α, IL-6 and IL-10 concentrations. Analysis of the MYMOP questionnaire for this patient suggested that this transient increase in pro-inflammatory cytokine levels correlated with a worsening of symptoms. However, towards the end of the trial the patient reported an improvement in their symptoms, which corresponded to a reduction in plasma cytokine concentration. Interestingly no significant change in the ESR was observed in these subjects. However, only three subjects presented with an elevated ESR before treatment, and these did show a reduction during the course of treatment.

Although the precise mechanism by which cupping therapy exerts its therapeutic effects cannot be determined from this study, the results indicate that cupping therapy is associated with significant changes in the levels of inflammatory cells and soluble markers, which suggests that this treatment can influence the inflammatory status of the patient leading to improved clinical outcome and that this effect therefore warrants further investigation (Fig. 16-1, Tables 16.2 and 16.3).

INTRODUCTION

Cupping is a therapeutic technique employed by many acupuncturists to treat Full, Mixed or Deficiency conditions. Despite its documented effectiveness, however, little is known from a Western scientific standpoint about the mechanisms by which cupping therapy yields its effects. In 2005, Ilkay Chirali published the results of a small trial conducted on 6 patients with musculoskeletal complaints. In this study, patients were treated every 2 days over a 2-week period and blood samples were taken and analysed before, during and after the treatment period. Analysis of the samples revealed a significant

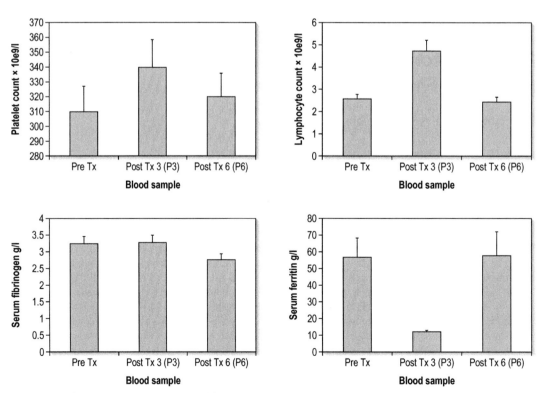

FIGURE 16-1 Changes in the platelet count ($p < 0.05$), lymphocyte count ($p = 0.05$) serum concentration of fibrinogen ($p < 0.001$) and ferritin ($p < 0.001$).

TABLE 16-2			MYMOP Results on Inflammatory Status of 14 Patients					
	Gender	Age	Complaint and Symptoms	Duration	TCM Diagnosis	Treatment	Medication	MYMOP
Pt 1	FM	26	L shoulder and neck pains+burning sensation	5 years	Bi syndrome Qi+Yin Xu	Light–Med cupping	Codeine Stopped medication	Symptom 1: 4-3-3-2-2-1 Symptom 2: 2-2-2-2-1 Activity: 4-4-2-2-2 Wellbeing: 2-2-2-2-2
Pt 2	FM	38	Lower-back pain+feeling hot	8 months	K-Qi+ Yin Xu	Med–Light cupping	None	Symptom 1: 4-4-4-3-3-2 Symptom 2: ------------ Activity: 6-6-6-6-6-6 Wellbeing: 3-2-5-5-5-3
Pt 3	FM	48	L hip pain+burning sensation	5 years+	Blood Xu K-Yang Xu Blood stasis	Light–Med cupping	Voltarol	Symptom 1: 3-3-3-5-3-1 Symptom 2: 5-4-4-4-3-3 Activity: 5-5-4-5-4-3 Wellbeing: 3-2-3-4-3-3
Pt 4	FM	49	R shoulder pain,+R sciatica pain	5 years	D-Heat Bi	Needle cupping Med cupping	Nurofen	Symptom 1: 4-4-4-3-2-1 Symptom 2: 4-3-5-2-2-1 Activity: 3-3-4-3-2-1 Wellbeing: 3-2-3-3-3-3
Pt 5	M	56	Achilles tendon pain+R toe swelling with pain	8 months	Bi syndrome	Needle cupping Moving cupping	None	Symptom 1: 5-5-5-3-4-4 Symptom 2: 5-6-5-4-4-3 Activity: 5-5-5-4-4-4 Wellbeing: 2-2-2-2-2-2
Pt 6	FM	52	Neck and shoulder pain	30 years	Yin Xu+ Bi syndrome	Medium cupping	Ramipril+ Zoton	Symptom 1: 5-3-3-1-2-1 Symptom 2: 5-3-3-1-1-1 Activity: 4-5-5-1-1-1 Wellbeing: 1-1-1-1-1-1
Pt 7	FM	51	R foot pain and stiffness	8-9 months	Liv-Qi stagnation+ Yin Xu	Needle cupping Med cupping	HRT+ Ramipril	Symptom 1: 2-2-2-3-2-1 Symptom 2: 3-1-3-3-2-2 Activity: 2-2-3-2-1-1 Wellbeing: 3-2-4-4-2-1
Pt 8	M	39	Poor balance when walking+lower back stiffness and pain	3 years	D-Heat+ K-Qi Xu	Med cupping+ Moving cupping	None	Symptom 1: 6-5-4-3-3-3 Symptom 2: 6-5-4-3-3-3 Activity: 5-5-4-2-3-3 Wellbeing: 0-0-0-0-0-0
Pt 9	FM	49	Osteoarthritis -upper back at T12 level	12 months D-Ht+	Yin Xu	Med cupping on Bladder channel	Glucosa- mine sulphate	Symptom 1: 4-1-3-2-4-1 Symptom 2: 3-1-1-4-2-1 Activity: 5-1-4-2-3-2 Wellbeing: 2-1-21-5-1
Pt 10	M	62	Lower back pain+R sciatica pain	4–5 years	K-Qi Xu	Med cupping Moving cupping	None	Symptom 1: 4-3-3-2-4-3 Symptom 2: 3-2-2-2-3-2 Activity: 4-2-2-1-3-2 Wellbeing: 1-1-1-1-1-4
Pt 11	FM	45	Lower back pains+stiffness across the back	8 years	Qi Xu	Cupping	None	Symptom1: 3-5-1-3-2-1 Symptom 2: 5-5-2-3-2-1 Activity: 4-5-2-2-2-1 Wellbeing: 3-3-2-2-2-1
Pt 12	M	53	Lower back pain with shooting pain inside leg	1 year	Blood+Qi stagnation	Med cupping	None	Symptom 1: 3-2-2-1-1-1 Symptom 2: 2-1-1-0-1-1 Activity: 3-2-1-1-1-0 Wellbeing: 3-3-3-1-1-1
Pt 13	M	37	R knee pain radiating to R calf muscle	1 year	Bi syndrome	Needle cupping	None	Symptom 1: 4-4-4-4-4 Symptom 2: 4-4-4-3-3 Activity: 4-4-4-4-3 Wellbeing: 3-3-2-3-3
Pt 14	FM	23	Both knees painful+lower back pain	5 years+	Blood+Qi Xu	Med cupping	None	Symptom 1: 2-5-2 Symptom 2: 4 Activity: 3-4 Wellbeing: 3

TABLE 16-3 Pathology Test Results for Portsmouth University Cupping Project

Date	Pt no.	Hb g/dL	RBC ×10¹²/L	WBC ×10⁹/L	Plt count ×10⁹/L	Neut ×10⁹/L	Lymph ×10⁹/L	Mono ×10⁹/L	Eos ×10⁹/L	Baso ×10⁹/L	ESR mm/h	Fibrinogen g/L	CRP mg/L	IgG screen g/L	Ferritin µg/L
06/11/2006	2	13.0	4.44	8.1	289	5.1	2.0	0.6	0.2	0.1	23	4.6	3	15.90	38.7
"	4	12.9	4.32	6.9	342	4.2	2.0	0.5	0.1	0.0	10	2.8	2	8.59	13.1
"	8	14.7	4.07	7.6	280	4.8	2.1	0.6	0.1	0.0	6	2.7	2	20.10	40.1
"	3	13.2	4.55	7.4	378	4.5	2.1	0.6	0.2	0.1	4	2.5	2	11.10	10.9
"	5	14.3	4.55	9.1	274	4.6	3.7	0.7	0.1	0.1	2	2.5	<1	10.60	172.6
"	6	13.9	4.24	9.5	265	6.0	2.9	0.5	0.1	0.0	8	3.4	4	13.50	78.7
"	7	13.7	4.44	10.6	268	7.2	2.6	0.7	0.1	0.1	4	3.3	3	12.90	92.6
07/11/2006	10	17.9	n/a	11.0	218	7.0	3.5	0.4	0.1	0.0	4	Insufficient	5	9.60	85.8
"	11	12.7	n/a	8.0	413	4.0	3.2	0.5	0.3	0.0	26	3.7	1	12.20	28.4
"	12	15.7	n/a	6.8	334	4.0	1.9	0.7	0.2	0.0	11	4.0	8	10.90	116.8
"	13	15.9	n/a	9.7	349	6.7	2.3	0.5	0.1	0.0	5	2.9	3	11.10	64.3
"	14	14.7	n/a	12.2	Clumped**	6.9	3.9	0.9	0.4	0.1	5	3.5	7	18.80	41.5
21/11/2006 &	2	12.4	4.24	6.4	258	4.7	1.1	0.6	0.0	0.0	27	4.5	60	14.50	66.6
22/22/2006	4	12.2	4.14	7.8	363	4.7	2.4	0.6	0.1	0.0	10	2.6	<5	8.78	12.6
"	8	14.4	4.38	6.3	320	3.7	2.0	0.5	0.0	0.0	6	2.9	2	18.90	36.4
"	3	12.7	4.46	9.3	488	6.6	2.0	0.3	0.3	0.1	5	2.6	<5	10.30	10.5
"	5	14.2	4.53	7.5	321	3.6	3.2	0.5	0.2	0.1	4	2.3	<1	9.70	147.9
"	6	14.5	4.46	7.6	295	4.4	2.6	0.5	0.1	0.0	8	4.0	5	13.10	82.4
"	7	13.2	4.34	9.8	346	6.8	2.2	0.7	0.1	0.1	6	3.5	<5	11.80	71.1
"	10	16.0	5.17	11.7	284	7.2	3.7	0.7	0.2	0.1	Clotted	Insufficient	<5	9.43	83.7
"	11	14.0	4.85	6.8	392	3.9	2.4	0.4	0.2	0.0	20	4.0	<5	12.90	19.3
"	12	15.7	4.59	7.2	339	4.4	2.0	0.6	0.2	0.0	4	3.2	2	12.20	132.9
"	13	14.8	4.76	11.3	336	8.5	1.9	0.8	0.1	0.0	6	3.2	8	9.90	59.4
"	14														
11/12/2006 &	9	12.6	4.30	4.7	373	2.6	1.8	0.3	0.0	0.0	16	3.7	4	8.60	104.8
12/12/2006	2	12.9	4.40	6.1	314	3.6	1.9	0.4	0.1	0.0	23	3.8	<5	17.60	27.8
"	4	12.5	4.24	7.4	346	4.9	1.9	0.5	0.1	0.0	8	2.4	<5	7.62	8.2
"	8	14.9	4.48	7.0	292	2.0	2.0	0.5	0.1	0.0	7	2.5	<5	22.30	150.2
"	3	12.8	4.45	6.9	393	4.2	2.0	0.4	0.2	0.0	5	1.9	<5	9.96	12.0
"	5	14.3	4.51	8.6	292	4.9	2.8	0.8	0.1	0.0	2	2.4	<5	8.97	????
"	6***	13.7	4.21	8.2	262	5.0	2.6	0.4	0.1	0.0	7	2.7	<5	9.61	72.3
"	7	13.7	4.45	9.9	280	6.6	2.5	0.7	0.1	0.0	2	3.3	<5	11.90	72.0
"	10	16.4	5.24	12.3	252	7.1	4.1	0.9	0.2	0.1	5	3.4	<5	9.27	74.3
"	11	13.0	4.52	8.4	416	4.8	2.9	0.5	0.2	0.0	23	2.9	8	13.90	15.5
"	12	16.0	4.60	5.7	359	3.0	1.8	0.6	0.2	0.1	8	3.3	<5	10.60	100.6
"	13	15.6	4.98	10.1	317	6.7	2.4	0.8	0.2	0.0	5	2.4	3	10.30	44.4
"	14														
"	9	13.2	4.50	4.6	383	2.5	1.8	0.3	0.0	0.0	14	3.1	<5	8.59	103.8

Normal ranges: CRP: <5 mg/mL; IgG: 5.4–16.1 g/L.
** Unsuitable for accurate count.
*** EDTA sample received unlabelled.

reduction in the erythrocyte sedimentation rate (ESR), a broad marker of inflammation. The aim of the current study was to identify inflammatory marker(s) whose plasma concentrations are altered during cupping therapy in the treatment of musculoskeletal disorders and which may account for changes in the ESR. This will provide biochemical evidence for the effectiveness of cupping therapy.

METHODS

Fourteen patients presenting with a range of chronic musculoskeletal complaints (diagnosed as Empty, Mixed and Full conditions) were recruited into the study. Full informed consent was obtained from each. A traditional diagnosis was then performed and the cupping treatment strategy determined accordingly. Each person then received six cupping treatments at weekly intervals. Prior to the first treatment and thereafter at weekly intervals, subjects completed a MYMOP questionnaire in order to assess clinical outcome. Venous blood samples were also obtained before treatment, after three treatments, after six treatments and 6 weeks post treatment. The following analyses were performed on blood samples: full blood count, haemoglobin concentration, erythrocyte sedimentation rate (ESR), serum concentration of fibrinogen, C-reactive protein (CRP), IgG and ferritin. Serum samples were also analysed for the concentration of inflammatory cytokines (IL-1β, IL-6, IL-10 and TNF-α). Data obtained were analysed by one-way ANOVA with matched values and Dunnett's Multiple Comparisons Test using Instat2 software.

RESULTS

Nine females (range 23–52 years) and 5 males (range 37–62 years) were recruited into the study. One female participant subsequently withdrew from the study at week 3. Analysis of MYMOP questionnaires indicated that 95% of patients reported improvements in their symptoms as a result of treatment and, overall, this improvement was found to significant.

Complete data sets from blood and serum analysis (before, during and after treatment) were obtained for 11 subjects. The 6-week post-treatment follow-up was 54%. Analysis of data revealed statistically significant increases in the platelet count ($p = 0.0373$) and lymphocyte count ($p = 0.0001$), and decreases in the serum concentration of fibrinogen ($p = 0.0008$) and ferritin ($p = 0.0024$). No changes were measured in the serum concentration of pro-inflammatory cytokines, with the exception of one patient where slight increases above normal levels were seen in TNF-α, IL-6 and IL-10 concentrations. Interestingly no significant change in the ESR was observed in these subjects, however, only three subjects presented with an elevated ESR before treatment.

DISCUSSION AND CONCLUSION

Ferritin and fibrinogen are inflammatory markers and their reduction during cupping therapy is concomitant with a reduction in the inflammatory status of the patient. Platelets and lymphocytes may increase as a result of local vascular damage from the cupping therapy itself or from a reduction in the adherence of these cells to areas of activated endothelium, which is associated with inflammation. With regard to the ESR, no overall significant change was observed in this study. However, only three patients presented with an elevated ESR prior to treatment. Furthermore, the ESR did decrease during the course of treatment in these subjects. In conclusion, although the precise mechanism by which cupping therapy exerts its therapeutic effects cannot be determined from the present study, the results indicate that cupping therapy is associated with significant changes in the levels of inflammatory cells and soluble markers, which suggests that this treatment can influence the inflammatory status of the patient leading to improved clinical outcome.

The Investigators

Ilkay Chirali is one of the foremost exponents of cupping in the UK and is the author of several publications on the subject. He has been a practitioner of acupuncture for over 20 years and currently practises from his clinic in Bexley Heath, Kent.

Dr Roslyn Gibbs, PhD is a Principal Lecturer in Biomedical Sciences at the University of Portsmouth where she specialises in immunology and molecular biology. She has been conducting research on aspects of immunology for approximately 14 years. She is also a practicing acupuncturist.

Mark Bovey is a practising acupuncturist and Co-ordinator of the Acupuncture Research Resource Centre at Thames Valley University. He is also a member of the British Acupuncture Council's Research Committee.

Dissemination of Research/Publications to Date

Poster presentation at the Society for Acupuncture Research (SAR) Conference, Baltimore, USA November 2007. Abstract from SAR presentation published in the *Journal of Complementary and Alternative Medicine*, Oct 2007, Vol 13. Invited presentation at the ARRC symposium, June 2008, London, UK. Powerpoint slides of this presentation will soon be available on the ARRC website.

Research Study 3   Cupping and Myofascial Pain Syndrome

Hossam Metwally

ABSTRACT

There is an increasing need to examine the effectiveness of traditional Chinese medicine and other alternative therapies for common conditions. However, little attention has been focused on cupping as a sole intervention for any illness.

Background. Cupping (Dry or Wet) has been used for a long time for treating acute and chronic illnesses including pain. Many doctors and practitioners in the field of pain management – including myself – have been using it as part of the management of several painful conditions; yet the effectiveness of this technique has not been evaluated according to Western standards.

Methods. A self-reported observational study of patients previously diagnosed with myofascial pain syndrome was conducted to investigate symptomatic improvement with Sliding (Dry) cupping. The objective was to evaluate the effectiveness of using cupping in clinical practice as a technique for managing myofascial pain syndrome and improving patients' quality of life.

Primary outcome measure: changes in the patients' quality of life using SF36 questionnaire. Secondary outcome measures: changes in anxiety and depression status using the Hospital Anxiety and Depression Score (HADS), changes in the pain interference with many variables according to the Brief Pain Inventory (BPI) score and changes in consumption of 'as-required' (PRN) pain medication as a result of cupping intervention.

Forty-two outpatients with myofascial pain syndrome, not previously treated with cupping and receiving treatment in the Chronic Pain Management Clinic, Diana Princess of Wales and Scunthorpe Hospitals, North East Lincolnshire and Goole NHS Trust were involved from January 2005 to March 2006. Each patient initially visited the therapist for an explanation, demonstration, discussion and to give consent. Each patient then visited the provider twice a week for 10 consecutive weeks. Only five to eight patients were assigned to each group and each could be seen twice per week; this entailed running the study over 15 months.

Different-sized plastic cups were applied according to the area of treatment and oil (baby oil) was used as a lubricant. The treatment was given twice a week for 3 to 20 minutes per session, the duration being guided by the appearance of the petechiae.

After the 10-week treatment, the effect was evaluated according to subjective symptoms, signs, and scores reported by the patients.

Initial and personal data were originally obtained from the Patient's Audit Collection System (PACS) in the pain service department. An average of HADS and BPI scores was calculated for every patient in the study. Each patient filled in a baseline form for the SF36, HADS and BPI before commencing the study, whilst sitting in the clinic before the first session. 'As required' (PRN) pain medication was tabulated for each patient and an average consumption of medication per week was recorded initially. Each patient was also given a diary to record the PRN medication plus any event that may interfere with pain, with the date and time.

All scores from before and after the intervention were presented to the statistician in a spreadsheet using Microsoft Excel; where a simple paired t-test was performed. The mean, standard deviation, standard error of the mean, t value and P value were calculated.

Results. All patients enrolled in this study showed an overall improvement as follows: SF36–Physical Health Score (PHS) = 33%, Mental Health Score (MHS) = 32.2%; Hospital Anxiety and Depression Score (HADS)–anxiety (AN) = 37.9%, depression (DEP) = 40.3%; Visual Analogue Score now (VASn) = 39.5%; pain interfering with general activity (GA) = 44.8%, pain interfering with normal work (NW) = 42.9%, pain interfering with mood (Mo) = 42.1%, pain interfering with relations with others = 30.2%, pain interfering with sleep (S) = 62.1%, pain interfering with walking ability (WA) = 44.7%, pain interfering with enjoyment with life (EOL) = 28%; PRN medications decreased by 56.2%.

Conclusion. Use of cupping (Dry, Sliding) technique to improve the condition of myofascial pain syndrome has shown promising results. The result obtained from this simple work suggests that cupping could have a place in the management of myofascial pain syndrome.

INTRODUCTION: EXAMINING THE EFFECT OF CUPPING ON THE MANAGEMENT OF MYOFASCIAL PAIN SYNDROME

There is an increasing need to examine the effectiveness of TCM and other alternative therapies for common conditions; however, little attention has focused on cupping as a sole intervention for any illness. Many patients in the pain clinic repeatedly report a pleasant experience after visiting complementary therapy practitioners as private clients and, amongst the interventions used, 'acupuncture' and 'cupping' have received the highest praises. Cupping (Dry or Wet) has been used for a long time for treating acute and chronic illnesses including pain. Wet cupping has been reported by many practitioners, as well as patients, to be particularly effective in such conditions as headache, migraine, trigeminal neuralgia, cervicobrachial syndrome, frozen shoulder, tennis elbow, sciatica, lower back pain and osteoarthritis; Sliding cupping has been reported to be effective in conditions such as myofascial pain as well as sciatica, lower back pain and general wellbeing.

In traditional terminology, its main effects are dredging the meridian system, activating Qi and removing Blood stasis. However, to the Western-trained physician, the diagnostic categories of traditional Chinese medicine (TCM) can appear mystifying and frequently seem to obfuscate more than clarify. Often, the conditions referred to in TCM appear to be bizarre descriptions of things considered irrelevant in conventional practice. Qi and Blood stagnation/excess/deficiency is a case in point. As physicians, we are confronted regularly with patients who have a mixture of chronic pain, numbness, or paraesthesias in association with and overlapping such systemic symptoms as fatigue, frustration and general malaise. Despite the best of intentions, physicians often have little idea how to categorize such patients, and such diagnostic confusion does not help formulate a coherent treatment plan.

Many doctors and practitioners in the field of pain management – including myself – have been using cupping as part of the management of several painful conditions; yet the effectiveness of this technique has not yet been evaluated according to Western standards. In this study, Dry cupping (Sliding technique) was offered to 50 patients suffering from myofascial pain syndrome. The aim was to evaluate its effect on their symptoms and their general health status. Forty-two patients agreed to try the technique and enrolled in a 10-week intervention. Twenty sessions in total were given to each patient, with two sessions taking place per week. The effect was evaluated as differences or changes in 'general health status' represented by SF36[1] questionnaire and 'psychological status' according to the Hospital Anxiety and Depression Score (HADS). The influence of pain on their normal 'daily life activities' was assessed by the Brief Pain Inventory (BPI). The consumption of pain-relieving medication was monitored to detect any increase or decrease in consumption due to the intervention.

METHODS

Objectives

- To probe into symptomatic improvement of myofascial pain syndrome with Sliding (Dry) cupping
- To determine the relationship between improvement and the course of disease as well as many other variables
- To evaluate the effectiveness of using cupping in our clinical practice as a technique for managing myofascial pain and to improve the quality of life.

Study Type

Self-reported observation on patients previously diagnosed with myofascial pain syndrome.

Project Type

Process.

Basis of Proposal

High volume.

Perceived Benefits to the Patient

- To improve the quality of life and if possible improve the pain score and decrease the quantity of painkillers required.

Perceived Benefits to the Organization

- To decrease the number of visits to and dependency on the pain service
- To decrease the number of procedures or surgical interventions to alleviate pain
- To decrease the amount of painkillers required with their high cost and unwanted side-effects
- To decrease the cost of running the pain service, through the above three.

Perceived Benefits to the Community

- Possible speedy return to work for susceptible patients
- Less dependence on community social and financial help and support
- Individuals with 'better quality of life' are less of a psychological and social burden on the society.

Standards Agreed

- Improvement in the quality of life by 30% or more in at least 50% of patients, in whom their scores were 'average' or lower as represented by SF36 questionnaire
- Improvement in anxiety and depression by 30% or more in at least 50% of patients, in whom their scores were 'average' or higher as represented by Hospital Anxiety and Depression Score (HADS)
- Improvement in pain scores by 30% or more in at least 50% of patients, in whom their scores were 'average' or higher as represented by Visual Analogue Score (VAS)
- Improvement in the degree of interference of pain in various aspects of daily life by 30% or more in at least 50% of patients, in whom their scores were 'average' or higher as represented by the Brief Pain Inventory Score (BPI)
- Decrease the rescue (PRN [pro re nata – i.e. as required]) medication required by 30% or more in at least 50% of patients.

References / Basis for Standards

Locally agreed standards.

Participants

A total of 42 outpatients with myofascial pain syndrome receiving treatment in the Chronic Pain Management Clinic, Department of Anaesthesia, Critical Care Division, Diana Princess of Wales and Scunthorpe Hospitals, North East Lincolnshire and Goole NHS trust were involved from January 2005 to March 2006.

Letters of invitation were sent to all adult patients with previously diagnosed myofascial pain syndrome who have been under the Chronic Pain Service in the Trust for 1 year or more, with no underlying pathology, and who met the following inclusion criteria.

INCLUSION CRITERIA

- Age between 18 and 70 years
- Still suffering from pain despite the use of medication and / or intervention.

EXCLUSION CRITERIA

- Patients with areas of skin that are inflamed, ulcerated, sores or have allergic skin conditions
- Cases of easy bleeding; pathological or if on any form of anticoagulant
- The abdominal area or lower back during pregnancy or in suspected pregnant ladies
- Areas on the face and cases of high fever and convulsions
- Patients with neurological symptoms or cramping
- Patients with signs of neuropathic pain
- Patients who have used cupping either currently or in the past.

PATIENT INTERVIEW. Patients who replied were invited to an interview with a member of the team.

PATIENT EXPECTATIONS. Patient expectations were analysed and no assurance was given regarding the result of the intervention.

Ethical Approval

Approval was obtained from the Directorate of Governance and Quality Improvement, supported by approval from the Audit Group within the trust.

Consent

All patients signed an informed consent form, after a detailed explanation about the proposed intervention. The consent form information highlighted the intended benefits and commonly occurring complications, for example 'marking'.

Patient's Explanation and Demonstration

- A demonstration was performed on a patient who had previously consented, or a volunteer from the newly recruited patients.
- The demonstration included technique, safety, maximum suction, maximum duration per treatment area, total duration per session and form filling.
- The aim was to give the patients an overall idea about cupping therapy and the degree of marking required for the intended benefit before they gave their consent.
- Pictures, diagrams and a plastic human skeleton were used during the demonstration.

Study Design

- Duration: 10 successive weeks of intervention
- Interval of intervention: twice per week
- Duration of each intervention: 3 to 20 minutes' cupping application depending on the degree of the petechiae produced
- Provider: I was the sole provider because I wanted to keep the intervention constant for all patients during all sessions.

Measurements

PRIMARY OUTCOME MEASURES
- Changes in functional health and wellbeing using the SF36 to identify the changes in physical health status (PHS) and mental health status (MHS).

SECONDARY OUTCOME MEASURES
- Changes in anxiety and depression status using the Hospital Anxiety and Depression Score (HADS)
- Changes in pain interference with many activities using the Brief Pain Inventory (BPI)
- Changes in PRN medication requirement due to cupping intervention.

EXTRA FINDINGS
- Reporting of any other findings that were not originally planned for.

Data Calculation, Analysis and Bias Prevention

- Double blinding was not appropriate in this type of intervention. The agreed blinding method to prevent bias was to prevent the study organizer and the provider from collecting or knowing the scores of any patient.
- The scoring of data was performed by two members of medical staff who are not part of the study group but had enough experience to perform calculations both manually (for HADS and PBI) and over the internet (for SF36). They had no contact with each other.
- Data were then recalculated by a third member of medical staff so as to establish whether there was any disparity between the first and second calculations.
- A different staff member designated the allocation of each patient's forms from 'before' and 'after' the intervention.

- Data calculation and analysis were performed by a member of the Department of Professional Development.
- Data statistical analysis was performed by a statistician from Sheffield University. The statistical output for the results and tables were provided in 'image' format with no possibility of editing results.

The Patient's Initial and Subsequent Visits

- Each patient initially visited the therapy provider for an explanation, demonstration, discussion and to give consent.
- Each patient then visited the provider twice a week for 10 consecutive weeks.
- Only five to eight patients were assigned to each group and each could be seen twice per week; this entailed running the study over 15 months.

Technique

EQUIPMENT

- Different-sized plastic cups were applied according to the area of treatment and oil (baby oil) was used as a lubricant.

INTERVENTIONS

- The patients were asked to position themselves in a relaxing prone or sitting position according to the site of intervention.
- Mechanical suction cupping – Sliding technique – was applied to the patient's affected painful area and/or tender points until petechiae appeared on the skin.
- The treatment was given twice a week for 3 to 20 minutes per session, the duration being guided by the appearance of the petechiae.
- After the 10-week treatment, the effect was evaluated according to subjective symptoms, signs, and the scores reported by the patients.

SAFETY

- The area of intervention was always prepared first.
- Each patient had his or her own private set of cups and was asked to bring them on every visit.
- Materials (size of cups, etc.) for each patient and each patient's condition were chosen before starting the cupping treatment.
- To ensure good hygiene, cups were checked to make sure there were no chips or cracks, and were cleaned.
- An appropriate suction pressure was determined; the rule was 'cupping should not hurt'.

Data Collection

- Initial and personal data were originally obtained from the Patient's Audit Collection System (PACS) in the pain service department. An average of the HADS and BPI scores was calculated for every patient in the study.
- Each patient filled in baseline SF36, HADS and BPI forms before commencing the study, whilst sitting in the clinic before the first session.
- PRN medication was recorded for each patient, with the initial average consumption per week.
- Patients were given a diary to record PRN medication plus any event that might have an effect on their pain, with a date and time.
- Each patient was twice allocated a number between 1 and 100, and his/her forms were identified only by these numbers. Two copies of each form were assigned to each patient, for 'before' and 'after' the intervention.

Data Calculations and Statistical Analysis

All scores, both baseline and post intervention, were presented to the statistician as a Microsoft Excel spreadsheet, in which a simple paired t-test was performed. The mean, standard deviation, standard error of the mean, t value and P value were calculated. (For initial patient analysis see Tables 16-4 to 16-12.)

TABLE 16-4 Gender of Patients

		Frequency	Percent	Valid Percent	Cumulative Percent
Valid	Female	16	38.1	38.1	38.1
	Male	26	61.9	61.9	100.0
	Total	42	100.0	100.0	

TABLE 16-5 Age of Patients

		Frequency	Percent	Valid Percent	Cumulative Percent
Valid	23	2	4.8	4.8	4.8
	25	1	2.4	2.4	7.1
	26	1	2.4	2.4	9.5
	27	2	4.8	4.8	14.3
	28	1	2.4	2.4	16.7
	29	1	2.4	2.4	19.0
	33	1	2.4	2.4	21.4
	34	2	4.8	4.8	26.2
	35	1	2.4	2.4	28.6
	36	2	4.8	4.8	33.3
	37	1	2.4	2.4	35.7
	39	2	4.8	4.8	40.5
	41	1	2.4	2.4	42.9
	42	1	2.4	2.4	45.2
	43	1	2.4	2.4	47.6
	44	1	2.4	2.4	50.0
	45	2	4.8	4.8	54.8
	46	3	7.1	7.1	61.9
	47	3	7.1	7.1	69.0
	48	3	7.1	7.1	76.2
	49	5	11.9	11.9	88.1
	54	2	4.8	4.8	92.9
	57	1	2.4	2.4	95.2
	58	1	2.4	2.4	97.6
	59	1	2.4	2.4	100.0
	Total	42	100.0	100.0	

TABLE 16-6 Patients' Duration of Pain

	< 2 yrs	2–<4 yrs	4–<6 yrs	6–<8 yrs	8–<10 yrs	10 yrs or more
Male	3	5	3	7	5	3
Female	3	2	4	3	0	4

TABLE 16-7 Patients' Duration in the Pain Clinic

	< 2 yrs	2–<4 yrs	4–<6 yrs	6–<8 yrs	8–<10 yrs	≥ 10 yrs
Male	5	4	8	5	4	0
Female	3	4	4	2	2	1

TABLE 16-8 Number of Regular Medications

	No Regular Medication	1 Regular Medication	2 Regular Medication	3 Regular Medication	4 Regular Medication	>4 Regular Medication
Male	0	3	6	7	2	8
Female	1	4	2	2	3	4

TABLE 16-9 Number of As Required (PRN) Medications

	No PRN Medication	1 PRN Medication	2 PRN Medication	3 PRN Medication	4 PRN Medication	>4 PRN Medication
Male	1	8	7	9	1	Nil
Female	1	4	2	2	3	4

TABLE 16-10 Number of Previous Procedures to Relieve Pain

	Nil	One	Two	Three	Four	>Four
Male	2	4	5	3	1	11
Female	2	2	2	0	4	6

TABLE 16-11 Baseline Patient Values: Paired Samples Statistics

		Mean	N	Std. Deviation	Std. Error Mean
Pair 1	ANa	8.50	42	2.725	.421
	ANb	13.71	42	3.424	.528
Pair 2	AVASa	4.05	42	1.561	.241
	AVASb	5.36	42	1.376	.212
Pair 3	DEPa	9.50	42	2.822	.435
	DEPb	15.88	42	2.752	.425
Pair 4	EOLa	5.12	42	1.966	.303
	EOLb	7.14	42	1.571	.242
Pair 5	GAa	3.95	42	1.847	.285
	GAb	7.14	42	1.539	.238
Pair 6	LVASa	3.00	42	1.913	.295
	LVASb	5.83	42	1.780	.275
Pair 7	MHSa	59.55	42	5.397	.833
	MHSb	45.00	42	7.622	1.176
Pair 8	Moa	4.07	42	2.017	.311
	Mob	7.12	42	1.953	.301
Pair 9	Nwa	4.12	42	2.144	.331
	NWb	7.21	42	1.389	.214
Pair 10	PHSa	57.93	42	6.190	.955
	PHSb	43.52	42	7.306	1.127
Pair 11	RWOa	4.60	42	1.726	.266
	RWOb	6.62	42	1.667	.257
Pair 12	Sa	3.00	42	1.562	.241
	Sb	8.05	42	1.710	.264
Pair 13	VASna	5.31	42	2.225	.343
	VASnb	7.45	42	1.565	.241
Pair 14	Waa	3.67	42	2.281	.352
	Wab	6.71	42	3.126	.482
Pair 15	WVASa	4.95	42	1.975	.305
	WVASb	7.98	42	1.522	.235

TABLE 16-12 Baseline Patient Values: Paired Samples Test

| | | | | | 95% CONFIDENCE INTERVAL OF THE DIFFERENCE | | | | |
		Mean	Std. Deviation	Std. Error Mean	Lower	Upper	t	df	P-value Sig. (2-tailed)
Pair 1	ANa - ANb	−5.2	2.0	.3	−5.8	−4.6	−17.156	41	.000
Pair 2	AVASa - AVASb	−1.3	1.5	.2	−1.8	−.9	−5.827	41	.000
Pair 3	DEPa - DEPb	−6.4	2.6	.4	−7.2	−5.6	−15.660	41	.000
Pair 4	EOLa - EOLb	−2.0	1.8	.3	−2.6	−1.5	−7.395	41	.000
Pair 5	GAa - GAb	−3.2	2.4	.4	−3.9	−2.4	−8.538	41	.000
Pair 6	LVASa - LVASb	−2.8	2.4	.4	−3.6	−2.1	−7.499	41	.000
Pair 7	MHSa - MHSb	14.5	5.2	.8	12.9	16.2	18.100	41	.000
Pair 8	Moa - Mob	−3.0	2.5	.4	−3.8	−2.3	−8.032	41	.000
Pair 9	Nwa - NWb	−3.1	2.2	.3	−3.8	−2.4	−9.183	41	.000
Pair 10	PHSa - PHSb	14.4	5.5	.8	12.7	16.1	17.043	41	.000
Pair 11	RWOa - RWOb	−2.0	1.8	.3	−2.6	−1.5	−7.176	41	.000
Pair 12	Sa - Sb	−5.0	2.3	.4	−5.8	−4.3	−13.936	41	.000
Pair 13	VASna - VASnb	−2.1	2.0	.3	−2.8	−1.5	−6.920	41	.000
Pair 14	Waa - Wab	−3.0	2.3	.4	−3.8	−2.3	−8.414	41	.000
Pair 15	WVASa - WVASb	−3.0	1.9	.3	−3.6	−2.4	−10.212	41	.000

RESULTS (SEE TABLES 16-13 TO 16-34)

Fifty patients were contacted initially; eight patients were excluded for different reasons. Each patient was randomly allocated two numbers, representing before and after intervention respectively. The practitioner was blinded as to the numbers corresponding to each patient.

Adherence to the Protocol

Adherence to the protocol was as follows:

- Filling out the forms (SF36, HADS, BPI): 100%
- Attending the cupping intervention sessions: 87%
- Recording PRN medication: 92%
- Recording any abnormal events: 79%.

Number of Patients Replied

Total: 42.

DISCUSSION

This study ran for 15 months. Every effort was made to ensure that patients would complete the 10-week course of cupping intervention.

Fifty patients were initially selected and interviewed. After an extensive discussion and explanation, eight patients were excluded. The main reason for this was the amount of marking that cupping causes (five patients), others were: expecting to conceive within the next few weeks or months (one young female) and an appointment for an elective surgical procedure within the next 2 months (two patients, with cholecystectomy and routine gynaecological procedures respectively) where interruption of cupping intervention and administration of analgesia, as well as the use of an anticoagulant as a prophylactic against deep vein thrombosis, would be unavoidable.

What Is the Overall Change due to Cupping Intervention?

It was agreed that the percentage of the improvement or deterioration would be calculated as: the change according to the intervention, divided by the initial score multiplied by a hundred (change/initial score×100). Table 16-13 represents the overall improvement or deterioration according to the intervention.

TABLE 16-13	Percentage of Overall Changes in Questionnaire Scores
Variable	**% of Change**
SF36 physical health status (PHS)	33
SF36 mental health status (MHS)	32.2
Anxiety (AN)	37.9
Depression (DEP)	40.3
Visual Analogue Score now (VASn)	39.5
Least Visual Analogue Score (LVAS)	48.2
Worst Visual Analogue Score (WVAS)	37.6
Average Visual Analogue Score (AVAS)	24.2
Pain interfering with general activity (GA)	44.8
Pain interfering with normal work (NW)	42.9
Pain interfering with mood (Mo)	42.1
Pain interfering with relation with others (RWO)	30.2
Pain interfering with sleep (S)	62.1
Pain interfering with walking ability (WA)	44.7
Pain interfering with enjoyment of life (EOL)	28

According to the statistical results, there were significant overall changes due to cupping intervention. From Table 16-13, the primary outcome measure, reflected by scores in the SF36 questionnaire showed a degree of improvement in physical health status (PHS) and mental health status (MHS) by 14.4 out of 70 (33%) and 14.5 out of 70 (32.2%), respectively, with standard deviations (st.d.) of 5.5 and 5.2, respectively. In simple terms this improvement, if applied evenly to the patient with the lowest physical and mental scores (31 out of 70) would shift the patient from having severe physical and mental impairment to a near average score.

Other values also showed high improvement markers; for example, the anxiety score improved, out of 21, by 5.2 (37.9%) and the depression score improved, out of 21, by 6.4 (40.3%) with standard deviations of 2.0 and 2.6 respectively. The mean anxiety and depression scores before the intervention were 13.71 and 15.8 out of 21 respectively; these are categorised as moderate to severe anxiety and depression. The improved scores achieved post intervention would be categorised as minor or insignificant in both cases.

The pain score also showed some improvement. For the Visual Analogue Scores (VAS) before and after the intervention (VASn) the improvement was 2.1 (39.5%), while the least VAS (LVAS) and the worst VAS (WVAS) improved by 2.8 and 3.0 (38.2% and 37.6%), respectively.

Pain interfering with general activity (GA) and normal work (NW) improved, out of 10, by 3.2 and 3.1 (44.8% and 42.9%) respectively. Mood (Mo) and enjoyment of life (EOL) scores also improved (out of 10) by 3.0 and 2.0 (42.1% and 28%), respectively, as did scores for normal work (NW) which improved by 3.1(42.9%), and walking ability (WA), which improved by 3.0 (44.7%). However, the best improvement was in the sleep score, which showed an improvement of 5.0 (62.1%) after the intervention. The p value was significant (less than 0.05) for all scores.

Which Gender Responded Better to the Intervention (Tables 16-14 to 16-17)?

It was notable from the initial scores before the intervention that female patients had slightly higher scores of anxiety and depression (14.1 and 16.3 respectively) compared with male patients (13.4 and 15.6). The improvement after cupping intervention amongst female patients was slightly better than in male patients. Anxiety and depression scores improved by 5.6 (39.7%) and 6.7 (41.4%) in female patients, compared with 4.9 (36.8%) and 6.1 (39.4%) in male patients.

The Visual Analogue Scores showed marked improvement in both genders, with a better response in the female patients as noted from the results:

VAS improvement: Female = 2.6 (34%); male = 1.8 (25.2%)
Least VAS improvement: Female = 3.4 (56.6%); male = 2.4 (43.2%)
Worst VAS improvement: Female = 4.0 (48.1%); male = 2.3 (30.9%).

However, the improvement of physical and mental health status measured by the SF36 showed almost no difference between male and female patients:

PHS: Female = 14.5 (33.8%); male = 14.3 (32.7)
MHS: Female = 15.7 (36.9%); male = 13.8 (29.8%).

TABLE 16-14   Overall Changes due to Cupping Intervention in Female Patients: Paired Samples Statistics[a]

		Mean	N	Std. Deviation	Std. Error Mean
Pair 1	ANa	8.50	16	3.011	.753
	ANb	14.13	16	3.594	.898
Pair 2	AVASa	3.81	16	1.601	.400
	AVASb	5.50	16	1.932	.483
Pair 3	DEPa	9.56	16	2.555	.639
	DEPb	16.31	16	2.845	.711
Pair 4	EOLa	5.00	16	1.713	.428
	EOLb	7.38	16	1.258	.315
Pair 5	GAa	3.50	16	1.826	.456
	GAb	7.63	16	1.258	.315
Pair 6	LVASa	2.63	16	2.187	.547
	LVASb	6.06	16	1.731	.433
Pair 7	MHSa	58.44	16	5.189	1.297
	MHSb	42.69	16	7.735	1.934
Pair 8	Moa	3.81	16	1.974	.493
	Mob	7.88	16	1.258	.315
Pair 9	Nwa	3.81	16	1.642	.410
	NWb	7.19	16	1.328	.332
Pair 10	PHSa	57.38	16	6.937	1.734
	PHSb	42.88	16	8.302	2.075
Pair 11	RWOa	4.63	16	1.821	.455
	RWOb	7.13	16	1.408	.352
Pair 12	Sa	2.75	16	1.238	.310
	Sb	8.44	16	1.209	.302
Pair 13	VASna	5.06	16	2.175	.544
	VASnb	7.69	16	1.621	.405
Pair 14	Waa	3.38	16	2.062	.515
	Wab	7.31	16	2.626	.656
Pair 15	WVASa	4.38	16	2.094	.523
	WVASb	8.44	16	1.459	.365

[a]Gender = Female

TABLE 16-15   Overall Changes due to Cupping Intervention in Female Patients: Paired Samples Test[a]

		PAIRED DIFFERENCES							
					95% CONFIDENCE INTERVAL OF THE DIFFERENCE				
		Mean	Std. Deviation	Std. Error Mean	Lower	Upper	t	df	Sig. (2-tailed)
Pair 1	ANa - ANb	−5.625	2.062	.515	−6.724	−4.526	−10.914	15	.000
Pair 2	AVASa - AVASb	−1.688	1.401	.350	−2.434	−.941	−4.818	15	.000
Pair 3	DEPa - DEPb	−6.750	2.793	.698	−8.238	−5.262	−9.668	15	.000
Pair 4	EOLa - EOLb	−2.375	1.928	.482	−3.402	−1.348	−4.928	15	.000
Pair 5	GAa - GAb	−4.125	1.893	.473	−5.134	−3.116	−8.716	15	.000
Pair 6	LVASa - LVASb	−3.438	2.159	.540	−4.588	−2.287	−6.368	15	.000
Pair 7	MHSa - MHSb	15.750	4.450	1.112	13.379	18.121	14.158	15	.000
Pair 8	Moa - Mob	−4.063	1.692	.423	−4.964	−3.161	−9.605	15	.000
Pair 9	Nwa - NWb	−3.375	1.928	.482	−4.402	−2.348	−7.003	15	.000
Pair 10	PHSa - PHSb	14.500	6.229	1.557	11.181	17.819	9.311	15	.000
Pair 11	RWOa - RWOb	−2.500	1.506	.376	−3.302	−1.698	−6.642	15	.000
Pair 12	Sa - Sb	−5.688	1.493	.373	−6.483	−4.892	−15.237	15	.000
Pair 13	VASna - VASnb	−2.625	1.668	.417	−3.514	−1.736	−6.294	15	.000
Pair 14	Waa - Wab	−3.938	1.806	.452	−4.900	−2.975	−8.720	15	.000
Pair 15	WVASa - WVASb	−4.063	1.526	.382	−4.876	−3.249	−10.648	15	.000

[a]Gender = Female

TABLE 16-16 Overall Changes due to Cupping Intervention in Male Patients: Paired Samples Statistics[a]

		Mean	N	Std. Deviation	Std. Error Mean
Pair 1	ANa	8.50	26	2.596	.509
	ANb	13.46	26	3.361	.659
Pair 2	AVASa	4.19	26	1.550	.304
	AVASb	5.27	26	.919	.180
Pair 3	DEPa	9.46	26	3.023	.593
	DEPb	15.62	26	2.714	.532
Pair 4	EOLa	5.19	26	2.136	.419
	EOLb	7.00	26	1.744	.342
Pair 5	GAa	4.23	26	1.840	.361
	GAb	6.85	26	1.642	.322
Pair 6	LVASa	3.23	26	1.728	.339
	LVASb	5.69	26	1.828	.358
Pair 7	MHSa	60.23	26	5.509	1.080
	MHSb	46.42	26	7.339	1.439
Pair 8	Moa	4.23	26	2.065	.405
	Mob	6.65	26	2.171	.426
Pair 9	Nwa	4.31	26	2.413	.473
	NWb	7.23	26	1.451	.285
Pair 10	PHSa	58.27	26	5.800	1.138
	PHSb	43.92	26	6.764	1.327
Pair 11	RWOa	4.58	26	1.701	.334
	RWOb	6.31	26	1.761	.345
Pair 12	Sa	3.15	26	1.736	.341
	Sb	7.81	26	1.939	.380
Pair 13	VASna	5.46	26	2.284	.448
	VASnb	7.31	26	1.543	.303
Pair 14	Waa	3.85	26	2.428	.476
	Wab	6.35	26	3.393	.666
Pair 15	WVASa	5.31	26	1.850	.363
	WVASb	7.69	26	1.517	.298

[a]Gender = Male

TABLE 16-17 Overall Changes due to Cupping Intervention in Male Patients: Paired Samples Test[a]

		PAIRED DIFFERENCES			95% CONFIDENCE INTERVAL OF THE DIFFERENCE				
		Mean	Std. Deviation	Std. Error Mean	Lower	Upper	t	df	Sig. (2-tailed)
Pair 1	ANa - ANb	−4.962	1.907	.374	−5.732	−4.191	−13.263	25	.000
Pair 2	AVASa - AVASb	−1.077	1.468	.288	−1.670	−.484	−3.742	25	.001
Pair 3	DEPa - DEPb	−6.154	2.572	.504	−7.193	−5.115	−12.200	25	.000
Pair 4	EOLa - EOLb	−1.808	1.674	.328	−2.484	−1.132	−5.507	25	.000
Pair 5	GAa - GAb	−2.615	2.562	.503	−3.650	−1.580	−5.204	25	.000
Pair 6	LVASa - LVASb	−2.462	2.580	.506	−3.504	−1.419	−4.864	25	.000
Pair 7	MHSa - MHSb	13.808	5.579	1.094	11.554	16.061	12.621	25	.000
Pair 8	Moa - Mob	−2.423	2.671	.524	−3.502	−1.344	−4.626	25	.000
Pair 9	Nwa - NWb	−2.923	2.348	.461	−3.872	−1.975	−6.347	25	.000
Pair 10	PHSa - PHSb	14.346	5.091	.998	12.290	16.402	14.370	25	.000
Pair 11	RWOa - RWOb	−1.731	1.971	.387	−2.527	−.935	−4.478	25	.000
Pair 12	Sa - Sb	−4.654	2.697	.529	−5.743	−3.564	−8.798	25	.000
Pair 13	VASna - VASnb	−1.846	2.167	.425	−2.721	−.971	−4.344	25	.000
Pair 14	Waa - Wab	−2.500	2.502	.491	−3.511	−1.489	−5.095	25	.000
Pair 15	WVASa - WVASb	−2.385	1.878	.368	−3.143	−1.626	−6.475	25	.000

[a]Gender = Male

Female patients showed a better response than male patients in all other scores, as noted from the results. These differences were more marked (almost twice as much) in general activity, mood and relations with others, but improvements in females were still higher than in males in walking ability, normal work, enjoyment of life and sleep.

What Pain Site / Sites Is / are Most Responsive to the Intervention?

The data on distribution of pain sites are summarized in Tables 16-18 to 16-20. The five main sites identified were: neck, shoulder(s), upper back, lower back and sacroiliac joint, while the sixth was considered as a mix of any of the above.

The results summarized in Tables 16-21 to 16-33 indicate that the response to the intervention was variable from site to site (e.g. the best improvement in VAS scores, pain affecting mood, relations with others and enjoyment of life were in the patients with neck pain). Their VAS scores were initially around average, but they responded significantly to the intervention. While walking ability scores notably decreased in those patients (by 64.2%), this should not be considered significant because their initial score was below average (4.67 out of 10).

TABLE 16-18　Site of Pain in Female Patients[a]

		Frequency	Percent	Valid Percent	Cumulative Percent
Valid	Neck	2	12.5	12.5	12.5
	Shoulders	1	6.3	6.3	18.8
	Upper back	1	6.3	6.3	25.0
	Lower back	5	31.3	31.3	56.3
	Mix of two or more of the above	7	43.8	43.8	100.0
	Total	16	100.0	100.0	

[a]Gender = Male

TABLE 16-19　Site of Pain in Male Patients[a]

		Frequency	Percent	Valid Percent	Cumulative Percent
Valid	Neck	1	3.8	3.8	3.8
	Shoulders	5	19.2	19.2	23.1
	Upper back	2	7.7	7.7	30.8
	Lower back	7	26.9	26.9	57.7
	Sacroiliac region	3	11.5	11.5	69.2
	Mix of two or more of the above	8	30.8	30.8	100.0
	Total	26	100.0	100.0	

[a]Gender = Male

TABLE 16-20　Site of Pain in all Patients

		Frequency	Percent	Valid Percent	Cumulative Percent
Valid	Neck	3	7.1	7.1	7.1
	Shoulders	6	14.3	14.3	21.4
	Upper back	3	7.1	7.1	28.6
	Lower back	12	28.6	28.6	57.1
	Sacroiliac region	3	7.1	7.1	64.3
	Mix of two or more of the above	15	35.7	35.7	100.0
	Total	42	100.0	100.0	

TABLE 16-21 Response to the Intervention According to Site of Pain – Neck: Paired Samples Statistics[a]

		Mean	N	Std. Deviation	Std. Error Mean
Pair 1	ANa	7.00	3	4.359	2.517
	ANb	11.00	3	4.583	2.646
Pair 2	AVASa	2.67	3	2.082	1.202
	AVASb	4.33	3	.577	.333
Pair 3	DEPa	8.33	3	4.163	2.404
	DEPb	13.00	3	2.000	1.155
Pair 4	EOLa	3.00	3	1.000	.577
	EOLb	7.33	3	2.082	1.202
Pair 5	GAa	2.67	3	1.155	.667
	GAb	7.00	3	1.000	.577
Pair 6	LVASa	1.33	3	2.309	1.333
	LVASb	5.00	3	1.000	.577
Pair 7	MHSa	63.00	3	4.000	2.309
	MHSb	50.00	3	2.646	1.528
Pair 8	Moa	2.67	3	2.517	1.453
	Mob	6.00	3	2.000	1.155
Pair 9	Nwa	3.33	3	1.528	.882
	NWb	7.00	3	1.000	.577
Pair 10	PHSa	61.00	3	4.583	2.646
	PHSb	46.67	3	4.041	2.333
Pair 11	RWOa	3.00	3	1.000	.577
	RWOb	7.33	3	1.155	.667
Pair 12	Sa	2.00	3	.000	.000
	Sb	8.67	3	2.309	1.333
Pair 13	VASna	3.33	3	2.517	1.453
	VASnb	6.00	3	1.000	.577
Pair 14	Waa	1.67	3	1.528	.882
	Wab	4.67	3	4.163	2.404
Pair 15	WVASa	2.33	3	2.309	1.333
	WVASb	7.00	3	1.732	1.000

[a]Site of pain = Neck

TABLE 16-22 Response to the Intervention According to Site of Pain – Neck: Paired Samples Test[a]

		PAIRED DIFFERENCES			95% CONFIDENCE INTERVAL OF THE DIFFERENCE				
		Mean	Std. Deviation	Std. Error Mean	Lower	Upper	t	df	Sig. (2-tailed)
Pair 1	ANa - ANb	−4.000	1.000	.577	−6.484	−1.516	−6.928	2	.020
Pair 2	AVASa - AVASb	−1.667	1.528	.882	−5.461	2.128	−1.890	2	.199
Pair 3	DEPa - DEPb	−4.667	2.309	1.333	−10.404	1.070	−3.500	2	.073
Pair 4	EOLa - EOLb	−4.333	1.528	.882	−8.128	−.539	−4.914	2	.039
Pair 5	GAa - GAb	−4.333	2.082	1.202	−9.504	.838	−3.606	2	.069
Pair 6	LVASa - LVASb	−3.667	2.517	1.453	−9.918	2.585	−2.524	2	.128
Pair 7	MHSa - MHSb	13.000	1.732	1.000	8.697	17.303	13.000	2	.006
Pair 8	Moa - Mob	−3.333	2.082	1.202	−8.504	1.838	−2.774	2	.109
Pair 9	Nwa - NWb	−3.667	2.309	1.333	−9.404	2.070	−2.750	2	.111
Pair 10	PHSa - PHSb	14.333	4.509	2.603	3.132	25.535	5.506	2	.031
Pair 11	RWOa - RWOb	−4.333	2.082	1.202	−9.504	.838	−3.606	2	.069
Pair 12	Sa - Sb	−6.667	2.309	1.333	−12.404	−.930	−5.000	2	.038
Pair 13	VASna - VASnb	−2.667	1.528	.882	−6.461	1.128	−3.024	2	.094
Pair 14	Waa - Wab	−3.000	3.000	1.732	−10.452	4.452	−1.732	2	.225
Pair 15	WVASa - WVASb	−4.667	.577	.333	−6.101	−3.232	−14.000	2	.005

[a]Site of pain = Neck

TABLE 16-23 Response to the Intervention According to Site of Pain – Shoulders: Paired Samples Statistics[a]

		Mean	N	Std. Deviation	Std. Error Mean
Pair 1	ANa	8.33	6	1.506	.615
	ANb	14.17	6	.408	.167
Pair 2	AVASa	5.00	6	1.789	.730
	AVASb	5.67	6	1.506	.615
Pair 3	DEPa	9.33	6	1.366	.558
	DEPb	16.67	6	2.338	.955
Pair 4	EOLa	4.33	6	1.862	.760
	EOLb	6.00	6	1.673	.683
Pair 5	GAa	5.17	6	1.602	.654
	GAb	5.83	6	2.639	1.078
Pair 6	LVASa	4.67	6	2.160	.882
	LVASb	5.50	6	1.871	.764
Pair 7	MHSa	60.17	6	4.355	1.778
	MHSb	43.33	6	8.892	3.630
Pair 8	Moa	4.50	6	2.429	.992
	Mob	6.00	6	3.286	1.342
Pair 9	Nwa	4.67	6	2.251	.919
	NWb	7.00	6	2.191	.894
Pair 10	PHSa	59.00	6	5.292	2.160
	PHSb	45.83	6	8.280	3.380
Pair 11	RWOa	4.67	6	1.862	.760
	RWOb	5.83	6	2.401	.980
Pair 12	Sa	3.67	6	2.251	.919
	Sb	7.33	6	2.805	1.145
Pair 13	VASna	6.00	6	1.897	.775
	VASnb	7.67	6	1.211	.494
Pair 14	Waa	3.00	6	2.608	1.065
	Wab	3.67	6	3.327	1.358
Pair 15	WVASa	5.83	6	1.472	.601
	WVASb	7.83	6	1.602	.654

[a]Site of pain = Shoulders

TABLE 16-24 Response to the Intervention According to Site of Pain – Shoulders: Paired Samples Test[a]

| | | PAIRED DIFFERENCES | | | | | | | |
| | | | | | 95% CONFIDENCE INTERVAL OF THE DIFFERENCE | | | | |
		Mean	Std. Deviation	Std. Error Mean	Lower	Upper	t	df	Sig. (2-tailed)
Pair 1	ANa - ANb	−5.833	1.472	.601	−7.378	−4.289	−9.707	5	.000
Pair 2	AVASa - AVASb	−.667	2.066	.843	−2.834	1.501	−.791	5	.465
Pair 3	DEPa - DEPb	−7.333	2.805	1.145	−10.277	−4.390	−6.404	5	.001
Pair 4	EOLa - EOLb	−1.667	1.633	.667	−3.380	.047	−2.500	5	.054
Pair 5	GAa - GAb	−.667	3.327	1.358	−4.158	2.824	−.491	5	.644
Pair 6	LVASa - LVASb	−.833	3.656	1.493	−4.670	3.003	−.558	5	.601
Pair 7	MHSa - MHSb	16.833	5.492	2.242	11.069	22.597	7.507	5	.001
Pair 8	Moa - Mob	−1.500	3.782	1.544	−5.468	2.468	−.972	5	.376
Pair 9	Nwa - NWb	−2.333	2.733	1.116	−5.201	.534	−2.092	5	.091
Pair 10	PHSa - PHSb	13.167	8.727	3.563	4.008	22.325	3.695	5	.014
Pair 11	RWOa - RWOb	−1.167	2.858	1.167	−4.166	1.832	−1.000	5	.363
Pair 12	Sa - Sb	−3.667	4.367	1.783	−8.249	.916	−2.057	5	.095
Pair 13	VASna - VASnb	−1.667	2.251	.919	−4.029	.696	−1.814	5	.129
Pair 14	Waa - Wab	−.667	3.011	1.229	−3.827	2.493	−.542	5	.611
Pair 15	WVASa - WVASb	−2.000	2.000	.816	−4.099	.099	−2.449	5	.058

[a] Site of pain = Shoulders

TABLE 16-25 Response to the Intervention According to Site of Pain – Upper Back: Paired Samples Statistics[a]

		Mean	N	Std. Deviation	Std. Error Mean
Pair 1	ANa	8.33	3	4.163	2.404
	ANb	12.00	3	5.292	3.055
Pair 2	AVASa	4.33	3	.577	.333
	AVASb	7.00	3	2.646	1.528
Pair 3	DEPa	7.67	3	1.155	.667
	DEPb	18.00	3	1.732	1.000
Pair 4	EOLa	4.00	3	1.000	.577
	EOLb	6.67	3	2.082	1.202
Pair 5	GAa	2.33	3	.577	.333
	GAb	7.33	3	2.309	1.333
Pair 6	LVASa	2.67	3	1.155	.667
	LVASb	7.33	3	3.055	1.764
Pair 7	MHSa	58.00	3	3.606	2.082
	MHSb	40.00	3	9.165	5.292
Pair 8	Moa	3.67	3	2.082	1.202
	Mob	6.00	3	3.464	2.000
Pair 9	Nwa	2.00	3	1.000	.577
	NWb	7.67	3	1.155	.667
Pair 10	PHSa	57.00	3	3.606	2.082
	PHSb	41.67	3	10.017	5.783
Pair 11	RWOa	4.00	3	1.000	.577
	RWOb	6.33	3	1.528	.882
Pair 12	Sa	1.67	3	.577	.333
	Sb	8.67	3	1.528	.882
Pair 13	VASna	4.67	3	1.528	.882
	VASnb	7.67	3	2.309	1.333
Pair 14	Waa	2.00	3	2.000	1.155
	Wab	4.00	3	5.292	3.055
Pair 15	WVASa	6.00	3	2.000	1.155
	WVASb	8.33	3	2.082	1.202

[a]Site of pain = Upper back

TABLE 16-26 Response to the Intervention According to Site of Pain – Upper Back: Paired Samples Test[a]

		PAIRED DIFFERENCES							
					95% CONFIDENCE INTERVAL OF THE DIFFERENCE				
		Mean	Std. Deviation	Std. Error Mean	Lower	Upper	t	df	Sig. (2-tailed)
Pair 1	ANa - ANb	−3.667	1.55	.667	−6.535	−.798	−5.500	2	.032
Pair 2	AVASa - AVASb	−2.667	3.055	1.764	−10.256	4.922	−1.512	2	.270
Pair 3	DEPa - DEPb	−10.333	1.528	.882	−14.128	−6.539	−11.717	2	.007
Pair 4	EOLa - EOLb	−2.667	3.055	1.764	−10.256	4.922	−1.512	2	.270
Pair 5	GAa - GAb	−5.000	1.732	1.000	−9.303	−.697	−5.000	2	.038
Pair 6	LVASa - LVASb	−4.667	4.163	2.404	−15.009	5.676	−1.941	2	.192
Pair 7	MHSa - MHSb	18.000	6.083	3.512	2.890	33.110	5.125	2	.036
Pair 8	Moa - Mob	−2.333	1.528	.882	−6.128	1.461	−2.646	2	.118
Pair 9	Nwa - NWb	−5.667	1.528	.882	−9.461	−1.872	−6.425	2	.023
Pair 10	PHSa - PHSb	15.333	6.506	3.756	−.829	31.496	4.082	2	.055
Pair 11	RWOa - RWOb	−2.333	2.082	1.202	−7.504	2.838	−1.941	2	.192
Pair 12	Sa - Sb	−7.000	1.000	.577	−9.484	−4.516	−12.124	2	.007
Pair 13	VASna - VASnb	−3.000	3.606	2.082	−11.957	5.957	−1.441	2	.286
Pair 14	Waa - Wab	−2.000	3.464	2.000	−10.605	6.605	−1.000	2	.423
Pair 15	WVASa - WVASb	−2.333	3.215	1.856	−10.319	5.652	−1.257	2	.336

[a]Site of pain = Upper back

TABLE 16-27 Response to the Intervention According to Site of Pain – Lower Back: Paired Samples Statistics[a]

		Mean	N	Std. Deviation	Std. Error Mean
Pair 1	Ana	8.42	12	2.392	.690
	ANb	14.17	12	3.040	.878
Pair 2	AVASa	3.83	12	1.403	.405
	AVASb	5.08	12	.793	.229
Pair 3	DEPa	9.83	12	2.623	.757
	DEPb	15.33	12	3.055	.882
Pair 4	EOLa	5.33	12	1.670	.482
	EOLb	7.08	12	1.165	.336
Pair 5	GAa	4.17	12	1.899	.548
	GAb	7.00	12	.853	.246
Pair 6	LVASa	2.67	12	1.723	.497
	LVASb	5.75	12	1.215	.351
Pair 7	MHSa	61.67	12	3.798	1.096
	MHSb	46.67	12	5.758	1.662
Pair 8	Moa	4.08	12	2.065	.596
	Mob	7.75	12	.965	.279
Pair 9	Nwa	4.17	12	1.642	.474
	NWb	7.08	12	.900	.260
Pair 10	PHSa	59.08	12	5.452	1.574
	PHSb	45.50	12	6.544	1.889
Pair 11	RWOa	4.75	12	1.422	.411
	RWOb	6.42	12	.996	.288
Pair 12	Sa	2.58	12	.996	.288
	Sb	7.67	12	1.155	.333
Pair 13	VASna	5.08	12	2.503	.723
	VASnb	7.25	12	1.658	.479
Pair 14	Waa	4.75	12	2.137	.617
	Wab	8.50	12	1.314	.379
Pair 15	WVASa	4.92	12	2.151	.621
	WVASb	8.08	12	1.165	.336

[a]Site of pain = Lower back

TABLE 16-28 Response to the Intervention According to Site of Pain – Lower Back: Paired Samples Test[a]

		PAIRED DIFFERENCES			95% CONFIDENCE INTERVAL OF THE DIFFERENCE				
		Mean	Std. Deviation	Std. Error Mean	Lower	Upper	t	df	Sig. (2-tailed)
Pair 1	ANa - ANb	−5.750	2.006	.579	−7.024	−4.476	−9.931	11	.000
Pair 2	AVASa - AVASb	−1.250	.965	.279	−1.863	−.637	−4.486	11	.001
Pair 3	DEPa - DEPb	−5.500	2.023	.584	−6.785	−4.215	−9.420	11	.000
Pair 4	EOLa - EOLb	−1.750	1.288	.372	−2.568	−.932	−4.706	11	.001
Pair 5	GAa - GAb	−2.833	1.586	.458	−3.841	−1.826	−6.189	11	.000
Pair 6	LVASa - LVASb	−3.083	1.564	.452	−4.077	−2.089	−6.828	11	.000
Pair 7	MHSa - MHSb	15.000	4.452	1.285	12.171	17.829	11.672	11	.000
Pair 8	Moa - Mob	−3.667	2.146	.620	−5.030	−2.303	−5.918	11	.000
Pair 9	Nwa - NWb	−2.917	1.832	.529	−4.081	−1.753	−5.515	11	.000
Pair 10	PHSa - PHSb	13.583	4.522	1.305	10.710	16.456	10.406	11	.000
Pair 11	RWOa - RWOb	−1.667	1.073	.310	−2.348	−.985	−5.380	11	.000
Pair 12	Sa - Sb	−5.083	1.443	.417	−6.000	−4.166	−12.200	11	.000
Pair 13	VASna - VASnb	−2.167	2.082	.601	−3.489	−.844	−3.606	11	.004
Pair 14	Waa - Wab	−3.750	1.913	.552	−4.965	−2.535	−6.791	11	.000
Pair 15	WVASa - WVASb	−3.167	1.992	.575	−4.433	−1.901	−5.506	11	.000

[a]Site of pain = Lower back

TABLE 16-29 **Response to the Intervention According to Site of Pain – Sacroiliac Region: Paired Samples Statistics**[b]

		Mean	N	Std. Deviation	Std. Error Mean
Pair 1	ANa	8.33[a]	3	.577	.333
	ANb	12.33[a]	3	.577	.333
Pair 2	AVASa	5.00	3	1.000	.577
	AVASb	5.67	3	.577	.333
Pair 3	DEPa	10.33	3	1.155	.667
	DEPb	14.00	3	1.000	.577
Pair 4	EOLa	6.00	3	3.000	1.732
	EOLb	8.00	3	1.732	1.000
Pair 5	GAa	5.33	3	1.155	.667
	GAb	6.67	3	1.155	.667
Pair 6	LVASa	4.00	3	1.000	.577
	LVASb	5.33	3	1.528	.882
Pair 7	MHSa	61.67	3	5.033	2.906
	MHSb	50.67	3	1.528	.882
Pair 8	Moa	5.33	3	1.155	.667
	Mob	6.67	3	.577	.333
Pair 9	Nwa	5.33	3	2.517	1.453
	NWb	7.00	3	1.732	1.000
Pair 10	PHSa	57.67	3	4.726	2.728
	PHSb	44.67	3	8.327	4.807
Pair 11	RWOa	5.33	3	1.155	.667
	RWOb	6.00	3	1.732	1.000
Pair 12	Sa	3.67	3	1.528	.882
	Sb	5.67	3	2.082	1.202
Pair 13	VASna	5.33	3	1.155	.667
	VASnb	6.33	3	.577	.333
Pair 14	Waa	5.33[a]	3	.577	.333
	Wab	9.33[a]	3	.577	.333
Pair 15	WVASa	5.00	3	1.000	.577
	WVASb	7.33	3	1.528	.882

[a]The correlation and t cannot be computed because the standard error of the difference is 0.
[b]Site of pain = Sacroiliac region

TABLE 16-30 **Response to the Intervention According to Site of Pain = Sacroiliac Region: Paired Samples Statistics**

		PAIRED DIFFERENCES							
					95% CONFIDENCE INTERVAL OF THE DIFFERENCE				
		Mean	Std. Deviation	Std. Error Mean	Lower	Upper	t	df	Sig. (2-tailed)
Pair 2	AVASa - AVASb	-0.667	1.155	0.667	-3.535	2.202	-1.000	2	0.423
Pair 3	DEPa - DEPb	-3.667	2.082	1.202	-8.838	1.504	-3.051	2	0.093
Pair 4	EOLa - EOLb	-2.000	1.732	1.000	-6.303	2.303	-2.000	2	0.184
Pair 5	GAa - GAb	-1.333	2.309	1.333	-7.070	4.404	-1.000	2	0.423
Pair 6	LVASa - LVASb	-1.333	2.309	1.333	-7.070	4.404	-1.000	2	0.423
Pair 7	MHSa - MHSb	11.000	4.359	2.517	0.172	21.828	4.371	2	0.049
Pair 8	Moa - Mob	-1.333	1.528	0.882	-5.128	2.461	-1.512	2	0.270
Pair 9	Nwa - NWb	-1.667	2.887	1.667	-8.838	5.504	-1.000	2	0.423
Pair 10	PHSa - PHSb	13.000	4.583	2.646	1.616	24.384	4.914	2	0.039
Pair 11	RWOa - RWOb	-0.667	0.577	0.333	-2.101	0.768	-2.000	2	0.184
Pair 12	Sa - Sb	-2.000	1.732	1.000	-6.303	2.303	-2.000	2	0.184
Pair 13	VASna - VASnb	-1.000	1.732	1.000	-5.303	3.303	-1.000	2	0.423
Pair 15	WVASa - WVASb	-2.333	2.309	1.333	1.333	3.404	-1.75	2	0.222

TABLE 16-31   Response to the Intervention According to Site of Pain – Mix of two or more of the above: Paired Samples Statistics[a]

		Mean	N	Std. Deviation	Std. Error Mean
Pair 1	Ana	9.00	15	3.229	.834
	ANb	14.33	15	4.082	1.054
Pair 2	AVASa	3.87	15	1.598	.413
	AVASb	5.27	15	1.486	.384
Pair 3	DEPa	9.73	15	3.615	.933
	DEPb	16.53	15	2.696	.696
Pair 4	EOLa	5.73	15	2.052	.530
	EOLb	7.53	15	1.598	.413
Pair 5	GAa	3.60	15	1.920	.496
	GAb	7.87	15	1.187	.307
Pair 6	LVASa	2.80	15	1.859	.480
	LVASb	6.00	15	2.070	.535
Pair 7	MHSa	56.80	15	6.581	1.699
	MHSb	43.20	15	8.825	2.279
Pair 8	Moa	4.00	15	1.964	.507
	Mob	7.60	15	1.595	.412
Pair 9	Nwa	4.20	15	2.569	.663
	NWb	7.40	15	1.549	.400
Pair 10	PHSa	56.20	15	7.984	2.061
	PHSb	40.53	15	7.298	1.884
Pair 11	RWOa	4.73	15	2.154	.556
	RWOb	7.13	15	1.885	.487
Pair 12	Sa	3.40	15	1.724	.445
	Sb	8.87	15	.743	.192
Pair 13	VASna	5.73	15	2.344	.605
	VASnb	8.00	15	1.558	.402
Pair 14	Waa	3.47	15	2.232	.576
	Wab	6.93	15	2.463	.636
Pair 15	WVASa	4.93	15	1.870	.483
	WVASb	8.20	15	1.740	.449

[a]Site of pain = Mix of two or more of the above

TABLE 16-32   Response to the Intervention According to Site of Pain – Mix of two or more of the above: Paired Samples Test[a]

		PAIRED DIFFERENCES							
					95% CONFIDENCE INTERVAL OF THE DIFFERENCE				
		Mean	Std. Deviation	Std. Error Mean	Lower	Upper	t	df	Sig. (2-tailed)
Pair 1	ANa - ANb	−5.333	2.350	.607	−6.635	−4.032	−8.789	14	.000
Pair 2	AVASa - AVASb	−1.400	1.183	.306	−2.055	−.745	−4.583	14	.000
Pair 3	DEPa - DEPb	−6.800	2.426	.626	−8.144	−5.456	−10.856	14	.000
Pair 4	EOLa - EOLb	−1.800	1.859	.480	−2.830	−.770	−3.749	14	.002
Pair 5	GAa - GAb	−4.267	1.907	.492	−5.323	−3.210	−8.664	14	.000
Pair 6	LVASa - LVASb	−3.200	1.859	.480	−4.230	−2.170	−6.666	14	.000
Pair 7	MHSa - MHSb	13.600	5.962	1.539	10.298	16.902	8.835	14	.000
Pair 8	Moa - Mob	−3.600	2.293	.592	−4.870	−2.330	−6.081	14	.000
Pair 9	Nwa - NWb	−3.200	2.042	.527	−4.331	−2.069	−6.068	14	.000
Pair 10	PHSa - PHSb	15.667	5.394	1.393	12.680	18.654	11.249	14	.000
Pair 11	RWOa - RWOb	−2.400	1.595	.412	−3.283	−1.517	−5.829	14	.000
Pair 12	Sa - Sb	−5.467	1.407	.363	−6.246	−4.687	−15.043	14	.000
Pair 13	VASna - VASnb	−2.267	1.831	.473	−3.281	−1.253	−4.795	14	.000
Pair 14	Waa - Wab	−3.467	1.885	.487	−4.510	−2.423	−7.124	14	.000
Pair 15	WVASa - WVASb	−3.267	1.624	.419	−4.166	−2.367	−7.789	14	.000

[a]Site of pain = Mix of two or more of the above

TABLE 16-33 Comparison of '% of Changes' in Different Pain Sites in Response to the Intervention

Variable	Neck (%)	Shoulder (%)	Upper Back (%)	Lower Back (%)	Sacroiliac (%)	Mix of any of the Above (%)	% of Total Change
PHS	30.7	28.7	36.8	29.8	29.1	38.6	33
MHS	26	38.8	45	32.1	21.7	31.5	32.2
AN	36.3	41	30.5	40.5	32.4	37.2	37.9
DEP	35.9	44	57.4	35.9	26.2	41.4	40.3
VASn	44.5	21.7	39.1	29.9	15.8	28.3	39.5
LVAS	73.3	15.1	63.7	53.6	25	53.3	48.2
WVAS	66.6	25.5	28	39.2	31.8	39.8	37.6
AVAS	38.4	11.7	38.1	24.6	11.8	26.6	24.2
GA	61.9	11.4	68.2	40.5	20	54.2	44.8
NW	52.3	33.3	73.9	41.2	23.8	43.2	42.9
Mo	55.5	25	38.9	47.3	20	47.4	42.1
RWO	59.1	20	36.9	25.9	11.1	33.7	30.2
S	76.8	50	80.7	66.3	35.2	61.6	62.1
WA	64.2	18.1	50	44.1	42.9	50	44.7
EOL	59	27.7	39.9	24.7	25	23.9	28

Patients with upper back pain showed the highest improvement in mental health status, depression score, general activity, normal work and sleep (see Table 16-33).

The sleep score showed the most improvement in all patients; it ranged from 35.2% in patients with sacroiliac pain to 80.7% in patients with upper back pain, with an average of 62.1% in all patients. Although patients with mixed pain and neck pain initially had the worst sleep scores, those with upper back pain reported the greatest improvement (7 out of 10) compared with those patients in the neck and mixed pain groups (6.6 and 5.4 out of 10 respectively).

Patients suffering from mixed pain demonstrated the best improvement in the physical health score (38.6%) and their anxiety scores, which improved by 37.2%; the improvement in anxiety was also greater in patients with shoulder pain (41%) compared with other patient groups. In most of the patients with mixed pain, the lower back and/or sacroiliac areas were involved. Physical improvement is reflected as a decrease in pain affecting walking ability (3.4 out of 10 = 50%) in this category of patients, as well as in patients with low back pain and sacroiliac pain (3.7 and 4.0 out of 10, = 44.1% and 42.9%, respectively).

The effect of cupping intervention on general activity scores for different pain sites needs some explanation. The best improvement was for the patients with upper back pain (5 out of 10 = 68.2%), whereas the change in patients with shoulder pain was almost unnoticeable (11.4%). This is because for the latter patients the pain did not initially interfere with the general activity as much as for those with neck pain or mixed pain (61.9% and 54.2%, respectively); accordingly there was not the room for noticeable improvement after the intervention.

Patients with upper back pain were the most depressed of the groups (score of 18 out of 21); after the intervention they also showed the greatest improvement (10.3 out of 21 = 57.4%).

It seems that pain affects each patient's score differently, depending on the site of pain and the quality of life that the patient used to have before suffering the pain. If he or she was young and active leading a normal life and had stopped some or all activities due to pain then the suffering level would be greater and the initial scores generally higher. Following the intervention, such a patient would respond better and the scores improve more than those of the other patients.

The greatest improvements in the mood score were in the patient groups with neck, lower back and mixed pain (more than 3 out of 10 on average, and 55.5, 47.3% and 47.4%, respectively); in contrast, the shoulder and upper back pain groups did not have such bad mood scores at baseline and their improvements were insignificant (25% and 20%, respectively).

Patients with upper back pain showed the most response in normal work scores. They had an initial score similar to the other groups (7 out of 10) but they showed a much greater improvement than the others (5.6 out of 10 = 73.9%).

Patients with lower back pain and mixed pain initially reported the worst mood scores (7.7 and 7.6 out of 10, respectively); after the intervention they responded very well and their scores improved by 47.3% and 47.4%, respectively.

In conclusion, all patients responded well to the intervention and this was reflected in all the scores as an improvement of more than 30%. The two exceptions were the average VAS (24.2%) and pain affecting enjoyment of life (28%). The simple explanation for this is that in most cases the average VAS is usually around the same or shows little difference, hence when statistical analysis is applied the percentage is small. Even so, the average VAS score was above average before the intervention (5.36 out of 10), but was below average after the intervention (4.05 out of 10) (see Table 16-33).

Overall Changes in PRN Medication per Week

In Table 16-34, the amount of PRN medication initially reported by all patients was 58.8 painkillers on average per patient per week: 50.8 for male patients and 71.7 for female patients. The highest consumption per week amongst the male patients was 76 tablets, whereas it was 116 tablets for the females. The lowest consumption was nil for both genders.

After the intervention, the average consumption per patient per week was 53.7 tablets (56.2% improvement). The average consumption for male patients was 22.7 tablets (55.4% improvement) whereas for females it was 31 tablets per week (56.8% improvement), thus giving an overall improvement of 55.9%.

What About Patients who Reported Deterioration in Pain Scores?

Only one male patient (number 20) reported deterioration in pain scores after the intervention, but noticeably his PRN medication had decreased during the same period by almost 50%. Anxiety and depression scores had also decreased by around 50%. His physical and mental health status showed a good improvement, from 37 to 58 and from 34 to 59 (out of 70) respectively. In the meantime, he carried on receiving cupping for 3 months after the intervention and his scores become as good as the rest of the group. So was this a delayed response? Or had the patient deliberately made the VAS score high for some reason (e.g. financial gain)? This idea is supported by the fact that his improved mental and physical health status was scored on the SF36 questionnaire, which uses indirect questions – unlike the BPI questionnaire, which uses direct questions!

Any Significant Events?

The patients did not report any important events during the intervention, and all the recorded events submitted to the study group revealed nothing of any significance. Possibly those events represented a big change to the individual patient who was able to perform a task that was not possible in the past, but nevertheless did not increase their painkiller consumption, nor did such events reflect badly on their overall scores.

Follow-up After 3, 6 and 9 Months

Twenty-six patients replied to the follow-up letter after a further 3 months; 12 of them were still having cupping on a regular basis. Six months after the end of the intervention, 16 patients replied of whom 5 were still using cupping. After 9 months, 9 patients further reported their scores, of whom 2 were still using cupping. Overall their improvement was reported as steady.

Those patients who did not continue using cupping did not specify an exact reason; most stated that they did not feel that they needed to maintain the treatment, as their condition was stable, while a few stated that they had forgotten about it! However, they all agreed that they would continue the therapy in the future if they felt the need to do so. Noticeably, however, those patients who did not continue

TABLE 16-34 **Changes of PRN Medication Per Week Due to the Intervention**					
	Total Male's Consumption Tablets Per Week	**Average Male's Consumption Tablets Per Week**	**Total Female's Consumption Tablets Per Week**	**Average Female's Consumption Tablets Per Week**	**Total All Patients Tablets Per Week**	**Average Per Patients Tablets Per Week**
Before	1321	50.8	1147	71.7	2468	58.8
After	591	22.7	497	31.1	1088	25.9
% of improvement	55.3	55.3	56.7	56.7	55.9	55.9

TABLE 16-35 Have we met the Standards?

Standards Agreed	Achieved
Improvement in quality of life by 30% or more in at least 50% of patients, in whom their scores were 'average' or lower, represented by SF36 questionnaire	**SF36:** Physical health score (PHS) = 33% Mental health score (MHS) = 32.2% In all patients
Improvement in anxiety and depression by 30% or more in at least 50% of patients, in whom their scores were 'average' or higher, represented by the Hospital Anxiety and Depression Score (HADS)	**HADS:** Anxiety = 37.9% Depression = 40.3% In all patients
Improvement in pain score by 30% or more in at least 50% of patients, in whom their scores were 'average' or higher represented by Visual Analogue Score (VAS)	**VAS** now = 39.5% In all patients
Improvement in the degree of interference of pain in various aspects of daily life by 30% or more in at least 50% of patients, in whom their scores were 'average' or higher, represented by the Brief Pain Inventory Score (BPI)	**BPI:** General activity = 44.8% Normal work = 42.9% Mood = 42.1% Relations with others = 30.2% Sleep = 62.1% Walking ability = 44.7% Enjoyment with life = 28% In all patients
Decrease the rescue (PRN) medication required by 30% or more in at least 50% of patients	**PRN medication:** Decreased by 56.2% In all patients

using cupping on a regular or as-required basis nevertheless reported a steady improvement in almost all scores. They also reported less PRN pain medication consumption compared with their requirement before commencing cupping treatment. Their scores were slightly higher than those immediately after the 10-week intervention.

Meanwhile, patients who continued using cupping on a regular or as-required basis stated that they continued using it because: (i) it made them 'feel better', or (ii) they 'were worried that the pain might come back', or (iii) they felt that they 'needed it as the pain was just starting again'. These statements are reflected in the scores the patients have reported and also in the PRN pain medications required: both have shown a slight increase in the overall scores after the 10 weeks of cupping – although they were still lower than the baseline scores.

Further Comments

Most, if not all, of the patients enjoyed the feeling of suction created by cupping. None of them complained of pain or discomfort due to the technique either during or after any session.

Have we Met the Agreed Standards?

Standards agreed upon and those achieved are compared in Table 16-35.

CONCLUSION

There is no stand-alone scoring system as a measure for the degree of pain or its influence on the patient's physical, mental or social status; this was always the challenge facing the chronic pain clinicians. To find an intervention or technique that proves useful in most aspects of a patient's life would be rather a dream, not a fact. Use of cupping (Dry, Sliding) technique to improve the condition of chronic myofascial pain syndrome has, however, shown promising results. The results obtained from this simple study suggest that cupping could have a place in the management of this condition. The improvement achieved by using cupping was actually higher than the standards originally agreed before the intervention (see Table 16-35). In fact, this improvement has been achieved whilst the consumption of PRN medication has decreased, which is another point in its favour.

If to this is added the simple fact that cupping is safe, non-painful, can be taught to and applied by non-medical professionals (relatives or friends) and can be used in the comfort of the patient's own home, it is then worth considering that this technique has a place in our practice.

It is well known amongst TCM practitioners that Wet cupping is more beneficial than the Dry technique. Wet cupping removes stagnant Blood from the body whereas the Dry technique moves it and frees the channels within the body. As the results of this study were achieved by using Dry cupping, it would be of interest to find out the magnitude of the effect of Wet cupping on the same patient groups. Nevertheless, additional prospective studies are needed to quantify the effectiveness of both Dry and Wet cupping and compare them with established Western approaches. Forthcoming studies should also critically analyse the costs of providing these techniques, to evaluate the financial benefits of the different interventions available.

(See also the Further Reading section at the end of the chapter for relevant studies and texts on myofascial pain syndrome.)

Research Study 4 A Systematic Literature Review of Clinical Evidence-Based Research

Hui-juan Cao / Jian-ping Liu

ABSTRACT

Background. Though cupping therapy has been used in China for thousands of years, there has been no systematic summary of clinical research on it. This review evaluates the therapeutic effect of cupping therapy using an evidence-based approach based on available clinical studies.

Methods. We included all clinical studies on cupping therapy for all kinds of diseases. We searched six electronic databases; all searches ended in December 2011. We extracted data on the type of cupping and type of diseases treated.

Results. 725 clinical studies published between 1958 and 2011 were identified, including 163 randomized controlled trials (RCTs), 30 clinical controlled trials, 419 case series, and 113 case reports. The number of RCTs has obviously increased during the last decades, but the quality of the RCTs has generally been poor, according to the risk of bias of the Cochrane standard for important outcomes within trials. The diseases in which cupping was commonly employed included herpes zoster, pain conditions, facial paralysis, etc. The meta-analysis showed that cupping therapy combined with other TCM treatments was significantly superior to other treatments alone in increasing the number of patients cured who were suffering from herpes zoster, facial paralysis, acne, cervical spondylosis, and prolapse of lumbar intervertebral disc. Wet cupping was used in the majority of studies, followed by Retained cupping, Moving cupping, Medicinal cupping, etc. No serious adverse effects were reported in the studies.

Conclusions. According to the above results, the quality and quantity of RCTs on cupping therapy in China appears to have improved over the past 50 years, and majority of studies show potential benefit on pain conditions, herpes zoster and other diseases. However, further rigorously designed trials in relevant conditions are warranted to support their use in practice.

INTRODUCTION

As was discussed in the early chapters of this book, cupping has been widely used in Chinese folk medicine, and the technique has been inherited by modern Chinese practitioners. In the 1950s, the clinical effect of cupping was confirmed by further research in China and acupuncturists from the former Soviet Union, and was established as an official therapeutic practice in hospitals all over the country. This activity substantially stimulated the development of further research into cupping.

As the process of systematically detecting, appraising and using contemporary research findings as the basis for clinical decision making, evidence-based medicine has been widely used in the health service and has served as a basis for achieving evidence-based practice in traditional medicine.[1]

Systematic review of well-designed randomized controlled trials is considered to be the top level of evidence. Five systematic reviews[2-6] on cupping therapy have so far been published, focusing respectively on pain conditions, stroke rehabilitation, hypertension and herpes zoster. The numbers of trials included in these reviews were quite small (between 1 and 8). Lee et al (2011)[7] conducted an overview of these five reviews and concluded that cupping is effective only as a treatment for pain, and even for this indication there are remaining doubts. Extensive searches did not find any further related reviews.

In the context of evidence-based medicine, we therefore need to evaluate therapeutic effect of cupping therapy by summarizing all available clinical evidence to inform this ancient practice.

METHODS

Objective

To evaluate the therapeutic effect of cupping therapy using an evidence-based approach on all available clinical studies.

Information Sources

We searched the China Network Knowledge Infrastructure (CNKI) (1911–1978, 1979–2011), Chinese Scientific Journal Database VIP (1989–2011), Wan Fang Database (1985–2011), Chinese Biomedicine (CBM) (1978–2011), PubMed (1966–2011) and the Cochrane Library (Issue 10, 2011), all the searches ended at December 2011. The search terms included 'cupping therapy', 'bleeding cupping', 'wet cupping', 'dry cupping', 'flash cupping', 'herbal cupping', 'moving cupping' or 'retained cupping'.

Selection Criteria

Any type of clinical studies were included – that is, randomized controlled trials (RCTs), clinical controlled trials (CCTs), case series (CSs), and case reports (CRs) identifying the therapeutic effect of cupping therapy, including one or more than two types of cupping methods, compared with no treatment, placebo or conventional medication. Combined therapy with cupping and other interventions compared with other interventions alone were also included. Cupping therapy combined with other TCM therapies (including acupuncture) compared with non-TCM therapies was excluded. There was no limitation on language and publication type. Multiple publications reporting the same patient data were excluded.

Data Extraction and Quality Assessment

The extracted data included authors and title of study, year of publication, study design (detail of randomization if the study was an RCT), type of disease, study size, age and sex of participants, type of cupping therapy, treatment process, detail of the control interventions, outcome (e.g. total effective rate) and adverse effect for each study. All data were extracted from the published studies.

Evidence from RCTs is considered as gold standard for therapeutic evaluation; we specifically evaluate the methodological quality of RCTs in this review. This assessment of methodological quality was carried out using criteria from the *Cochrane Reviewers' Handbook*.[8] We assessed studies according to the risk of bias for each important outcome within included trials, including adequacy of generation of the allocation sequence, allocation concealment, blinding and outcome reporting. The quality of all the included trials was categorized into low/unclear/high risk of bias. Trials that met all criteria were categorized to low risk of bias, trials that met none of the criteria were categorized to high risk of bias, and other trials were categorized to unclear risk of bias if insufficient information to make a judgement was acquired.

Data Analysis and Statistical Methods

Data were extracted using Microsoft Access, and all the information and data were transferred into Excel worksheet form for frequency calculation. The numbers of studies on cupping therapy were summarized by study type and publication date. The constituent ratio of types of cupping therapy and mapping of top 20 diseases/conditions treated by cupping therapy were reported. For RCTs, outcome data were summarized as risk ratios (RR) with 95% confidence intervals (CI) for binary outcomes, or mean difference (MD) with 95% CI for continuous outcomes. Revman5.0.20 software was used for data analysis. Meta-analysis was used to estimate the therapeutic effect of cupping therapy if the trials had a good homogeneity of study design, participants, interventions, control, and outcome measures. Publication bias was explored by funnel plot analysis.

RESULTS

Basic Information about Studies

After primary searches in six databases, 8328 citations were identified, of which the majority was excluded because of obvious ineligibility after reading the title/abstract; the full-text papers of 725 studies were then retrieved. All of these final 725 studies were included in this review, comprising 719 studies published in Chinese and 6 studies published in English (Fig. 16-2). All the included studies were published between 1958 and 2011, including 163 RCTs,[9-171] 30 CCTs, 419 CSs, and 113 CRs; 584 of these studies (80.55%) were published between 1994 and 2011, and the number of studies has obviously increased over the course of five decades (Fig. 16-3). The first RCT was published in 1993 and over half of them were reported between 2009 and 2011.

Amongst the included studies, 435 (59.72%) used Bleeding cupping as the main intervention, 130 (17.93%) used Retained cupping, 51 (7.17%) used Moving cupping, 34 studies (4.69%) used Medicinal cupping, 18 (2.34%) used Flash cupping, 5 (0.69%) used Water cupping, and 3 (0.41%) used Needle cupping; combined cupping that used at least two types of cupping method was used in 52 studies (7.03%) (Fig. 16-4).

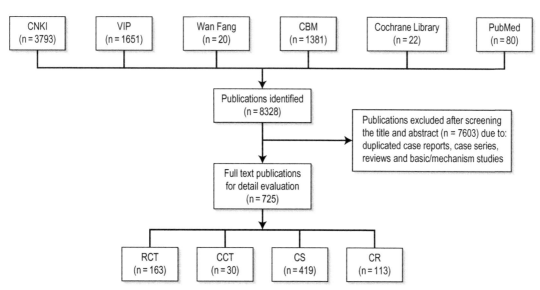

FIGURE 16-2 The process of study selection.

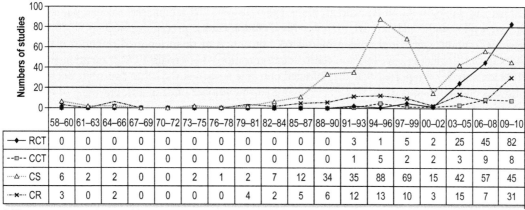

RCT: randomised controlled trial; CCT: clinical controlled trial; CS: case studies; CR: case report

FIGURE 16-3 Numbers of studies on cupping therapy by study type between 1958 and 2011.

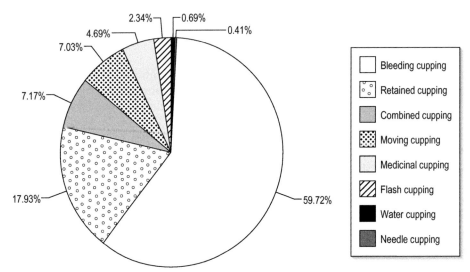

FIGURE 16-4 Constituent ratio of types of cupping therapy.

More than 50 kinds of diseases or symptoms were treated by cupping therapy, according to the included studies. The top 20 diseases/conditions in which cupping was commonly employed were herpes zoster (84 studies), pain conditions (including prolapse of lumbar intervertebral disc, non-specific lower back pain, etc. [62 studies]), cough or asthma (50 studies), acne (37 studies), facial paralysis (29 studies), common cold (24 studies), cervical spondylosis (22 studies), lateral femoral cutaneous neuritis (19 studies), lumbar sprain (18 studies), scapulohumeral periarthritis (18 studies), urticaria (13 studies), mastitis (11 studies), headache (11 studies), soft tissue injury (10 studies), arthritis (10 studies), neurodermatitis (8 studies), myofascitis (8 studies), wound and sinus (7 studies), Bi syndrome (Wind, Cold and Dampness invading the body [which is caused by changeable climate and alternate cold and heat, dwelling in damp places, wading or being caught in the rain] and lingering in channels and joints resulting in stagnation of Qi and Blood [6 studies]) and sciatica (5 studies). A further 273 studies were concerned with other diseases treated by cupping therapy (see Table 16-36, in Appendix).

Meta-analyses were conducted on five diseases/conditions: herpes zoster, facial paralysis (Bell's palsy), acne, cervical spondylosis and prolapse of lumbar intervertebral disc. (Characteristics of the RCTs involving these diseases are presented in Tables 16-37 to 16-41, in Appendix.) Due to the insufficient number of included trials and heterogeneity of the relevant RCTs of the remaining 15 diseases/conditions, meta-analyses could not be completed.

Methodological Quality of RCTs

According to our predefined quality criteria, all of the 163 included trials were evaluated as 'high risk of bias' (see Table 16-42, in Appendix). Six of the trials reported sample size calculation, including 3 that were pilot studies. Thirty-five trials described randomization procedures (such as random number table or computer-generated random numbers), but only 6 of them reported methods of allocation concealment (including envelope and central randomization). Four trials[14,53,109,116] mentioned blinding, of which only 2[53,109] reported that they blinded outcome assessors; the other two trials did not report who was blinded. Seven trials[9,41,51,84,93,135,136] reported the number of dropouts, but none of these used intention-to-treat analysis.

There were 124 (76.07%) trials that reported comparability of baseline data, 54 (33.13%) trials specified the inclusion criteria, 52 (31.90%) trials specified the exclusion criteria, and 124 (76.07%) trials described diagnostic criteria. The efficacy standard was reported in 154 (94.51%) trials, but 130 of these used composite outcome measures, which categorized treatment efficacy into four grades (cured, markedly effective, effective, and ineffective) according to changes in symptoms; the other 24 trials used a single outcome measure for therapeutic effect. Symptom changes were commonly used as outcome measures.

Estimated Effects of RCTs with Cupping

Due to the insufficient number of RCTs and the variations in study quality, participants, intervention, variable control, and outcome measures, the results of most of the studies could not be synthesized by quantitative methods. Although 161 of the 163 included studies showed that cupping therapy, as well as cupping combined with another treatment, was significantly effective for certain diseases (see Table 16-43, in Appendix), interpretation of the positive findings from these individual studies needs to be incorporated with the clinical characteristics of the included studies and the evidence power. Therefore, the reported beneficial effects of cupping therapy need to be confirmed by large and rigorously designed RCTs. In this study we conducted meta-analyses to evaluate therapeutic effect of cupping therapies only for herpes zoster, facial paralysis, acne, cervical spondylosis and prolapse of lumbar intervertebral disc (see Table 16-41).

Estimated Effects of RCTs with Cupping for Herpes Zoster

In a meta-analysis of 22 RCTs to evaluate the efficacy of Wet cupping therapy for herpes zoster, Wet cupping was found to be superior to pharmaceutical medications, such as antivirals, in effecting a cure (RR 2.05, 95%CI 1.80 to 2.34, $p<0.00001$, 7 trials, $I^2 = 22\%$, fixed model) (Fig. 16-5), and in lowering the incidence rate of post-herpetic neuralgia (RR 0.12, 95%CI 0.06 to 0.28, $p<0.00001$, 4 trials, $I^2 = 0\%$, fixed model).[18,20,29,32,35,39,45,48,68,70–72,78,88,92,95,109,120,121,143,148,169] Eight trials reported the number of patients with improved symptoms; five of them showed Wet cupping to be better than medication on this outcome, though the application of meta-analysis was inadequate due to heterogeneity of these trials ($I^2 = 91\%$). Wet cupping in combination with pharmaceutical medication was significantly better than medication alone in effecting a cure (RR 1.64, 95%CI 1.27 to 2.13, $p=0.0002$, 7 trials, $I^2 = 78\%$, random model), but no difference in symptom improvement was observed (RR 1.03, 95%CI 0.98 to 1.08, $p=0.30$, 5 trials, $I^2 = 66\%$, random model) (Fig. 16-6). Wet cupping combined with acupuncture was superior to acupuncture alone, both in effecting a cure (RR 1.65, 95%CI 1.08 to 2.53, $p=0.02$, 3 trials, $I^2 = 49\%$, random model) and in improving symptoms (RR 1.13, 95%CI 1.01 to 1.26, $p=0.02$, 3 trials, $I^2 = 0\%$, fixed model). Four trials reported the average cure time as an outcome; the meta-analysis showed Wet cupping used singly (MD –0.69, 95%CI –1.08 to –0.30, $p=0.0006$, 2 trials, $I^2 = 0\%$, fixed

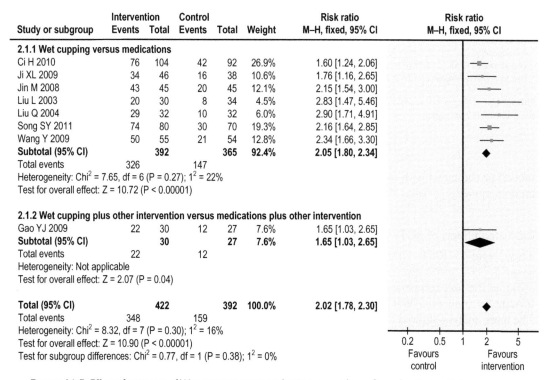

FIGURE 16-5 Effect of estimates of Wet cupping versus medication on numbers of cured patients with herpes zoster.

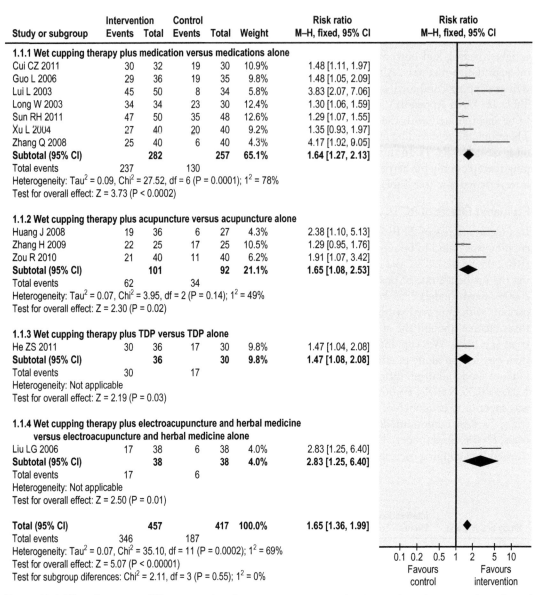

FIGURE 16-6 Effect of estimates of Wet cupping plus other interventions versus other interventions alone on numbers of cured patients with herpes zoster.

model) or combined with medication (MD −3.30, 95%CI −6.16 to −0.43, $p = 0.02$, 2 trials, $I^2 = 68\%$, random model) was better than medication alone in reducing average time to cure.

Estimated Effects of RCTs with Cupping for Facial Paralysis

There were 19 RCTs that assessed the therapeutic effect of cupping therapy for facial paralysis.[25,28,41,42,52,55–57,66,80,82,87–89,93,104,155,163,171] Two of these trials[51,56] were excluded from the meta-analysis owing to the non-comparability of their treatment and control groups. Six trials used Flash cupping therapy, 10 trials used Wet cupping, and 1 trial used Medicinal cupping as the main intervention. The meta-analysis showed Flash cupping combined with acupuncture (RR 1.42, 95%CI 1.23 to 1.65, $p < 0.00001$, 5 trials, $I^2 = 0\%$, fixed model) and Wet cupping combined with acupuncture (RR 1.56, 95%CI 1.34 to 1.83, $p < 0.00001$, 8 trials, $I^2 = 0\%$, fixed model) were markedly better than acupuncture alone in effecting a cure (Fig. 16-7). In addition, cupping in combination with medication (such as neurotrophic drugs) was superior to medication alone in reducing the average time to cure (MD −6.05, 95%CI −9.83 to −2.27, $p = 0.002$, 2 trials, random model).

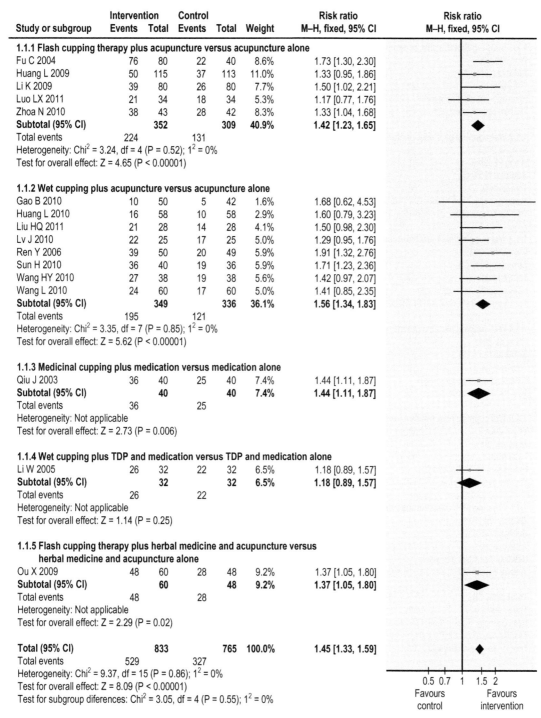

Study or subgroup	Intervention Events	Total	Control Events	Total	Weight	Risk ratio M–H, fixed, 95% CI
1.1.1 Flash cupping therapy plus acupuncture versus acupuncture alone						
Fu C 2004	76	80	22	40	8.6%	1.73 [1.30, 2.30]
Huang L 2009	50	115	37	113	11.0%	1.33 [0.95, 1.86]
Li K 2009	39	80	26	80	7.7%	1.50 [1.02, 2.21]
Luo LX 2011	21	34	18	34	5.3%	1.17 [0.77, 1.76]
Zhoa N 2010	38	43	28	42	8.3%	1.33 [1.04, 1.68]
Subtotal (95% CI)		**352**		**309**	**40.9%**	**1.42 [1.23, 1.65]**
Total events	224		131			

Heterogeneity: Chi^2 = 3.24, df = 4 (P = 0.52); I^2 = 0%
Test for overall effect: Z = 4.65 (P < 0.00001)

1.1.2 Wet cupping plus acupuncture versus acupuncture alone						
Gao B 2010	10	50	5	42	1.6%	1.68 [0.62, 4.53]
Huang L 2010	16	58	10	58	2.9%	1.60 [0.79, 3.23]
Liu HQ 2011	21	28	14	28	4.1%	1.50 [0.98, 2.30]
Lv J 2010	22	25	17	25	5.0%	1.29 [0.95, 1.76]
Ren Y 2006	39	50	20	49	5.9%	1.91 [1.32, 2.76]
Sun H 2010	36	40	19	36	5.9%	1.71 [1.23, 2.36]
Wang HY 2010	27	38	19	38	5.6%	1.42 [0.97, 2.07]
Wang L 2010	24	60	17	60	5.0%	1.41 [0.85, 2.35]
Subtotal (95% CI)		**349**		**336**	**36.1%**	**1.56 [1.34, 1.83]**
Total events	195		121			

Heterogeneity: Chi^2 = 3.35, df = 7 (P = 0.85); I^2 = 0%
Test for overall effect: Z = 5.62 (P < 0.00001)

1.1.3 Medicinal cupping plus medication versus medication alone						
Qiu J 2003	36	40	25	40	7.4%	1.44 [1.11, 1.87]
Subtotal (95% CI)		**40**		**40**	**7.4%**	**1.44 [1.11, 1.87]**
Total events	36		25			

Heterogeneity: Not applicable
Test for overall effect: Z = 2.73 (P = 0.006)

1.1.4 Wet cupping plus TDP and medication versus TDP and medication alone						
Li W 2005	26	32	22	32	6.5%	1.18 [0.89, 1.57]
Subtotal (95% CI)		**32**		**32**	**6.5%**	**1.18 [0.89, 1.57]**
Total events	26		22			

Heterogeneity: Not applicable
Test for overall effect: Z = 1.14 (P = 0.25)

1.1.5 Flash cupping therapy plus herbal medicine and acupuncture versus herbal medicine and acupuncture alone						
Ou X 2009	48	60	28	48	9.2%	1.37 [1.05, 1.80]
Subtotal (95% CI)		**60**		**48**	**9.2%**	**1.37 [1.05, 1.80]**
Total events	48		28			

Heterogeneity: Not applicable
Test for overall effect: Z = 2.29 (P = 0.02)

Total (95% CI)		**833**		**765**	**100.0%**	**1.45 [1.33, 1.59]**
Total events	529		327			

Heterogeneity: Chi^2 = 9.37, df = 15 (P = 0.86); I^2 = 0%
Test for overall effect: Z = 8.09 (P < 0.00001)
Test for subgroup diferences: Chi^2 = 3.05, df = 4 (P = 0.55); I^2 = 0%

0.5 0.7 1 1.5 2
Favours control — Favours intervention

FIGURE 16-7 Effect of estimates of cupping combined with other interventions versus other interventions alone on numbers of cured patients with facial paralysis (Bell's palsy).

Estimated Effects of RCTs with Cupping for Cervical Spondylosis

Eight trials evaluated the efficacy of cupping therapy for cervical spondylosis.[15,91,101,105,108,134,138,167] Cupping therapy, especially Wet cupping on Du-14 and Ashi points, combined with other treatment including acupuncture and traction, was better than other treatments alone in effecting a cure (RR 1.69, 95%CI 1.36 to 2.08, $p < 0.00001$, 7 trials, I^2 = 39%, random model) (Fig. 16-8) and in ameliorating symptoms (RR 1.14, 95%CI 1.07 to 1.22, $p < 0.0001$, 8 trials, I^2 = 37%, fixed model). One trial[138] compared Wet cupping with flunarizine for symptom improvement, and found no difference between the two groups (RR 1.18, 95%CI 0.60 to 2.32, $p = 0.63$, 1 trial).

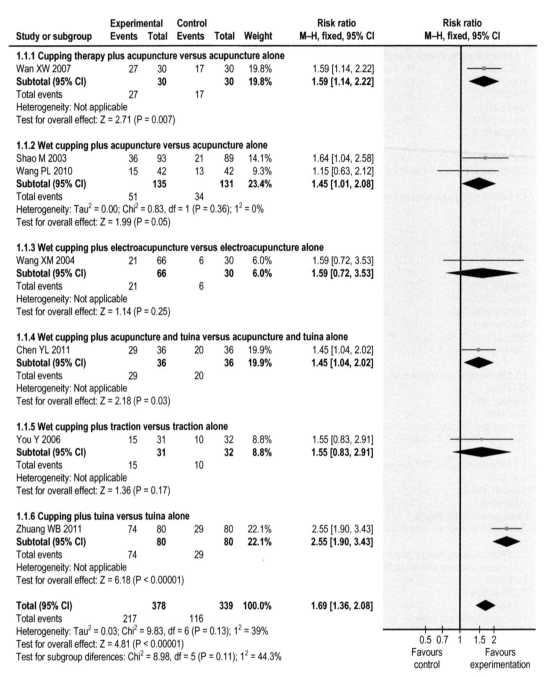

FIGURE 16-8 Effect of estimates of cupping combined with other interventions versus other interventions alone on numbers of cured patients with cervical spondylosis.

Estimated Effects of RCTs with Cupping for Acne

Seven trials evaluated the efficacy of cupping therapy for acne[36,40,65,106,111,113,147]. The meta-analysis showed that, for improving the cure rate, Wet cupping therapy was significantly better than medication such as tanshinone, tetracycline and ketokonazole (RR 2.07, 95%CI 1.22 to 3.52, $p=0.007$, 3 trials, $I^2 = 37\%$, random model) (Fig. 16-9). Furthermore, cupping therapy combined with other interventions was superior to other interventions alone (RR 1.88, 95%CI 1.40 to 2.52, $p<0.0001$, 4 trials, $I^2 = 0\%$, fixed model).

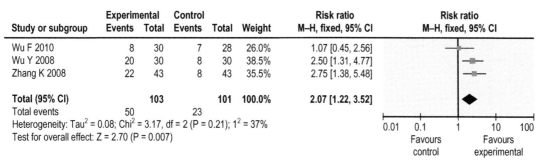

FIGURE 16-9 Effect of estimates of cupping therapy versus medication on numbers of cured patients with acne.

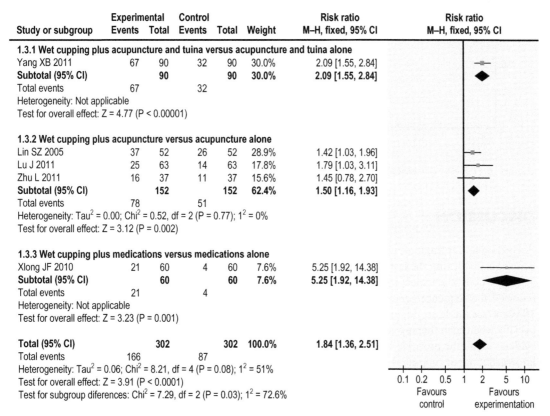

FIGURE 16-10 Effect of estimates of cupping combined with other interventions versus other interventions alone on numbers of cured patients with lumbar disc herniation.

Estimated Effects of RCTs with Cupping for Prolapse of Lumbar Intervertebral Disc

Five trials evaluated the efficacy of cupping therapy for lumbar disc herniation.[62,76,118,130,164] The meta-analysis showed that cupping therapy combined with other interventions was superior to other interventions alone (RR 1.84, 95%CI 1.36 to 2.51, $p<0.0001$, 5 trials, $I^2=51\%$, random model) for improving the cure rate (Fig. 16-10).

Funnel Plot Analysis

A funnel plot analysis of 39 trials was performed to examine outcomes for the number of cured patients irrespective of disease; the result showed potential asymmetry (Fig. 16-11).

Adverse Events

No serious adverse effects were reported in any of the 163 included trials.

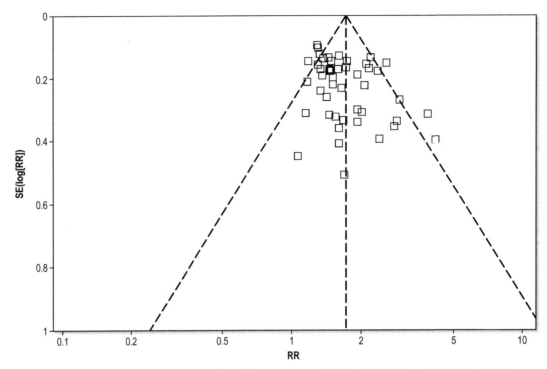

FIGURE 16-11 Funnel plot assessing outcomes of cured patients reported in 49 randomized controlled trials on five diseases.

DISCUSSION

According to our findings, clinical studies on cupping therapy have obviously improved in either number or quality during the last 50 years. Although the methodological quality of the included RCTs was generally poor, the inclusion of certain items of information – such as the number of the RCTs that reported the sequence generation of randomization – indicated that it has improved during the last 10 years (see Table 16-36, in Appendix). Cupping therapy may have an effect in several conditions, especially when such therapy is combined with another treatment (although only poor quality, provisional evidence could be provided by this systematic review). The long-term effect of cupping therapy is not known, but use of cupping is generally considered safe, based on long-term clinical use and reports from the reviewed clinical trials.

All these trials leave much scope for trials that are well designed, conducted and reported. We have included 163 RCTs in this review, but the majority of these had a high risk of bias. According to the Consolidated Standards of Reporting Trials (CONSORT Group, 2001),[172] the randomization methods need to be clearly described and fully reported. Although double blinding is always a big challenge for the manual healing therapies such as acupuncture, massage and cupping therapy, a sham cupping device was recently developed by introducing a small hole in the cup to reduce the negative pressure after suction, so that the pressure inside could not be maintained. A pilot RCT[173] conducted to testify the validity of this sham control method (Lee et al, 2010) found this new sham cupping device seemed to provide a credible control for real cupping therapy by producing little or no negative pressure, but more rigorous research was warranted regarding its use.

Although blinding of cupping therapy might be very difficult, blinding of outcome assessors and statistics should be attempted as much as possible to minimize performance and assessment biases. Sample size calculation and analysis of outcomes based on intention-to-treat principle are important. Also, as cupping therapy, like acupuncture, is a treatment using meridians and acupoints, researchers may refer to the *Revised STandards for Reporting Interventions in Clinical Trials of Acupuncture* (STRICTA) report[174] – therefore, details of the cupping treatment should be reported, such as the type of cups, experience of the practitioners, period and frequency of the treatment.

As we have mentioned, 79.75% of the included trials used a composite outcome measure that categorized the effect of the treatment into four grades. The classification of 'cure', 'markedly effective', 'effective' or 'ineffective' is not internationally recognized, however, making it hard to interpret the treatment effect, and this may increase the clinical heterogeneity within such categories. We suggest that future trials chose and comply with international standards in the evaluation of treatment effect.

We have also conducted an overall funnel plot test to examine whether the association between the effect of cupping therapy and the standard error of this effect (a measure of study size) is greater than might be expected to occur by chance. The funnel plot of 49 RCTs for the outcome of number of cured patients of five diseases showed potential asymmetry (see Fig. 16-11). The funnel plot asymmetry may be caused by publication bias, small study effects or even heterogeneity in intervention effects. For the asymmetric funnel plot in our meta-analysis, it seemed that the asymmetry was most probably caused by the small study sample sizes. However, as we didn't include the unpublished studies, there was also high potential that our review might have a publication bias. We strongly suggest that researchers should calculate sample sizes for randomized controlled trials to make sure the trial has the adequate statistical power.

CONCLUSION

Although the number of RCTs on treatment using cupping therapy is small in terms of any specific disease, and existing trials are of small size and low methodological quality, meta-analysis of a combination of cupping therapy with other treatments (such as acupuncture or medications) has nevertheless demonstrated significant benefit compared with other treatments alone in curing patients with herpes zoster, acne, facial paralysis, cervical spondylosis and prolapse of lumbar intervertebral disc. However, we evaluated almost all the included trials as having a high risk of bias, so consider it to be worthwhile (and, indeed, necessary) to conduct further high-quality RCTs of larger sample size in order to assess fully the effectiveness of cupping therapy for those common conditions that most benefited from cupping therapy according to this review's findings. In addition, we suggest that the study design and report should be standardized, and the study protocol registered with an authoritative organization[175,176] such as WHO International Clinical Trial Registration Platform (WHO ICTRP).

APPENDIX

TABLE 16-36   Mapping of Top 20 Diseases/Conditions by Study Type Between 1994 and 2011

Diseases/Conditions	RCT	CCT	CS	CR	RCT	CCT	CS	CR	RCT	CCT	CS	CR	RCT	CCT	CS	CR	RCT	CCT	CS	CR	RCT	CCT	CS	CR	Sum
Herpes zoster	0	2	9	2	0	1	1	1	0	1	0	0	3	0	4	2	6	1	12	0	11	3	19	4	84
Pain conditions	0	0	9	4	1	1	4	3	1	1	0	1	2	0	4	4	3	1	9	4	5	0	4	1	62
Cough and asthma	0	0	9	7	1	0	10	1	0	0	2	0	0	0	2	0	1	1	3	1	4	0	3	4	50
Acne	0	0	4	0	0	0	2	0	0	0	1	0	0	0	4	0	6	1	5	1	4	0	6	3	37
Facial paralysis	0	0	1	0	0	0	3	0	0	0	0	0	2	0	1	2	1	0	0	2	14	2	2	0	29
Common cold	1	0	3	0	0	0	2	2	0	0	2	0	1	0	4	2	0	0	2	2	0	0	3	2	24
Cervical spondylosis	0	0	3	0	0	0	1	0	0	0	2	1	2	0	2	0	3	0	2	1	3	0	1	1	22
Lateral femoral cutaneous neuritis	0	0	2	1	0	0	0	0	0	0	0	0	0	0	0	0	1	0	0	0	0	0	1	1	19
Strain of lumbar muscles	0	0	3	0	0	0	5	2	0	0	1	0	0	0	0	1	1	0	1	0	0	0	1	1	18
Scapulohumeral periarthritis	0	0	3	0	0	0	5	1	0	0	0	0	0	0	0	2	0	0	1	0	2	0	1	0	18
Urticaria	0	1	3	1	0	0	3	1	0	0	0	1	0	1	0	0	0	0	1	0	1	0	2	1	13
Mastitis	0	1	4	0	0	0	2	1	0	0	1	0	0	0	1	0	0	0	1	0	0	0	1	0	11
Headache	0	1	1	0	0	0	1	1	0	1	2	0	0	0	1	1	0	0	0	2	0	0	0	1	11
Soft tissue injury	0	0	1	3	0	0	1	1	0	0	2	0	0	0	0	0	0	0	0	1	1	0	0	0	10
Arthritis	0	0	4	0	0	0	0	0	0	1	0	0	0	0	1	3	2	0	1	1	1	2	0	0	10
Nero dermatitis	0	0	2	1	0	0	1	0	0	0	0	0	0	0	0	1	0	0	1	0	0	0	1	1	8
Myofascitis	0	0	1	0	0	0	0	0	0	0	1	0	0	0	0	1	1	0	1	0	0	0	1	0	8
Wound and sious	0	0	1	0	0	0	0	0	0	0	0	0	0	0	2	0	0	0	0	0	1	0	0	0	7
Bi syndrome	0	0	2	0	0	0	1	1	0	0	0	0	0	0	0	0	0	0	0	0	0	0	0	1	6
Sciatica	0	0	1	1	0	0	1	0	1	0	0	0	1	0	0	1	0	0	0	0	0	0	0	0	5
Summary	1	4	64	20	4	1	49	17	3	1	12	7	12	2	29	20	24	4	41	11	51	7	47	21	452
Year	1994–1996				1997–1999				2000–2002				2003–2005				2006–2008				2009–2011				

TABLE 16-37   Characteristics of 23 Included Trials on Cupping for Herpes Zoster

Trials	PATIENTS (M/F) Treatment	PATIENTS (M/F) Control	Average Age (yrs)	Diagnostic Criteria	INTERVENTIONS Cupping Treatment	INTERVENTIONS Control	Duration of Treatment	Outcome Measure
Ci 2010[18]	48/56	42/50	51.6	Criteria in text book in China	Prick with common needle on lesion then cupping on the same place for 10 min, once every 2 days	Aciclovir 0.5 g plus 250 mL normal saline intravenous drip twice daily	12 days	**Cure, markedly effective, ineffective
Cui & Chen 2011[20]	19/13	17/13	18–72	Criteria in text book in China	Prick with triangle-edged needle and cupping on lesion for 10 min, once every 2 days; plus aciclovir cream for external use and aciclovir 0.2 g five times daily	Aciclovir cream for external use and aciclovir 0.2 g five times daily	10 days	**Cure, markedly effective, effective, ineffective
Gao & Liu 2009[29]	19/11	17/10	45.6	Postherpetic neuralgia	Prick with triangle-edged needle and cupping on lesion for 10 minutes, once every two days, plus electroacupuncture 30 min, once daily	Carbamazepine 0.1 g three times daily, mecobalamine 500 µg twice daily, plus electroacupuncture 30 min, once daily	20 days	Pain relief
Guo 2006[32]	19/17	17/18	Unclear	Chinese criteria for diagnosis	Prick with triangle-edged needle and cupping on lesion for 10 minutes, once every 2 days, plus aciclovir 200 mg 3 times daily, vit B₁ 100 mg, vit B₁₂ 250 mg injection once daily	Aciclovir 200 mg 3 times daily, vit B₁ 100 mg, vit B₁₂ 250 mg injection once daily	10 days	*Cure, improve, ineffective Average time of cure
He 2011[35]	20/16	16/14	42.96	Criteria in text book in China	Prick with plum-blossom needle on lesion then cupping on the same place for 3–5 min, once daily, plus TDP 10 min once daily	TDP 10 min once daily	7 days	*Cure, improve, ineffective
Huang & Li 2008[39]	11/25	9/18	58.6	Criteria in text book in China	Prick with plum-blossom needle on lesion then cupping on the same place for 2–3 min, once daily, plus acupuncture 30 min once daily	Acupuncture 30 min once daily	10 days	*Cure, improve, ineffective
Ji & Guo 2009[45]	11/35	17/21	48.6	Unavailable	Prick with triangle-edged needle and cupping on lesion for 10 minutes once every 2 days	Aciclovir injection 5 mg/kg/d, once per 8 hours	14 days	**Cure, markedly effective, effective, ineffective Average time of cure Average dry-up time of lesion Average time of pain disappear Incidence rate of PHN

Continued

TABLE 16-37 Characteristics of 23 Included Trials on Cupping for Herpes Zoster (Continued)

Trials	PATIENTS (M/F) Treatment	PATIENTS (M/F) Control	Average Age (yrs)	Diagnostic Criteria	INTERVENTIONS Cupping Treatment	INTERVENTIONS Control	Duration of Treatment	Outcome Measure
Jin et al 2008[48]	26/19	25/20	55.5	Professional criteria in China	Prick with seven-star needle and cupping on the lesion for 10–15 min, once daily for first 3 days, then once every 2 days and last for 4 days	Aciclovir capsule 0.2g five times daily, cimetidine 0.2g three times daily, indomethacin tablet 50mg three times daily, mecobalamin tablets 0.5 mg three times daily, washout with aciclovir and use aciclovir cream	10 days	*Cure, improve, ineffective; Incidence rate of post-herpetic neuralgia (PHN)
Liu & Li 2003[68]	28/22	19/15	55.1 54.2	Criteria in text book in China	Group 1: prick with plum-blossom needle on lesion then cupping on the same place for 10–15 min, once every 2 days, plus aciclovir 0.2g five times daily, vit B_1 20mg three times daily, vit B_{12} 500mg injection once every 2 days, 2–3% aciclovir cream for external use	Aciclovir 0.2g five times daily, vit B_1 20mg three times daily, vit B_{12} 500mg injection once every 2 days, 2–3% aciclovir cream for external use	10 days	**Cure, markedly effective, effective, ineffective; Average time of cure; Incidence rate of PHN
	16/14	19/15			Group 2: prick with plum-blossom needle on lesion then cupping on the same place for 10–15 min, once every 2 days	Aciclovir 0.2g five times everyday, vit B_1 20mg three times everyday, vit B_{12} 500mg injection once every 2 days, 2–3% acyclovir cream for external use		
Liu et al 2006b[70]	27/11	25/13	20–71	Criteria in text book in China	Prick with triangle-edged needle and cupping on lesion for 3 minutes, once daily, plus electroacupuncture 30min, once daily, and herbal decoction 50mL 3–5 times daily	Electroacupuncture 30 min, once daily, and herbal decoction 50mL 3–5 times daily	7 days	**Cure, markedly effective, effective, ineffective; Change of pain intensity
Liu & Chang 2004[71]	32	32	55.6	Unavailable	Prick with triangle-edged needle and cupping on lesion	Aciclovir 1.2g five times every day, poly 1-C injection 2mg once every 2 days	10 days	**Cure, markedly effective, effective, ineffective
Long & Liu 2003[72]	34	30	44.5	Unavailable	Prick with plum needle on lesion then cupping on the same place plus ultraviolet radiation once every 2 days	Ultraviolet radiation once every 2 days	10 days	Times of treatment for *cured

Study	Sample size	Group	Age	Diagnostic criteria	Treatment group	Control group	Duration	Outcomes
Luan & Tang 2011[78]	30/20	23/27	20–82	Professional criteria in China	Prick with plum needle on lesion then cupping on the same place for 10–15 min, once every 2 days, plus acupuncture 30 min once daily, aciclovir injection 0.1–0.2 g twice daily, vit B_{12} 500 μg injection once daily	Acupuncture 30 min once daily, aciclovir injection 0.1–0.2 g twice daily, vit B_{12} 500 μg injection once daily, plus tramadol one tablet twice daily	Unclear	**Cure, markedly effective, effective, ineffective
Song & Zhang 2011[92]	50/30	40/30	27–70	Criteria in text book in China	Prick with triangle-edged needle and cupping on lesion for 10 minutes once daily	Aciclovir injection 5 mg/kg/d, once per 8 hours	7 days	**Cure, markedly effective, effective, ineffective
Sun et al 2011[95]	50	48	41.2	Criteria in text book in China	Prick with plum-blossom needle on lesion then cupping on the same place for 10–15 min, once every 2 days, plus aciclovir injection 5 mg/kg/d, once per 8 hours, and mecobalamin 0.5 mg three times daily	Aciclovir injection 5 mg/kg/d, once per 8 hours, and mecobalamin 0.5 mg three times daily	7 days	**Cure, markedly effective, effective, ineffective
Wang et al 2009[109]	55	54	Unclear	Criteria in text book in China	Prick with common needle on lesion then cupping on the same place for 5–10 min, once daily for first 3 days, then once every 2 days	Valaciclovir 0.3 g twice daily	9 days	*Cure, improve, ineffective; Scores given by patients according to their symptom of disease; Average dry up time of lesion; average time of pain disappear
Xiong SY et al 2007[119]	56	56	52	Professional criteria in China	Prick with plum needle on lesion then cupping on the same place 10–15 min, once daily, plus herbal decoction twice daily	Herbal decoction twice daily	Until pain disappear	Time of pain disappearance
Xiong ZL et al 2007[120]	20/28	16/24	49	Criteria in text book in China	Prick on lesion and cupping for 5 minutes	Aciclovir plus normal saline 250 mL intravenous drip once daily	7 days	Incidence rate of PHN
Xu & Yang 2004[121]	20/20	21/19	Unclear	Unavailable	Prick with triangle-edged needle and cupping on lesion for 15 min, aciclovir cream for external use plus aciclovir 0.5 g and glucose 250 mL intravenous drip twice daily	Aciclovir cream for external use plus aciclovir 0.5 g and glucose 250 mL intravenous drip twice daily	7 days	*Cure, improve, effective, ineffective; Scores given by patients according to their symptom of disease; Average dry up time of lesion; average time of pain disappear

Continued

TABLE 16-37 Characteristics of 23 Included Trials on Cupping for Herpes Zoster (Continued)

Trials	PATIENTS (M/F) Treatment	PATIENTS (M/F) Control	Average Age (yrs)	Diagnostic Criteria	INTERVENTIONS Cupping Treatment	INTERVENTIONS Control	Duration of Treatment	Outcome Measure
Zhang et al 2009[143]	10/15	12/13	Unclear	Professional criteria in China	Prick with plum-blossom needle and cupping on lesion for 5–10 minutes, plus electroacupuncture 30 min, once daily	Electroacupuncture 30 min once daily	10 days	*Cure, improve, effective, ineffective Pain relief Average time of pain lasting and starting relief
Zhang et al 2008[148]	14/26	12/28	Unclear	Criteria in text book in China	Aciclovir 200 mg five times daily, acupuncture beside the lesion 30 min once daily, plus prick with triangle-edged needle on Dazhui, Feishu (double), Ganshu (double) and cupping for 10 min once every 2 days, bloodletting on auditive apex twice every week	Aciclovir 200 mg five times daily, acupuncture beside the lesion 30 min once daily	14 days	*Cure, improve, effective, ineffective
Zou et al 2010[169]	14/26	13/27	43.9	Criteria in text book in China	Prick with plum-blossom needle and cupping on lesion for 5–10 minutes, plus electroacupuncture 30 min, once daily	Electroacupuncture 30 min once daily	10 days	*Cure, improve, effective, ineffective Average time of pain to disappear Average dry-up time of lesion

Definitions of 'cure', 'markedly effective', 'effective', and 'ineffective':

*Cure: rash totally faded, the clinical symptoms are disappeared, no accompanying pain; markedly effective: rash faded more than 70% (including 70%), the accompanying pain was almost disappeared; improved: rash faded 30–69%, the accompanying pain was obviously alleviated; ineffective: rash faded less than 30%, no alleviation of the accompanying pain.

**Cure: rash totally fade, no accompanying pain; markedly effective: rash faded more than 50%, the accompanying pain was almost disappeared; effective: rash faded 10–50%, the accompanying pain was alleviated a little; ineffective: rash faded less than 10%, no alleviation of the accompanying pain.

TABLE 16-38   Characteristics of 18 Included Trials on Cupping for Facial Paralysis (Bell Palsy)

Trials	PATIENTS (M/F) Treatment	PATIENTS (M/F) Control	Average Age (yrs)	Diagnostic Criteria	INTERVENTIONS Cupping Treatment	INTERVENTIONS Control	Duration of Treatment	Outcome Measure
Fu & Bai 2004[25]	80	40	Unclear	Unclear	Flash cupping on relevant points and retained for 10 min plus acupuncture for 30 min, once daily	Acupuncture for 30 min once daily	30 days	Cure, markedly improved, effective, ineffective
Gao 2010[28]	26/24	22/20	39,42	Criteria in text book in China	Prick with triangle-edged needles and cupping on relevant acupoints for 10 min, once every 2 days, plus acupuncture for 30 min once daily, and mecobalamine intramuscular injection once every 2 days	Acupuncture for 30 min once daily, and mecobalamine intramuscular injection once every 2 days	20 days	Cure, markedly improved, effective, ineffective
Huang et al 2009[41]	71/49	73/47	40.73	Criteria in text book in China	Flash cupping on relevant points for 5 min plus acupuncture for 30 min, once daily	Acupuncture for 30 min once daily	30 days	Cure, markedly improved, effective, ineffective
Huang et al 2010[42]	27/31	30/28	Unclear	Criteria in text book in China	Prick with common needles and cupping on relevant acupoints until 3–5 mL bleeding for 5 days, plus acupuncture for 30 min once daily	Acupuncture 30 min once daily	30 days	Cure, markedly improved, effective, ineffective
Liu 2009[65]	80	80	40.2	Criteria in text book in China	Flash cupping on relevant points for 5 min plus acupuncture for 30 min, once daily	Acupuncture for 30 min once daily	20 days	Cure, markedly improved, effective, ineffective
Li 2005[57]	24/8	22/10	42.3	Criteria in text book in China	Prick with plum-blossom needle and cupping on relevant points for 5 min, once daily, plus TDP for 20 min and antivirus drug, neurotrophic medicine once daily	TDP for 20 min and antivirus drug, neurotrophic medicine once daily	20 days	Cure, markedly improved, effective, ineffective
Liu & Zhang 2011[66]	19/9	16/12	25–72	Chinese criteria for diagnosis	Prick with common needles and cupping on relevant acupoints 5 min once every 2 days, plus acupuncture for 30 min once daily	Acupuncture for 30 min once daily	20 days	Cure, markedly improved, effective, ineffective
Luo & Lou 2011[80]	18/16	20/14	12–74	Criteria in text book in China	Flash cupping on relevant points plus acupuncture for 30 min, once daily	Acupuncture for 30 min once daily	20 days	Cure, markedly improved, effective, ineffective
Lü 2010[82]	14/11	15/10	46.8	Unclear	Prick with plum-blossom needles and cupping on relevant acupoints once every two days, plus electroacupuncture for 30 min once daily	Electroacupuncture for 30 min once daily	40 days	Cure, effective, ineffective

Continued

TABLE 16-38 Characteristics of 18 Included Trials on Cupping for Facial Paralysis (Bell Palsy) (Continued)

Trials	PATIENTS (M/F) Treatment	Control	Average Age (yrs)	Diagnostic Criteria	INTERVENTIONS Cupping Treatment	Control	Duration of Treatment	Outcome Measure
Ou & Xu 2009[87]	60	48	48.6	Criteria in text book in China	Flash cupping on relevant points plus herbal decoction twice daily and acupuncture for 30 min, once daily	Plus herbal decoction twice daily and acupuncture for 30 min, once daily	30 days	Cure, effective, ineffective
Qiu et al 2003[88]	40	40	Unclear	Unclear	Medicinal cupping (mixture of ginger, mustard, and dimethyl sulfoxide) on relevant acupoints for 30 min, once daily, plus neurotrophic medicine once daily	Neurotrophic medicine once daily	30 days	Cure, markedly improved, effective, ineffective; average time of cured
Ren 2006[89]	26/24	25/24	Unclear	Chinese criteria for diagnosis	Prick with plum needles and cupping on Yifeng acupoints for 10 min once daily, plus acupuncture for 30 min	Acupuncture for 30 min once daily	30 days	Cure, effective, ineffective
Sun & Li 2010[93]	28/12	25/11	44.6	Unclear	Prick with plum-blossom needles and cupping on Yifeng acupoints for 10 min once every 2 days, plus acupuncture for 30 min once daily	Acupuncture for 30 min once daily	15 days	Cure, markedly improved, effective, ineffective
Wang HY 2010[171]	23/15	26/12	1.5–78	Criteria in text book in China	Prick with plum-blossom needles and cupping on relevant acupoints for 7–8 min, plus acupuncture for 30 min once daily	Acupuncture for 30 min once daily	45 days	Cure, markedly improved, effective, ineffective
Wang L 2010[103]	32/28	34/26	unclear	Chinese criteria for diagnosis	Prick with plum needles and cupping on relevant acupoints until 3–5 mL bleeding once every 2 days, plus acupuncture for 30 min once daily	Acupuncture for 30 min once daily	30 days	Cure, markedly improved, effective, ineffective
Zhao et al 2010[155]	27/16	25/17	unclear	Symptoms	Flash cupping on relevant points for 5 min plus acupuncture for 30 min, once daily	Acupuncture for 30 min once daily	30 days	Cure, markedly improved, effective, ineffective
Zhu et al 2009[163]	20/14	18/16	33.1	Unclear	Prick with plum-blossom needle and flash cupping on relevant points for 3 min, once daily, after 7 days plus acupuncture once daily	Antiviral drug, neurotrophic medicine once daily, after 7 days plus acupuncture once daily	30 days	Cure, markedly improved, effective, ineffective

TABLE 16-39   Characteristics of 8 Included Trials on Cupping for Cervical Spondylosis

| Trials | PATIENTS (M/F) | | Average Age (y) | Diagnostic Criteria | INTERVENTIONS | | Duration of Treatment | Outcome Measure |
	Treatment	Control			Cupping Treatment	Control		
Chen et al 2011[15]	22/14	23/13	38.6	Criteria in text book in China	Prick with plum-blossom needle on Jiaji, Jianyu, and Jianwaishu points then cupping on the same place for 10–15 min, once every 2 days, plus electroacupuncture 30 min, tuina 10 min once daily, and medicinal injection twice daily	Electroacupuncture 30 min, tuina 10 min once daily, and medicinal injection twice daily	20 days	*Cure, markedly effective, ineffective; pain intensity (VAS); average treatment duration
Shao & Liu 2003[91]	40/53	41/48	47.5	Chinese criteria for diagnosis	Prick with seven-star needle and cupping on Dazhui points for 8–10 minutes, plus acupuncture on Jiaji points for 20 minutes, twice weekly	Acupuncture on Jiaji points for 20 minutes, twice weekly	35 days	*Cure, markedly effective, ineffective
Wan 2007[101]	19/11	18/12	29.9	Chinese criteria for diagnosis	After needling the points (Fengchi, Ex-B2 and *Ashi*),each needle hole was applied immediate cupping therapy with appropriate vacuum glass jar and last for 3–5 min, needles remained for 10 min, once daily	Acupuncture on Fengchi, Ex-B2 and *Ashi* points for 10 minutes, once daily	30 days	*Recovery, improvement, failure; treatment course; relapse rate
Wang 2010[105]	42	42	45.7	Criteria in text book in China	Prick with plum needle on Dazhui, Jiaji, Jianjing, Tianzong, and *Ashi* points then cupping on the same place for 10–15 min, once daily, plus acupuncture abdominal acupoints for 30 minutes once daily	Acupuncture abdominal acupoints for 30 minutes once daily	30 days	*Cure, markedly effective, effective, ineffective

Continued

TABLE 16-39 Characteristics of 8 Included Trials on Cupping for Cervical Spondylosis (Continued)

Trials	Patients (M/F) Treatment	Patients (M/F) Control	Average Age (y)	Diagnostic Criteria	Interventions Cupping Treatment	Interventions Control	Duration of Treatment	Outcome Measure
Wang 2004[108]	29/37	13/17	Unclear	Unclear	Electroacupuncture on Dazhui, Dazhui, Jiaji, et al. Prick with triangle-edged needle and cupping on same points for 10-15 minutes, once every 2 days	Electroacupuncture on Dazhui, Dazhui, Jiaji, et al once every 2 days	30 days	*Cure, markedly effective, effective, ineffective
You et al 2006a[134]	18/12 (1 drop-out)	17/13 (2 drop-out)	45.25	Local government criteria for diagnosis	Prick with plum-blossom needle and cupping on Hand-Sanjiao and Hand-Taiyang Meridian points for 5 minutes, plus 30 minutes traction once daily	30 minutes traction once daily	20 days	*Cure, markedly effective, ineffective
Zeng et al 2007[138]	40	40	47	Chinese criteria for diagnosis	Prick with triangle-edged needle and cupping on Dazhui and C6 level points for 8 minutes, then acupuncture and moxibustion at Fengchi, Bailao points once daily	Acupuncture and moxibustion at Fengchi, Bailao points once daily	20 days	**Markedly effective, ineffective; specific viscosity of blood; hemorrheological parameters
	40	40			Prick with triangle-edged needle and cupping on Dazhui and C$_6$ level points for 8 minutes, once daily	Flunarizine 5 mg once daily		
Zhuang et al 2011[167]	41/39	42/38	47.95	Chinese criteria for diagnosis	Prick with plum-blossom needle and cupping on ashi points for 5 min, moving the cups along the Du Mai and Jiaji points, plus tuina once every 2 days	Tuina once every 2 days	20 days	*Cure, markedly effective, ineffective

Definition of 'cure', 'markedly effective', 'effective', and 'ineffective': *cure*: the clinical symptoms are disappeared, the cervical or limb functions restored to normal; *markedly effective*: the symptoms obviously alleviated and improvement of the cervical and limb function; *effective*: the symptoms alleviated but the cervical or limb functions still could not restored to normal; *ineffective*: the symptoms and signs remain unchanged after the treatment.

TABLE 16-40   Characteristics of 7 Included Trials on Cupping for Acne

Trials	PATIENTS (M/F) Treatment	PATIENTS (M/F) Control	Average Age (y)	Diagnostic Criteria	INTERVENTIONS Cupping Treatment	INTERVENTIONS Control	Duration of Treatment	Outcome Measure
Hong & Wu 2011[36]	8/11	7/11	23.51	Criteria in text book in China	Prick with needles on Du-14, and 3 Back-Shu points then cupping on the same place for 10–15 min, twice per week Plus herbal medicinal mask 30 min twice per week	Herbal medicinal mask 30 min twice per week	35 days	*Cure, markedly effective, effect, ineffective
Huang et al 2010[40]	76	50	23	Chinese criteria for diagnosis	Prick with triangle-edged needle and cupping on 5 Back-Shu points for 5–10 min, twice weekly, plus herbal preparation 50 mL, three times daily, external facial cream	Herbal preparation 50 mL, three times daily plus external facial cream	Unclear	*Cure, markedly effective, ineffective
Liu et al 2009[65]	14/29	39	23.8	Chinese criteria for diagnosis	Flash cupping on lesion until face flush, plus acupuncture for 30 min, once daily at first 10 days, then once every 2 days for another 10 days	Acupuncture for 30 minutes, once daily at first 10 days, then once every two days for another 10 days	30 days	*Cure, markedly effective, ineffective Number of popular, and pustule
Wang & Wang 2007[106]	30	30	Unclear	Criteria in text book in China	Prick with plum-blossom needle on 5 Back-Shu points then cupping on the same place for 5–10 min, once every 3 days, plus moving cupping on back and acupuncture for 30 minutes once daily	Acupuncture 30 min once daily	30 days	*Cure, markedly effective, ineffective
Wu 2010[111]	30	28	Unclear	Unclear	Prick with triangle-edged needle and cupping on 2 Back-Shu points for 5–10 min, once every 5–7 days	Tanshinone 1 g, three times daily	30 days	*Cure, markedly effective, ineffective
Wu 2008[113]	9/21	7/23	25.5	Criteria in text book in China	Prick with triangle-edged needle and cupping on back ashi points to get 5–7 mL bleeding, once daily	Tetracycline 0.25 g four times daily, plus 0.2% ketoconazole external cream once daily	10 days	*Cure, markedly effective, ineffective
Zhang & Song 2008[147]	25/18	28/15	Unclear	Chinese criteria for diagnosis	Prick with triangle-edged needle and cupping on back ashi points for 10–15 minu, once every 2 days	Tetracycline 500 mg, three times daily, plus external cream twice daily	15 days	**Cure, markedly effective, ineffective

Definition of 'cure', 'markedly effective', 'effective', and 'ineffective': *cure*: lesion totally faded (or more than 95%), the clinical symptoms are disappeared, left mild pigmentation and scars; *markedly effective*: lesion faded more than *70% (**60%), the severity obviously alleviated; *effective*: lesion faded *30%–69% (**20%–59%), the severity of lesion was reduced; *ineffective*: lesion faded less than *30% (**20%), or even worse.

TABLE 16-41 Characteristics of 5 Included Trials on Cupping for Prolapse of Lumbar Intervertebral Disc

Trials	PATIENTS (M/F) Treatment	PATIENTS (M/F) Control	Average Age (y)	Diagnostic Criteria	INTERVENTIONS Cupping Treatment	INTERVENTIONS Control	Duration of Treatment	Outcome Measure
Lin 2005[62]	27/25	28/24	44.89 ± 11.72	Chinese criteria for diagnosis	Prick with plum-blossom needle and cupping on Du Maipoints, Jiaji and BL-40 for 10 min, plus 30 minutes electroacupuncture on ashi, Jiaji points once daily	30 min electroacupuncture on ashi, Jiaji points once daily	20 days	*Cure, effective, ineffective
Lu & Wang 2007[76]	32/21	33/30	38.95	Chinese criteria for diagnosis	Prick with plum-blossom needle and cupping on 2 points of BL-23, BL-25, Du-4, Du-3, GB-30, BL-36, BL-58 for 10 minutes, plus 30 minutes electroacupuncture on BL-23, Jiaji points once daily	30 min electroacupuncture on BL23, Jiaji points once daily	20 days	*Cure, markedly improve, effective, ineffective
Xiong 2010[118]	39/21	37/23	40.5	Chinese criteria for diagnosis	Prick with plum-blossom needle and cupping on BL-23, BL-28, BL-25, ashi, GB-34, BL-57, GB-30 and BL-40 for 5 min, once every 3 days, plus Bloven sustained-release tablet 1 tablet twice daily and Xiao Huo Luo Pill 1 pill twice daily	Bloven sustained release tablet 1 tablet twice daily and Xiao Huo Luo Pill 1 pill twice daily	21 days	*Cure, markedly improve, effective, ineffective
Yang 2011[130]	46/44	48/42	50.25	Chinese criteria for diagnosis	Prick with triangle-edges needle and cupping on BL-23, BL-25, Du-4, Du-3, GB-30, BL-36, BL-58 once daily, plus 30 min acupuncture on BL-23, Jiaji points, etc, tuina and moxibustion once daily	30 min acupuncture on BL-23, Jiaji points, etc., tuina and moxibustion once daily	10 days	*Cure, markedly improve, effective, ineffective
Zhu et al 2011[164]	37	37	22–79	Chinese criteria for diagnosis	Prick with plum-blossom needle and cupping on ashi, once every 2–3 days, plus 30 min acupuncture on BL-23, BL-25, GB-30 three times per week	30 min acupuncture on BL-23, BL-25, GB-30 three times per week	30 days	*Cure, markedly improve, effective, ineffective

Definition of 'cure', 'markedly effective', 'effective', and 'ineffective'; *cure*: the clinical symptoms are disappeared, the cervical or limb functions restored to normal; *markedly effective*: the symptoms obviously alleviated and improvement of the lumbar function; *effective*: the symptoms alleviated but the lumbar functions still could not restored to normal; *ineffective*: the symptoms and signs remain unchanged after the treatment.

TABLE 16-42   Reporting of Five Quality Components in Randomized Clinical Trials on Cupping Therapy

Publication Year	No. of Randomized Controlled Trials	Adequate Sequence Generation (%)	Adequate Allocation Concealment (%)	Blinding Method Reported (%)	Incomplete Outcome Data (yes, %)	Selective Outcome Reporting (yes, %)	Comparability of Baseline (yes, %)	Sample Size Estimation (yes, %)	Inclusive Criteria (yes, %)	Exclusive Criteria (yes, %)	Diagnostic Standard (yes, %)
1992	2	0	0	0	0	0	0	0	0	0	0
1993	1	1(100%)	0	0	0	0	0	0	0	0	0
1994	1	0	0	0	0	0	0	0	0	0	0
1995	—	—	—	—	—	—	—	—	—	—	—
1996	—	—	—	—	—	—	—	—	—	—	—
1997	2	0	0	0	0	0	0	0	0	0	0
1998	1	0	0	0	0	0	0	0	0	0	0
1999	2	0	0	0	0	0	1 (50%)	0	0	0	1 (50%)
2000	1	0	0	0	0	0	1 (100%)	0	0	1 (100%)	1 (100%)
2001	—	—	—	—	—	—	—	—	—	—	—
2002	—	—	—	—	—	—	—	—	—	—	—
2003	7	0	0	0	0	0	2 (28.57%)	0	0	1 (14.29%)	4 (57.14%)
2004	9	0	0	0	0	0	5 (55.56%)	0	3 (33.33%)	2 (22.22%)	4 (44.44%)
2005	10	2 (20%)	0	1 (10%)	0	0	7 (70%)	0	6 (60%)	5 (50%)	8 (80%)
2006	18	5 (27.78%)	0	1 (5.56%)	1 (5.56%)	0	15 (83.33%)	1 (5.56%)	4 (22.22%)	4 (22.22%)	14 (77.78%)
2007	15	4 (26.67%)	0	0	2 (13.33%)	0	12 (80%)	0	3 (20%)	3 (20%)	11 (73.33%)
2008	12	6 (50%)	0	1 (8.33%)	1	0	11 (91.67%)	0	5 (41.67%)	5 (41.67%)	10 (83.33%)
2009	29	5 (17.24%)	3 (10.34%)	1 (3.45%)	1 (3.45%)	1 (3.45%)	25 (86.21%)	3 (10.34%)	12 (41.38%)	13 (44.83%)	23 (79.31%)
2010	31	3 (9.68%)	0	0	1 (3.23%)	2 (6.45%)	27 (87.10%)	0	9 (29.03%)	8 (25.81%)	27 (87.10%)
2011	22	9 (40.91%)	3 (13.64%)	0	1 (4.55%)	0	18 (81.82%)	2 (9.09%)	12 (54.55%)	10 (45.45%)	20 (90.91%)
Total	163	35 (21.47%)	6 (3.68%)	4 (2.45%)	7 (4.29%)	3 (1.84%)	124 (76.07%)	6 (3.68%)	54 (33.13%)	52 (31.90%)	124 (76.07%)

TABLE 16-43 **Characteristics of Randomized Controlled Trials outside Meta-analysis**

Type of Intervention	Included Disease	No. of Trials	No. of Participants	Methodological Quality	Main Finding
Cupping versus no treatment	Branchialgia paraesthetica nocturna	1	10/10	Unclear risk of bias	Wet cupping therapy is better than no treatment in symptom improvement according to change of VAS scores
	Non-specific lower back pain	2	43/35	High risk of bias	Wet cupping therapy is significantly better than waiting list in pain relief
Cupping versus usual care	Wound and sinus	4	370/339	High risk of bias	Cupping therapy is significantly better than usual care in symptom improvement
	Non-specific lower back pain	3	110/108	Unclear risk of bias	Cupping therapy is significantly better than usual care in pain relief
	Cough and asthma	3	640/381	High risk of bias	Cupping therapy is significantly better than usual care on symptom improving
	Acute sprain lumbar muscle	3	108/106	High risk of bias	Cupping therapy is significantly better than usual care in pain relief
	Common cold	2	130/80	High risk of bias	Cupping therapy is significantly better than usual care on symptom improvement
	Chronic obstructive pneumonia	2	72/70	High risk of bias	Cupping therapy is significantly better than usual care in symptom improvement
	External humeral epicondylitis	1	60/60	Unclear risk of bias	No significant difference between cupping and usual care in symptom improvement
	Lateral femoral cutaneous neuritis	1	77/71	High risk of bias	Cupping therapy is significantly better than usual care in symptom improvement
	Cancer pain	1	30/30	High risk of bias	Cupping therapy is significantly better than usual care in pain relief
	Cerebral infarction	1	40/40	High risk of bias	Cupping therapy is significantly better than usual care in symptom improvement
	Insomnia	1	20/20	High risk of bias	Cupping therapy is significantly better than usual care on symptom improvement
	Obesity	1	42/33	High risk of bias	Cupping is superior to usual care in reducing waist circumference but has similar effective in reducing weight
	Carpal tunnel syndrome	1	26/26	Unclear risk of bias	Cupping therapy is significantly better than usual care in symptom improvement
	Venosmous snake bite	1	50/50	High risk of bias	Cupping therapy is significantly better than usual care in symptom improvement
	Nausea/vomiting	1	30/30	High risk of bias	Cupping therapy is significantly better than usual care in symptom improvement
	Osteoarthritis	1	90/45	High risk of bias	Cupping therapy is significantly better than usual care in symptom improvement
	Rheumatoid arthritis	1	80/80	High risk of bias	Cupping therapy is significantly better than usual care in relieving pain of knee

	Upper-back myofascitis	1	45/45	High risk of bias	Cupping therapy is significantly better than usual care in symptom improvement
	Oedema of the upper extremity after surgery	1	34/33	High risk of bias	Cupping therapy is significantly better than usual care on symptom improvement
	Chronic gastritis	1	56/56	High risk of bias	Cupping therapy is significantly better than usual care on symptom improvement
	Postoperative retention of urine	1	40/40	High risk of bias	Cupping therapy is significantly better than usual care in symptom improvement
	Pain in waist and lower extremities	1	46/41	High risk of bias	Cupping therapy is significantly better than usual care in pain relief
	Atherosclerosis	1	22/20	High risk of bias	Cupping therapy is significantly better than usual care on symptom improvement
	Inflammation of superior clunial nerves	1	80/75	High risk of bias	Cupping therapy is significantly better than usual care in symptom improvement
	Prolapsed lumbar intervertebral disc	1	60/60	High risk of bias	Cupping therapy is significantly better than usual care in symptom improvement
	Chronic neck pain	1	25/25	High risk of bias	Cupping therapy is significantly better than usual care in pain relief
Cupping versus medications	Flat wart	1	48/45	High risk of bias	Cupping therapy is significantly better than medications in symptom improvement
	Bronchial asthma	1	24/24	High risk of bias	Cupping therapy is significantly better than medications in symptom improvement, no difference is fund between two groups in lung function improvement
	Non-specific lower back pain	1	60/30	High risk of bias	Cupping therapy is significantly better than medications in pain relief
Combination of cupping and herbal medicine versus herbal medicine alone	Leucoderma	1	40/40	High risk of bias	Combination of cupping therapy and herbal medicine is significantly better than herbal medicine alone in symptom improvement
	Cough and asthma	1	30/28	High risk of bias	Combination of cupping therapy and herbal medicine is significantly better than herbal medicine alone in symptom improvement
	Perimenopausal syndrome	1	30/30	High risk of bias	Combination of cupping and herbal medicine is significantly better than herbal medicine alone in symptom improvement

Continued

TABLE 16-43 Characteristics of Randomized Controlled Trials outside Meta-analysis (Continued)

Type of Intervention	Included Disease	No. of Trials	No. of Participants	Methodological Quality	Main Finding
Combination of cupping and acupuncture versus acupuncture alone	Facial paralysis	2	82/70	High risk of bias	Combination of cupping and acupuncture is significantly better than acupuncture alone in symptom improvement
	Obesity	6	233/231	High risk of bias	Five of them showed cupping plus acupuncture had significant effect in reducing weight, another one showed no significant effect for combination treatment group compared with acupuncture alone
	Chloasma	3	148/110	High risk of bias	Combination of cupping and acupuncture is significantly better than acupuncture alone in symptom improvement
	Prolapsed lumbar intervertebral disc	1	30/30	High risk of bias	Combination of cupping and acupuncture is significantly better than acupuncture alone in symptom improvement
	Shoulder–hand syndrome	3	95/95	High risk of bias	Combination of cupping and acupuncture is significantly better than acupuncture alone in symptom improvement
	Scapulohumeral periarthritis	2	90/88	High risk of bias	Combination of cupping and acupuncture is significantly better than acupuncture alone in symptom improvement
	Insomnia	1	50/50	High risk of bias	Combination of cupping and acupuncture is significantly better than acupuncture alone in symptom improvement
	Facial spasm	1	25/23	High risk of bias	Combination of cupping and acupuncture is significantly better than acupuncture alone in symptom improvement
	Osteoarthritis	1	20/30	High risk of bias	Combination of cupping and acupuncture is significantly better than acupuncture alone on symptom improvement
	Acute ankle sprain	1	46/46	High risk of bias	Combination of cupping and acupuncture is significantly better than acupuncture alone in symptom improvement
	Functional dyspepsia	1	42/33	High risk of bias	Combination of cupping and acupuncture is significantly better than acupuncture alone in symptom improvement
	Chronic diarrhoea	1	30/30	High risk of bias	Combination of cupping and acupuncture is significantly better than acupuncture alone in symptom improvement
	Health under par	1	32/30	High risk of bias	Combination of cupping and acupuncture is significantly better than acupuncture alone in symptom improvement
	Diabetic peripheral neuropathy	1	33/32	High risk of bias	Combination of cupping and acupuncture is significantly better than acupuncture alone in symptom improvement
	Sciatica	1	48/38	High risk of bias	Combination of cupping and acupuncture is significantly better than acupuncture alone in symptom improvement
	Knee pain	1	34/38	High risk of bias	Combination of cupping therapy and acupuncture is significantly better than acupuncture alone in pain relief
	Nausea/vomiting	1	16/16	High risk of bias	Combination of cupping therapy and acupuncture is significantly better than acupuncture alone in symptom improvement
	Depression	2	68/68	High risk of bias	Combination of cupping and acupuncture is superior to acupuncture alone on improving the symptoms of depression according to the change of Hamilton Depression Scale

Combination of cupping and medications versus medications alone	Cough and asthma	4	183/171	High risk of bias	Combination of cupping and medication is significantly better than medication alone in symptom improvement
	Herpes zoster	1	22/19	High risk of bias	Combination of cupping and medication is significantly better than medication alone on symptom improvement
	Chronic obstructive pneumonia	2	76/76	High risk of bias	Combination of cupping and medication is significantly better than medication alone in symptom improvement
	Acute myelitis	1	24/15	High risk of bias	Combination of cupping and medication is significantly better than medication alone in symptom improvement
	Diabetes mellitus	1	35/35	High risk of bias	Combination of cupping and medication is significantly better than medication alone in symptom improvement
	Intracranial hypertension	1	40/40	High risk of bias	Combination of cupping and medication is significantly better than medication alone in symptom improvement
Combination of other TCM treatment versus other TCM treatment alone	Shoulder pain	1	23/23	High risk of bias	Combination of cupping and rehabilitation training is significantly better than rehabilitation training in pain relief
	Ulcerative colitis	1	15/15	High risk of bias	Combination of cupping and moxibustion is significantly better than moxibustion alone in symptom improvement
	Cervical spondylosis	1	30/30	High risk of bias	Combination of cupping and traction are significantly better than traction alone in symptom improvement
	Prolapsed lumbar intervertebral disc	2	61/60	High risk of bias	Combination of cupping and traction is significantly better than traction alone in symptom improvement
	Vertigo	1	50/47	High risk of bias	Combination of cupping and manual traction is significantly better than manual traction in symptom improvement

ENDNOTES

1. The SF-36® is a comprehensive short form questionnaire with only 36 questions that yields an 8-scale health profile as well as summary measures of health-related quality of life. As documented in more than 2000 publications, the SF-36® has proven useful in monitoring general and specific populations, comparing the burden of different diseases, differentiating the health benefits produced by different treatments, and in screening individual patients.

REFERENCES

1. Rosenberg, W., Donald, A., 1995. Evidence based medicine, an approach to clinical problem solving. Br. Med. J. 310, 1122–1126.
2. Cao, H.J., Zhu, C.J., Liu, J.P., 2010. Wet cupping therapy for treatment of herpes zoster: a systematic review of randomized controlled trials. Altern. Ther. Health Med. 16, 48–54.
3. Kim, J.I., Lee, M.S., Lee, D.H., et al., 2011b. Cupping for treating pain: a systematic review. Evid. Based Complement. Alternat. Med. doi:10.1093/ecam/nep035.
4. Kwon, Y.D., Cho, H.J., 2007. Systematic review of cupping including bloodletting therapy for musculoskeletal diseases in Korea. Korean Journal of Oriental Physiology and Pathology 21, 789–793.
5. Lee, M.S., Choi, T.Y., Shin, B.C., et al., 2010a. Cupping for stroke rehabilitation: a systematic review. Journal of Neurological Science 294, 70–73.
6. Lee, M.S., Choi, T.Y., Shin, B.C., et al., 2010b. Cupping for hypertension: a systematic review. Clin. Exp. Hypertens. 32, 423–425.
7. Lee, M.S., Kim, J.I., Ernst, E., 2011. Is cupping an effective treatment? An overview of systematic reviews. J. Acupunct. Meridian Stud. 4 (1), 1–4.
8. Higgins, J.P.T., Green, S. (Eds.), 2009. Cochrane Handbook for Systematic Reviews of Interventions (Version 5.0.2). The Cochrane Collaboration. Online. Available: http://www.mrc-bsu.cam.ac.uk/cochrane/handbook502/front_page.htm.
9. Bu, T.W., Tian, X.L., Wang, S.J., et al., 2007. Comparison and analysis of therapeutic effects of different therapies on simple obesity. Chinese Acupuncture and Moxibustion 27, 337–340 (in Chinese).
10. Chen, J., Xu, H.Y., 1993. Wet cupping therapy on 50 patients with herpes zoster. Chinese Journal of Dermatovenereology 5, 252 (in Chinese).
11. Chen, J.J., 2009. Clinical observation of therapeutic effect of combination of electroacupunture and wet cupping therapy for scapulohumeral periarthritis. Journal of Complementary and Alternative Medicine 25 (1), 27–28 (in Chinese).
12. Chen, L.A., 2010. Zhi Zhi Heng Tui massage in treating 150 cases with strain of lumbar muscles by syndrome differentiation. Jiangxi Journal of Traditional Chinese Medicine 41 (328), 62–63 (in Chinese).
13. Chen, M.X., Huang, D.J., 2000. Clinical Study on Combination of Cupping Therapy and Moxibustion for Treatment of Asthenic Splenonephro-Yang Type of Colitis Gravis. (in Chinese) (Master's thesis), Chengdu University of Traditional Chinese Medicine.
14. Chen, Y.L., Liu, X.L., Xia, J.Z., 2008. Clinical observation of wet cupping combined with acupuncture, tuina and traction on 30 patients with blood stasis type of prolapse of lumbar intervertebral disc. Jiangsu Journal of Traditional Chinese Medicine 40 (8), 47–48 (in Chinese).
15. Chen, Y.L., Zhang, X.L., Xia, J.Z., et al., 2011. Clinical observation of wet cupping combined with acupuncture and tuina for 36 patients with blood stasis syndrome of cervical spondylosis. Jiangsu Journal of Traditional Chinese Medicine 43 (3), 64–65 (in Chinese).
16. Cheng, G., 2000. Clinical report of observation of cupping therapy on lumbocrural pain caused by degenerative spondylolisthesis. Journal of Clinical Acupuncture and Moxibustion 16 (7), 33–34 (in Chinese).
17. Chi, F.L., Liu, G.L., 1987. Clinical observation of therapeutic effect of cupping therapy on wound healing. Chinese Primary Health Care 1 (9), 24–25 (in Chinese).
18. Ci, H.F., 2010. Clinical observation of therapeutic effect of combination of acupuncture and cupping therapy on 104 cases with acute herpes zoster. Modern Medicine and Health 26, 1550–1551 (in Chinese).
19. Cramer, H., Lauche, R., Hohmann, C., et al., 2011. Randomized controlled trial of pulsating cupping (pneumatic pulsation therapy) for chronic neck pain. Forsch. Komplementarmed. 18 (6), 327–334.
20. Cui, C.Z., Chen, D.H., 2011. Integrative Chinese and western medicine in treating 62 cases of herpes zoster. Chinese Medicine Modern Distance Education of China. 9 (3), 76 (in Chinese).
21. Dai, J.Y., Shao, J., Wang, Y.H., et al., 2006. Clinical comparative observations on acupuncture treatment of 200 simple obesity patients by syndrome differentiation. Shanghai Journal of Acupuncture and Moxibustion 25 (10), 13–15 (in Chinese).
22. Fang, X., Jin, Y., 2006. Clinical observation of medicinal cupping therapy on indirectly contusion injuries of temporomandibular joint. Modern Journal of Integrated Traditional Chinese and Western Medicine 15, 734 (in Chinese).
23. Farhadi, K., Schiwebel, D.C., Saeb, M., et al., 2009. The effectiveness of wet-cupping for nonspecific low back pain in Iran: a randomized controlled trial. Complement. Ther. Med. 17, 9–15.
24. Feng, W.M., 2004. Clinical observation of instant and forward analgesic effect of wet cupping therapy on 156 patients with soft tissue injury. Chinese Journal of Traditional Medical Science and Technology 11 (3), 180 (in Chinese).
25. Fu, C.A., Bai, Z.Q., 2004. Clinical observation of comparison of acupuncture and acupuncture combined with cupping therapy on facial paralysis. Journal of Yanan University (Medical Science) 2 (3), 59 (in Chinese).
26. Fu, L., Liu, W.A., Wu, Q.M., et al., 2009. Observation on the efficacy of acupuncture plus pricking-cupping bloodletting in treating postapoplectic shoulder-hand syndrome. Shanghai Journal of Acupuncture and Moxibustion 28, 132–134 (in Chinese).

27. Fu, Y., Jin, J.L., 2005. Clinical Observation of Therapeutic effect of Moving Cupping Therapy Combined with Herbal Medicine on Perimenopausal Syndrome. (in Chinese) (Master's thesis), Tianjin University of Traditional Chinese Medicine.

28. Gao, B.B., 2010. Combination of acupuncture and wet cupping therapy on treating 92 cases with idiopathic facial palsy. China Journal of Guang Ming Chinese Medicine 25, 1244–1245 (in Chinese).

29. Gao, Y.J., Liu, H.S., 2009. Combination of acupuncture and wet cupping therapy on treating 30 cases with post-herpetic neuralgia. Journal of External Therapy of TCM 18 (6), 34–35 (in Chinese).

30. Ge, J.J., Sun, L.H., Li, W.L., 2003. Clinical observation of 48 cases on sciatica by retaining the needle and cupping. Chinese Journal of the Practical Chinese with Modern Medicine 3, 823–824 (in Chinese).

31. Guo, J.M., Xu, C.J., 1997. Wet cupping therapy on Tanzhong (RM17) for schizophrenia. Shandong Journal of Traditional Chinese Medicine 16 (2), 74 (in Chinese).

32. Guo, L.X., 2006. Clinical observation of therapeutic effect of pricking cupping bloodletting therapy on herpes zoster. Shanxi Journal of Traditional Chinese Medicine 22 (3), 41 (in Chinese).

33. Guo, X.L., Wang, X.J., Zuo, W.Y., 1992. Clinical observation of pricking–cupping bloodletting therapy on mastitis. Zhen Jiu Xue Bao [vol unknown] 2, 34–35 (in Chinese).

34. Han, L.X., Wang, Y.Y., 1998. Observation of therapeutic effect of cupping therapy on muscle pain caused by wind-pathogen. Tianjin Journal of Traditional Chinese Medicine 15 (3), 122 (in Chinese).

35. He, Z.S., 2011. The therapeutic effect of tapped cupping with laser exposure therapy in the treatment of herpes zoster: an analysis of 36 cases. Journal of Clinical Acupuncture and Moxibustion. 27 (8), 44–45 (in Chinese).

36. Hong, T.T., Wu, L.X., 2011. Combined pricking cupping and Chinese medicinal mask for treating acne. Shanghai Journal of Acupuncture and Moxibustion 30 (6), 387–388 (in Chinese).

37. Hong, Y.F., Wu, J.X., Wang, B., 2006. The effect of moving cupping therapy on nonspecific low back pain. Chinese Journal of Rehabilitation Medicine 21, 340–343 (in Chinese).

38. Huang, G.Q., Li, F.Y., Huang, Y., 2004. Clinical observation on therapeutic effect of moving cupping therapy on wind-cold type of common cold. Chinese Journal of Current Clinical Medicine 2, 1680–1681 (in Chinese).

39. Huang, J., Li, W.J., 2008. Clinical observation on acute posterior ganglionitis by method of surrounding puncture method and percussopunctator combined with cupping cup. Journal of Liaoning University of Traditional Chinese Medicine 10, 168–169 (in Chinese).

40. Huang, J., Wei, D., Wu, J.D., 2010a. Venesection and cupping treating acne in 76 cases. China Bio-Beauty 1, 19–21 (in Chinese).

41. Huang, L.P., Cao, R.L., Bi, Y.F., et al., 2009. Combination of flash cupping and acupuncture on treating of 115 cases with peripheral facial paralysis. Shanxi Journal of Traditional Chinese Medicine 30, 597–599 (in Chinese).

42. Huang, L.P., Cao, R.L., Zhang, X.X., 2010b. Wet cupping therapy on Yifeng (SJ17) for 58 cases with acute peripheral facial paralysis. Shanxi Journal of Traditional Chinese Medicine 31, 473–474 (in Chinese).

43. Huang, Z.F., Li, H.Z., Zhang, Z.J., et al., 2006. Observations on the efficacy of cupping for treating 30 patients with cancer pain. Shanghai Journal of Acupuncture and Moxibustion 25 (8), 14–15 (in Chinese).

44. Ji, J., 1992. Observation on clinical effect of vitiligo treated with medicinal cupping. Chinese Acupuncture and Moxibustion 12 (3), 11–12 (in Chinese).

45. Ji, X.L., Guo, H.Q., 2009. The clinical observation on belt-shaped herpes cases treated by Ciluo fa. Inner Mongolia Medicine Journal 41 (6), 698–699 (in Chinese).

46. Jiang, H., Hu, D., Chen, H.Y., 2006. Observation and nursing for cupping along the channels of TCM to treatment chronic bronchitis with acute pulmonary infection. Journal of Nursing Science 21 (1), 48–49 (in Chinese).

47. Jiang, X.Y., Zhuo, R., 2008. Therapeutic effect of blood-letting puncture and cupping on upper-limb edema after mastectomy for breast cancer. Journal of Nursing Science 23 (8 Surgery Edition), 37–38 (in Chinese).

48. Jin, M.Z., Xie, Z.Q., Chen, X.W., et al., 2008. Observations on the efficacy of blood-letting puncture and cupping in treating middle-aged and senile herpes zoster. Shanghai Journal of Acupuncture and Moxibustion 27 (3), 20–21 (in Chinese).

49. Kang, H.Q., Li, M., 2005. Clinical observation of wet cupping on 48 patients with erysipelas. Journal of Emergency Traditional Chinese Medicine 14 (1), 51 (in Chinese).

50. Kim, J.I., Kim, T.H., Lee, M.S., et al., 2011a. Evaluation of wet-cupping therapy for persistent non-specific low back pain: a randomized, waiting list controlled, open-label, parallel-group pilot trial. Trials 12, 146–152.

51. Lauche, R., Cramer, H., Choi, D.E., et al., 2011. The influence of a series of five dry cupping treatments on pain and mechanical thresholds in patients with chronic non-specific neck pain – a randomized controlled pilot study. BMC Complement. Altern. Med. 11, 63–73.

52. Li, H.T., Liu, J.H., 2005. Clinical observation on treatment of peripheral facial paralysis with acupuncture and pricking-cupping therapy. Journal of Chinese Integrated Medicine 3 (1), 18 69 (in Chinese).

53. Li, J.C., Fan, Y.S., 2008. Clinical observations on treatment of subhealth with acupuncture and moxibustion plus moving cupping on the back. Shanghai Journal of Acupuncture and Moxibustion 27 (2), 8–9 (in Chinese).

54. Li, J.Y., Chen, W.T., 2009. Clinical observation of wet cupping therapy for non-specific low back pain. Inner Mongolia Journal of Traditional Chinese Medicine 7, 31–32 (in Chinese).

55. Li, K.Z., 2009. Clinical observation on treatment of 80 cases of peripheral facial paralysis with acupuncture and flash cupping therapy. Journal of Qiqihar Medical College 30 (24), 3091 (in Chinese).

56. Li, P., 2010. Clinical observation on treatment of 60 cases of acute peripheral facial paralysis with acupuncture and flash cupping therapy. Journal of Shanxi College of Traditional Chinese Medicine 33 (4), 83–84 (in Chinese).

57. Li, W.H., 2005. Clinical observation on plum-blossom needle therapy combined with cupping for treatment of acute facial paralysis. Chinese Acupuncture and Moxibustion 25, 765–767 (in Chinese).

58. Li, X., 2006. Therapeutic effect of plum-blossom needle tapping and moving cupping on lateral thigh skin neuritis: a clinical study. Practical New Medicine 7, 702–703 (in Chinese).

59. Liang, S.Y., 2009. Wet cupping therapy plus massage on treatment of 50 cases with pivot joint disturbance vertigo. Fujian Journal of Traditional Chinese Medicine 40 (1), 28–29 (in Chinese).

60. Liang, Y.L., Lu, L.Q., Yang, X.Q., et al., 2009. Clinical observation of wet cupping therapy plus acupuncture on treatment of insomnia. Nursing Practice and Research 6 (6), 79–80 (in Chinese).

61. Liao, F.R., 2009. Observations on the efficacy of pricking bloodletting plus cupping in treating cervical vertigo. Shanghai Journal of Acupuncture and Moxibustion 28, 399–400 (in Chinese).

62. Lin, S.Z., 2005. Observation of wet cupping combined with electroacupuncture on 52 patients with prolapse of lumbar intervertebral disc. Traditional Chinese Medicine Research 18 (11), 47–49 (in Chinese).

63. Liu, B.X., Xu, M., Huang, C.J., et al., 2008. Therapeutic effect of balance cupping therapy on non-specific low back pain. Chinese Journal of Rehabilitative Theory and Practice 14, 572–573 (in Chinese).

64. Liu, B.X., Xu, M., Huang, C.J., et al., 2010. Clinical observation on the treatment of lateral humeral epicondylitis using self-made herbal decoction cupping therapy. Journal of Zhejiang University of Traditional Chinese Medicine 34, 409–410 (in Chinese).

65. Liu, H.P., Liang, B., He, J.B., 2009a. Therapeutic effect of acupuncture combined with flash cupping for acne vulgaris. Liaoning Journal of Traditional Chinese Medicine 36, 1395–1397 (in Chinese).

66. Liu, H.Q., Zhang, L.C., 2011. Combined wet cupping therapy and acupuncture in treating 28 cases facial paralysis. Journal of Changchun University of Traditional Chinese Medicine. 27 (4), 255–256 (in Chinese).

67. Liu, J., Zhao, Y., Zeng, R., 2005. Randomized controlled trial on observation of wet cupping therapy on sore pain of keen joint of African people. Chinese Journal of Clinical Rehabilitation 9 (47), 135–136 (in Chinese).

68. Liu, L., Li, Z.L., 2003. Curative effect observation on treating herpes zoster by Zhong Xi Medicine. Chinese Journal of the Practical Chinese with Modern Medicine 3, 1088–1089 (in Chinese).

69. Liu, L., Li, W.L., Man, W., 2006a. Clinical observation of wet cupping combined with auricular therapy on chloasma. Journal of Hebei Traditional Chinese Medicine and Pharmacology 21 (2), 30–31 (in Chinese).

70. Liu, L.G., Liu, L., Lu, M., 2006b. Clinical observation of therapeutic effect of wet cupping therapy combined with electro acupuncture for herpes zoster. Zhongguo Zhen Jiu (Supplement), 21–22 (in Chinese).

71. Liu, Q.W., Chang, H.S., 2004. Integrative Chinese and western medicine for herpes zoster. Journal of External Therapy of Traditional Chinese Medicine 13 (5), 53 (in Chinese).

72. Long, W.H., Liu, H., 2003. 34 cases observation of combined therapy for herpes zoster. Journal of Medical Theory and Practice 16, 1170 (in Chinese).

73. Liu, Y.Z., 2007. Combination of moving cupping and electro acupuncture in treating of 51 cases with obesity. Zhongguo Zhen Jiu (Supplement)12 (in Chinese).

74. Liu, Y.Z., Liu, J.R., Liu, L.S., et al., 2009b. Clinical study of Wang Yan Xun Jing medicinal cupping therapy for cerebral infarction. China Foreign Medical Treatment 2, 113–114.

75. Lu, H.M., Ding, S., 2009. Clinical observation of therapeutic effect of combination of electroacupuncture and wet cupping therapy for shoulder-hand syndrome. Journal of Practical Traditional Chinese Medicine 25, 320–321 (in Chinese).

76. Lu, J., Wang, Y., 2007. Acupuncture combined with wet cupping therapy on 63 cases of prolapse of lumbar intervertebral disc. Journal of Clinical Acupuncture and Moxibustion 23 (3), 16–17 (in Chinese).

77. Lu, Z.X., Jin, H.L., Zhang, P., 2009. Cupping for preventing nausea and vomiting after laparoscopic gallbladder resection. Journal of Zhejiang College of Traditional Chinese Medicine 33, 862–863 (in Chinese).

78. Luan, R.F., Tang, J., 2011. Clinical observation of wet cupping therapy combined with electroacupuncture for 50 cases of herpes zoster. Chinese Community Doctors. 13 (287), 174 (in Chinese).

79. Ludtke, R., Albrecht, U., Stange, R., 2006. Brachialgia paraesthetica nocturna can be relieved by 'wet cupping' – results of a randomized pilot study. Complement. Ther. Med. 14, 247–253.

80. Luo, L.X., Lou, L.L., 2011. The clinical curative effect observation on acute peripheral facial paralysis treatment in needling combined with rapid cupping 34 cases. Journal of Practical Traditional Chinese Internal Medicine 25 (1), 89–90 (in Chinese).

81. Luo, X.X., Ma, L.S., 2010. Clinical observation of effect of balance cupping for acute strain of lumbar muscle. Chinese Journal of Information on TCM 17 (9), 75–76 (in Chinese).

82. Lü, J.C., 2010. Combination of electroacupuncture and wet cupping therapy for intractable facial paralysis accompany with sensory disturbance of facial nerve. China Higher Medical Education 10, 136–137 (in Chinese).

83. Lü, S.Q., 2011. Clinical observation on acupuncture plus moving cupping for depression. Shanghai Journal of Acupuncture and Moxibustion 30 (11), 735–737 (in Chinese).

84. Ma, C.T., Zhang, J., 2006. Clinical Observation of Moving Cupping Therapy on Excess Pattern Depression. (in Chinese) (Master's thesis), Beijing University of Chinese Medicine.

85. Michalsen, A., Bock, S., Ludtke, R., et al., 2009. Effects of traditional cupping therapy in patients with carpal tunnel syndrome: a randomized controlled trial. Journal of Pain 10, 601–618.

86. Ni, M.L., 2010. 48 cases clinical observation of acupuncture plus flash cupping therapy on treating facial muscle spasm. Heilongjiang Medicine Journal 23, 453 (in Chinese).

87. Ou, X.H., Xu, S.C., 2009. Sixty cases of refractory facial paralysis treated with traditional Chinese medicine using acupuncture and flash tank. Journal of Chengdu University of Traditional Chinese Medicine 32 (3), 37–38 (in Chinese).

88. Qiu, J.Z., Fan, C.M., Wei, F.Y., et al., 2003. Clinical observation of therapeutic effect of medicinal cupping on acute facial neuritis. China Journal of Modern Medicine 13 (21), 146 (in Chinese).

89. Ren, Y.J., 2006. Observation of wet cupping combined with acupuncture on 50 patients with facial paralysis. Shanxi Journal of Traditional Chinese Medicine 27, 480–481 (in Chinese).

90. Rui, X.G., 2010. Observations on the efficacy of acupuncture plus cutaneous needle tapping in treating inflammation of superior cluneal nerves. Shanghai Journal of Acupuncture and Moxibustion 29, 515–516 (in Chinese).

91. Shao, M., Liu, T.Y., 2003. Clinical observations on the treatment of 93 cervical spondylopathy by Dazhui blood-letting puncturing and cupping. Shanghai Journal of Acupuncture and Moxibustion 22 (8), 20–21 (in Chinese).

92. Song, S.Y., Zhang, X.L., 2011. Wet cupping therapy for 80 cases of herpes zoster. Shanxi Journal of Traditional Chinese Medicine 32 (7), 892–893 (in Chinese).

93. Sun, H.W., Li, L., 2010. Observation of wet cupping therapy on treating 40 cases with post- auricular pain after peripheral facial palsy. China Journal of Guang Ming Chinese Medicine 25, 1674 (in Chinese).

94. Sun, L.J., Xu, X.D., 2007. Clinical observation of therapeutic effect of moving cupping on back shu points combined with acupuncture on 30 patients with simple obesity. China Practical Medicine 2 (32), 138–139 (in Chinese).

95. Sun, R.H., Wang, J., Hong, L.J., 2011. Combination of western medication and wet cupping therapy for herpes zoster. Chinese Community Doctors 13 (293), 191 (in Chinese).

96. Sun, S.Q., Xu, S.X., 2006. 67 cases suffered from erysipelas on lower legs cured by means of integration of traditional Chinese medicine and western medicine. Journal of Chinese Practical Medicine 1 (5), 109–110 (in Chinese).

97. Tang, C.R., 2003. Acupuncture combined with moving cupping therapy for diabetic peripheral neuropathy. Sichuan Journal of Traditional Chinese Medicine 21 (7), 89–90 (in Chinese).

98. Tang, Y.Q., Liang, A.J., Wang, Y.J., 2010. Observations on the efficacy of medicated cupping plus functional training in treating rheumatoid arthritis. Shanghai Journal of Acupuncture and Moxibustion 29 (9), 596–597 (in Chinese).

99. Tao, Q., Lu, H.X., 2007. Clinical observation of electroacupuncture combined with wet cupping therapy on abdominal aorta calcification related to lumbar intervertebral disc prolapse. Journal of Clinical Acupuncture and Moxibustion 23 (8), 46–47 (in Chinese).

100. Wan, X.W., 2005. Clinical observation on acupuncture combined with cupping therapy for treatment of ankylosing spondylitis. Chinese Acupuncture and Moxibustion 25, 551–552 (in Chinese).

101. Wan, X.W., 2007. Clinical observation on treatment of cervical spondylosis with combined acupuncture and cupping therapies. Journal of Acupuncture and Tuina Science 5, 345–347 (in Chinese).

102. Wang, J., 2010b. Combination of acupuncture and moving cupping therapy for 42 cases with functional dyspepsia. China Science and Technology Information 15, 176 (in Chinese).

103. Wang, L., 2010c. Clinical observation of flash cupping for treating chronic obstructive pulmonary disease in remission. Chinese General Nursing 8, 1574–1575 (in Chinese).

104. Wang, L.R., Liu, H.F., Li, Q.Y., 2010. Observation on the clinical efficacy of meridian cupping plus acupuncture in treating 60 cases of acute peripheral facial paralysis. Sichuan Journal of Traditional Chinese Medicine 28 (1), 110–112.

105. Wang, P.L., 2010d. Clinical observation on therapeutic effects of abdominal acupuncture combined with blood-letting acupuncture and cupping for treating nerve-root cervical spondylosis. Clinical Journal of Chinese Medicine 9 (2), 15–17.

106. Wang, Q.F., Wang, G.Y., 2007. Observation on the efficacy of acupuncture and moxibustion plus blood-letting puncture and moving cupping in treating acne. Shanghai Journal of Acupuncture and Moxibustion 26 (12), 20–21 (in Chinese).

107. Wang, S.P., 2009. Observation of cupping therapy in treating 62 cases of bronchial asthma. Guiding Journal of Traditional Chinese Medicine and Pharmacology 15 (10), 56 (in Chinese).

108. Wang, X.M., Zhou, Z.X., 2004. Electroacupuncture combined with wet cupping therapy on 66 patients with cervical spondylotic radiculopathy. Shanxi Journal of Traditional Chinese Medicine 25 (1), 60–61 (in Chinese).

109. Wang, Y.H., Huang, S.X., Liu, B.Y., et al., 2009. Clinical observation of therapeutic effect of acupuncture for herpes zoster. Chinese Journal of Basic Medicine in Traditional Chinese Medicine 15, 774–777 (in Chinese).

110. Wang, Z.L., 2011. 36 cases observation of moving cupping therapy for infant bronchial pneumonia. Chinese Pediatrics Integrative of Traditional Chinese and Western Medicine 3 (1), 46–47 (in Chinese).

111. Wu, F.F., Yang, S.Q., Zhang, S.J., 2010a. Wet cupping therapy on back shu points on treatment of acne. Journal of Qiqihar Medical College 31, 1596 (in Chinese).

112. Wu, P.X., Ma, W.L., Zhao, X.X., 2010b. Clinical observation of acupuncture plus cupping therapy for chronic urticaria. Guiding Journal of Traditional Chinese Medicine and Pharmacology 16 (11), 79 (in Chinese).

113. Wu, Y.T., 2008. Therapeutic effects on acne by bloodletting with cupping therapy on the back. Journal of Practical Traditional Chinese Internal Medicine 22 (10), 61–62 (in Chinese).

114. Wu, Z.Y., Huang, W., 2011. Clinical observation of wet cupping therapy combined with rehabilitation for shoulder pain after stroke. Journal of Zhejiang Chinese Medical University 35 (3), 425–426 (in Chinese).

115. Xiao, W., Wang, Y., Kong, H.B., et al., 2009. Observation of cupping therapy on back-shu points for chronic obstructive pulmonary disease. Chinese Journal of Traditional Chinese Medicine 21, 420–421 (in Chinese).

116. Xiao, W., Wang, Y., Kong, H.B., et al., 2010. Effect of cupping at back-shu acupoints on immunologic function in patients with chronic obstructive pulmonary disease during stable stage. Journal of Anhui College of Traditional Chinese Medicine 29 (5), 37–39 (in Chinese).

117. Xin, K.P., 2006. Cupping on Dazhui on 30 children with fever caused by heat stroke. Jiangxi Journal of Traditional Chinese Medicine 37 (285), 53–54 (in Chinese).

118. Xiong, J.F., 2010. Observation of wet cupping therapy for 60 cases with acute prolapse of lumbar intervertebral disc. Journal of External Therapy of Traditional Chinese Medicine 19 (5), 28–29 (in Chinese).

119. Xiong, S.Y., Hu, Y., Gong, L.P., 2007. Observation of therapeutic effect of cupping therapy on herpes zoster pain. Journal of Nurses Training 22, 948–949 (in Chinese).

120. Xiong, Z.L., Zhang, G.H., 2007. Cupping therapy combined with acupuncture on 48 patients with acute herpes zoster. Journal of Clinical Acupuncture and Moxibustion 23 (7), 38–39 (in Chinese).

121. Xu, L., Yang, X.J., 2004. Therapeutic effect of acyclovir in combination with meridian acupuncture and cupping in the treatment of 40 cases of herpes zoster. Tianjin Pharmacy 16 (3), 23–24 (in Chinese).

122. Xu, M., Liu, B.X., Huang, C.J., et al., 2009. The therapeutic effects of balance cupping therapy on chronic lumbar muscle strain. Liaoning Journal of Traditional Chinese Medicine 36, 1007–1008 (in Chinese).

123. Xu, M.Y., 2006. Clinical observation of therapeutic effect of cupping on Zhong Ji (RM3) in the treatment of post-operative uroschesis. Liaoning Journal of Traditional Chinese Medicine 33, 719 (in Chinese).

124. Xu, S.W., 2008. Observation on the therapeutic effect of acupuncture on generalized osteoarthritis. Shanghai Journal of Acupuncture and Moxibustion 27 (4), 11–12 (in Chinese).

125. Xu, S.X., 1999. Application of cupping therapy in treatment of furuncles. The Chinese Journal of Dermatoneurology 21 (2), 21–22 (in Chinese).

126. Xu, W.D., Zhang, Y.J., Yang, J., et al., 2006. Cupping on back shu points for acute bronchitis. Journal of Clinical Acupuncture and Moxibustion 22 (8), 39–40 (in Chinese).

127. Xu, Y., Ge, H.Z., 2010. Clinical observation on treating acute lumbar sprain by cupping plus acupuncture. Clinical Journal of Chinese Medicine 10 (2), 70–71.

128. Xue, W.H., Wang, J.L., Wang, G.R., 2005. Clinical observation of wet cupping therapy on rotaviral enteritis. Liaoning Journal of Traditional Chinese Medicine 32, 826 (In Chinese).

129. Yang, J.H., Guo, L.Z., Xiong, J., 2007. Clinical observation on the treatment of 46 cases of acute ankle sprain with acupuncture combined with venesection and ventouse. Guiding Journal of Traditional Chinese Medicine 13 (4), 57–58 (in Chinese).

130. Yang, X.B., 2011. Clinical observation of acupuncture and moxibustion combined with tuina and wet cupping for 90 patients with prolapse of lumbar intervertebral disc 28 (2), 54–56 (in Chinese).

131. Yao, H.X., Chai, Y., Wang, W.S., 2011. Clinical effectiveness of adjunctive therapy using cupping in treating patients with obesity and type 2 diabetes mellitus. Chinese General Practice 14 (5C), 1723–1725 (in Chinese).

132. Yao, X., 2006. Clinical observation of cupping therapy combined with acupuncture on chronic diarrhea. Jilin Medical Journal 27, 1403–1404 (in Chinese).

133. Yin, G.Z., Zheng, L.J., 2009. Observation of 72 cases of psoriasis treated by wet cupping therapy. Xinjiang Journal of Traditional Chinese Medicine 27 (5), 13–15 (in Chinese).

134. You, Y., Lan, C.Y., Liang, W., et al., 2006a. Wet cupping combined with traction for prolapse of lumbar vertebral disc. Chinese Journal of Convalescent Medicine 15 (1), 14–15 (in Chinese).

135. You, Y., Yang, Z.H., Sun, D.Z., 2006b. Effect of plum-blossom needle therapy and cupping therapy combined with traction on cervical spondylosis of vertebral artery type. Chinese Journal of Rehabilitative Theory and Practice 12, 1037–1038 (in Chinese).

136. Yu, X.Y., Geng, L.M., 2008. The clinical research on asthma treated of chronicity-persistent period with pricking meridian and ventouse, (in Chinese). (Dissertation for Master's degree of Hebei Medical College.).

137. Yu, Y.C., Li, H.B., 2011. Clinical observation of wet cupping therapy on improving recovery of muscle strength of patients with acute myelitis 35 (4), 331–332 (in Chinese).

138. Zeng, H.W., Nie, B., Huang, N.B., 2007. Analysis of the efficacy of blood-letting puncture and cupping plus warming acupuncture for treating cervical spondylopathy of vertebral artery type. Shanghai Journal of Acupuncture and Moxibustion 26 (6), 8–10 (in Chinese).

139. Zha, B.G., Wang, Z.Y., 2005. Cupping therapy on accelerating thenar wound healing: clinical trial of 28 cases. Hunan Journal of Traditional Chinese Medicine 21 (3), 81 (in Chinese).

140. Zhang, D.D., Li, J.B., 2009. Combination of wet cupping therapy and acupuncture on treatment of post-stroke shoulder-hand syndrome. Jilin Journal of Traditional Chinese Medicine 29, 796–797 (in Chinese).

141. Zhang, F.Y., Liu, X.H., 2006. Acupuncture combined with moving cupping therapy on 30 cases of simple obesity and hyperlipidemia. Journal of External Therapy of Traditional Chinese Medicine 15 (5), 42–43 (in Chinese).

142. Zhang, H.B., 2010. Clinical observation of acupuncture combined with venesection and ventouse on periarthritis of the shoulder: report of 60 cases. Shanxi Journal of Traditional Chinese Medicine 26 (10), 28–29 (in Chinese).

143. Zhang, H.X., Liu, Y.N., Huang, G.F., et al., 2009. Observation of different types of acupuncture on pain reduction of herpes zoster of the head and face. Journal of Emergency Traditional Chinese Medicine 18, 1979–1981 (in Chinese).

144. Zhang, J.P., 2011. Observations on the efficacy of plum-blossom needle tapping plus cupping in treating flat wart. Shanghai Journal of Acupuncture and Moxibustion. 30 (3), 173–174 (in Chinese).

145. Zhang, J.W., Wang, X.L., Zhou, S.H., 2004. Clinical observation of combination of acyclovir and acupuncture in the treatment of 41 cases of herpes zoster. Chinese General Practice 7, 1179–1180 (in Chinese).

146. Zhang, J.X., Diao, J., Yu, S.P., 2007. Traditional cupping therapy with syndrome differentiation on insomnia. Chinese Journal of Clinical Medicinal Professional Research 13, 3444 (in Chinese).

147. Zhang, K.X., Song, S.J., 2008. Clinical observation of wet cupping therapy on back shu points for acne. World Health Digest 5, 193–194 (in Chinese).

148. Zhang, Q., Liang, X.S., Guo, T.Z., et al., 2008. Observation on treatment of head-face herpes zoster. Liaoning Journal of Traditional Chinese Medicine 35, 602 (in Chinese).

149. Zhang, Q.L., Fu, X.H., 2009. Clinical observation of cupping therapy plus electroacupuncture on treatment of lumbar vertebral disc prolapse with blood stasis syndrome. Acta Chinese Medicine and Pharmacology 37 (5), 79–80 (in Chinese).

150. Zhang, X.Y., 2009. Sixteen cases with refractory hiccup treated by moving cupping on back shu points. Journal of the Chinese Acupuncture and Moxibustion 25 (7), 45–46 (in Chinese).

151. Zhang, Y.B., Yan, C.Y., 2010. Clinical observation of medicinal cupping therapy on treating chronic gastritis. Guangxi Journal of Traditional Chinese Medicine 33 (2), 17–18.

152. Zhang, Y.C., Yan, X.Y., 2004. Clinical observation of and nursing care for the treatment of bronchiolitis by auxiliary glass cupping. Journal of Qilu Nursing 10 (1), 28 (in Chinese).

153. Zhang, Y.D., 2005. Observation of moving and retained cupping therapy on 30 pediatric cases with recurrent respiratory tract infection. Journal of External Therapy of Traditional Chinese Medicine 14 (6), 40–41 (in Chinese).

154. Zhao, J., 2010. Combination of cupping therapy and antibiotic treatment of 220 pediatric cases with cough after acute upper respiratory infection. Shanxi Journal of Traditional Chinese Medicine 26 (8), 34 (in Chinese).

155. Zhao, N.X., Shi, H.J., Ren, T.Y., et al., 2010. Observation of flash cupping therapy for acute peripheral facial neuritis. Journal of Guiyang College of Traditional Chinese Medicine 32 (2), 72–73 (in Chinese).

156. Zhao, X.Q., Zheng, J.H., Wang, G.C., et al., 2003. Treatment of 40 cases of intracranial hypertension syndrome by pricking GV14 acupoint plus cupping. Chinese Acupuncture and Moxibustion 23 (2), 75–76 (in Chinese).

157. Zheng, L., 2008. Clinical observation of wet cupping therapy on osteoarthritis. Chinese Journal of Traditional Medical Traumatology and Orthopedics 16 (10), 27–28 (in Chinese).

158. Zheng, Z.H., Liu, Q.Q., Xiao, Y.L., et al., 1999. Clinical observation of therapeutic effect of medicinal cupping therapy on prevention and treatment of bronchial asthma. Hebei Journal of Traditional Chinese Medicine 14 (2), 29–30 (in Chinese).

159. Zhong, J.R., Zhao, Y.S., Liang, Q.S., et al., 2010. Observation of ventouse therapy immediately following venomous snake bite. China Modern Medicine 17 (4), 19–21 (in Chinese).

160. Zhou, L.W., 2007. Moving cupping therapy on 45 cases of myofasciitis causing rigidity of the neck and back. Clinical Journal of Traditional Chinese Medicine 19, 170–171 (in Chinese).

161. Zhou, Y., Wu, R.M., Cao, Y., 2010. Observation of cupping therapy for pneumonia. Journal of Guiyang College of Traditional Chinese Medicine 32 (4), 54–55 (in Chinese).

162. Zhou, Y.M., 1994. Moving cupping therapy on 100 cases of common cold. Chinese Acupuncture and Moxibustion 14 (S1), 292 (in Chinese).

163. Zhu, F., Chen, S.J., Feng, D.R., et al., 2009. Observation of wet cupping therapy on treatment of acute peripheral facial neuritis. Journal of Emergency Traditional Chinese Medicine 18, 702–703 (in Chinese).

164. Zhu, L., Yang, D.H., Tan, Y.F., 2011. Clinical study of wet cupping therapy combined with acupuncture for prolapse of lumbar intervertebral disc. Jilin Journal of Traditional Chinese Medicine 31 (12), 1214–1215 (in Chinese).

165. Zhu, Y., Zhang, F.X., 2009. Observation of wet cupping therapy plus auricular acupressure for chloasma. Chinese Medicine Modern Distance Education of China 7 (3), 97 (in Chinese).

166. Zhu, Y., 2010. Combination of acupuncture and wet cupping therapy for 50 cases of chloasma. Shanxi Journal of Traditional Chinese Medicine 31, 476–478 (in Chinese).

167. Zhuang, W.B., Zhuang, L.H., Wu, H.M., 2011. Combination of wet cupping and tuina for 80 patients with nerve root type cervical spondylosis. Chinese Journal of Ethnomedicine and Ethnopharmacy 5, 111–112 (in Chinese).

168. Zou, L.Y., Hu, J.Y., 2009. Cupping therapy on treatment of 40 cases with acute lumbar muscle strain. Henan Traditional Chinese Medicine 29, 802–803 (in Chinese).

169. Zou, R., Zhang, H.X., Huang, G.F., et al., 2010. Analgesic effect of electroacupuncture at EX-B2 combined with press needles and ventouse for patients with herpes zoster. Chinese Journal of Rehabilitation 25, 205–206 (in Chinese).

170. Xu, J., Ma, Q.J., 2011. Combination of acupuncture and cupping therapy for 50 cases of obesity. Shangdong Journal of Traditional Chinese Medicine 30 (2), 106–107 (in Chinese).

171. Wang, H.Y., 2010a. Acupuncture combined with pricking blood therapy for treatment of 76 cases of peripheral facial paralysis. Liaoning Journal of Traditional Chinese Medicine 37 (9), 1799–1800 (in Chinese).

172. CONSORT Group. CONSORT Statement 2001 – Checklist: Items to Include When Reporting a Randomized Trial. Online. Available: http://www.consort-statement.org.

173. Lee, M.S., Kim, J.I., Kong, J.C., et al., 2010c. Developing and validating a sham cupping device. Acupuncture Medicine 28, 200–204.

174. MacPherson, H., Altman, D.G., Hammerschlag, R., et al., 2010. Revised STandards for Reporting Interventions in Clinical Trials of Acupuncture (STRICTA): extending the CONSORT Statement. PLoS Med. 7 (6), e1000261. doi:10.1371/journal.pmed.1000261.

175. Laine, C., Horton, R., DeAngelis, C.D., et al., 2007. Clinical trial registration looking back and moving ahead. New England Journal of Medicine 356, 2734–2736.

176. Viergever, R.F., Ghersi, D., 2011. The Quality of Registration of Clinical Trials. PLoS ONE 6 (2), e14701.

FURTHER READING

Aiwen, L., 1996. The use of warm needle acupuncture plus cupping therapy for chronic low back pain involving osteoarthritic hyperostosis. American Journal of Acupuncture 24 (1), 5–10.

Bennett, R.M. (Ed.), 1986. The fibrositis/fibromyalgia syndrome: current issues and perspectives, symposium. American Journal of Medicine 81 (3A), 1–115.

Bennett, R.M., 1990. Myofascial pain syndromes and the fibromyalgia syndrome: a comparative analysis. In: Fricton, J.R., Awad, E.A. (Eds.), Myofascial Pain and Fibromyalgia: Advances in Pain Research and Therapy, vol. 17. Raven Press, New York, pp. 43–65.

Bonci, A.S., Oswald, S., 1993. Barrier trigger points and muscle performance. National Strength and Conditioning Association Journal 15 (6), 39–43.

Campbell, S.M., 1989. Regional myofascial pain syndromes. Rheum. Dis. Clin. North Am. 15 (1), 31–44.

Cupping. Online. Available: http://www.cancer.org/treatment/treatmentsandsideeffects/complementaryandalternativemedicine/herbsvitaminsandminerals/cupping?sitearea=ETO (accessed 17.10.13.).

Fomby, E.W., Mellion, M.B., 1997. Identifying and treating myofascial pain syndrome. The Physician and Sports Medicine 25 (2). Online. Available: https://physsportsmed.org/doi/10.3810/psm.1997.02.1674.

Fricton, J.R., Kroening, R., Haley, D., et al., 1985. Myofascial pain syndrome of the head and neck: a review of clinical characteristics of 164 patients. Oral Surgery, Oral Medicine and Oral Pathology 60 (6), 615–623.

Gerwin, R.D., 1991. Myofascial aspects of low back pain. Neurosurgery of Clinics of North America 2 (4), 761–784.

Goldenberg, D.L., 1992. Fibromyalgia, chronic fatigue, and myofascial pain syndromes. Current Opinion in Rheumatology 4 (2), 247–257.

Goldman, L.B., Rosenberg, N.L., 1991. Myofascial pain syndrome and fibromyalgia. Semin. Neurol. 11 (3), 274–280.

Greenwood, M., 2005. Psychosomatic compartmentalization, the root of Qi and Blood Stagnation. Online. Available: http://members.shaw.ca/paradoxpublishing/pdf/articles/aama/vol-13-1-qiBloodStag.pdf (accessed 13.07.05.).

Kemper, K.J., Sarah, R., Silver-Highfield, E., 2000. On pins and needles? Pediatric pain patients' experience with acupuncture. Pediatrics 105 (4 Pt 2), 941–947.

Liu, X., Liu, G., Zhang, H., 2005. Symptomatic improvement of cervical spondylosis by sliding cupping and its relation to disease course and age. Zhongguo Linchuang Kangfu 22, 230–232, also in: Chinese Journal of Clinical Rehabilitation 9(22):232-232.

Prudden, B., 1980. Pain Erasure: The Bonnie Prudden Way. Evans, New York City.

Rachlin, E.S., 1994. History and physical examination for regional myofascial pain syndrome. In: Rachlin, E.S. (Ed.), Myofascial Pain and Fibromyalgia: Trigger Point Management. CV Mosby, St Louis, pp. 159–172.

Sherman, K.J., Cherkin, D.C., Hogeboom, C.J., 2001. The diagnosis and treatment of patients with chronic low-back pain (LBP) by traditional Chinese medical acupuncturists. Journal of Alternative and Complementary Medicine 7 (6), 641–650.

Simons, D.G., Travell, J.G., 1983. Myofascial origins of low back pain 1: principles of diagnosis and treatment. Postgraduate Medicine 73 (2), 66–73.

Simons, D.G., 1988. Myofascial pain due to trigger points. In: Goodgold, J. (Ed.), Rehabilitation Mmedicine. CV Mosby, St Louis, pp. 686–723.

Sola, A.E., Rodenberger, M.L., Gettys, B.B., 1955. Incidence of hypersensitive areas in posterior shoulder muscles: a survey of two hundred young adults. American Journal of Physical Medicine 34 (6), 585–590.

Song, Y., 2004. Observations on the therapeutic efficacy of treating 318 patients with sciatic pain with warm needle and cupping. Gan Su Zhong Yi (Gansu Chinese Medicine) 5, 27. Online. Available: http://caod.oriprobe.com/order.htm?id=7822237&ftext=base (accessed 17.10.13.).

Travell, J.G., Simons, D.G., 1983. Myofascial Pain and Dysfunction: The Trigger Point Manual. Williams & Wilkins, Baltimore.

Wolfe, F., Smythe, H.A., Yunus, M.B., et al., 1990. The American College of Rheumatology 1990 criteria for the classification of fibromyalgia: report of the multicenter criteria committee. Arthritis Rheumatology 33 (2), 160–172.

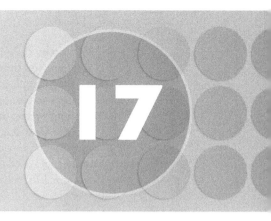

FREQUENTLY ASKED QUESTIONS AND PRECAUTIONS AND CONTRAINDICATIONS

17

CHAPTER CONTENTS

FREQUENTLY ASKED QUESTIONS (FAQS), 311

PRECAUTIONS AND CONTRAINDICATIONS, 312

FREQUENTLY ASKED QUESTIONS (FAQS)

Is it safe?
All cupping methods described in the book are safe to practice when performed by an experienced or trained practitioner.

Can I do cupping on myself?
Yes, self-cupping on the frontal aspect of the body is quite possible.

Does it hurt?
In most methods of cupping therapy a 'pulling' sensation is experienced rather than 'pain'. Only Moving cupping and Strong cupping may cause painful sensations in some people.

Do cupping marks always happen?
Following cupping treatment, some degree of marking on the skin is inevitable. However, these marks fade within a day or two and sometimes never occur.

How long do cupping marks last?
Cupping marks can last between 1 and 15 days, depending on the severity of the application.

Is there any bleeding from the cupping location?
If acupuncture has been performed in the same location before cupping treatment, a small amount of blood (a few drops) is normally sucked into the cup. Also of course, during the application of the Bleeding cupping method, a desired amount of blood is drawn into the cup. Otherwise no bleeding takes place during cupping treatment.

Does cupping cause skin lesion or any kind of damage to the skin?
Definitely not! A pinkish or reddening appearance of the skin surface is expected owing to increased blood circulation to the area.

What if I blister during the cupping?
Sometimes Strong cupping methods, if left on the skin for a long time, can cause a blister to appear. There is no need to panic if this happens. Using an acupuncture needle, burst the blister and drain the fluid out. Using sterilized gauze, cover the area and keep it dry for few days.

How many cups are used in one session?
Western practitioners use between 5 and 12 cups during one session. In the Far East, however, it is normal to see up to 60 cups being used during one session!

Can I cup over the eyes?
No, cupping over the eyes is contraindicated.

Can I cup on the face?
Yes, the Light cupping technique is normally used on the face.

Can I cup on the genitals?

No, cupping on the genitalia (male or female) is contraindicated.

How long is each cupping session?

Cupping sessions can last anywhere from 5 minutes to a massive 40-minute session!

Will cupping treatment interfere with my prescribed medication?

Not really. Cupping therapy is one of the safest treatment modalities I have come across in my 40 years of cupping practice!

Should I feel tired after the treatment?

It is normal to feel slightly tired or light-headed immediately after the treatment. A short rest should rectify this.

Can I go swimming or to the gym after the cupping session?

A 'rest' in a warm environment is recommended rather than 'activity', especially where it can be cold or windy! Following cupping treatment, the pores on the skin open. Any exposure to wind or cold at this stage will certainly be damaging to the Wei Qi (Defensive Qi), therefore should be avoided.

Can I go for run after the cupping session?

It is not recommended, for the same reason as above.

Can I receive cupping treatment during menstruation?

Yes, cupping during or leading up to the menstrual cycle is normal.

When is the best time for cupping treatment?

It can be done any time of the day.

Can I have a bath after the cupping treatment?

Yes – as a matter of fact, cupping was often performed in the Ottoman hamams and in Roman and Greek baths, to 'strengthen' the body as well as to 'get rid of colds'.

Is there a particular period in a month to avoid cupping?

No.

Is there a particular period in a month to favour cupping?

Only in Muslim traditional medicine, where Bleeding cupping (Hejama) is recommended during the 'full moon', as the 'bodily fluids also rise'; therefore the therapy is considered to be more 'effective'.

What is best, cupping on an empty stomach or on a full stomach?

Neither, as both conditions can cause Qi or Blood irregularities, as well as channel blockage.

If someone is fasting, especially during the month of Ramadan, is cupping therapy possible?

Cupping therapy, especially Dry cupping, is possible. Wet cupping should be avoided as indicated above.

Can one obtain strong suction using small cups?

Suction strength depends on two factors: the size of the cup and the size of the flame! Both factors help to determine the suction strength on the skin. However, one can easily create strong pulling action even with the small cup providing the flame inserted into the cup is large enough.

PRECAUTIONS AND CONTRAINDICATIONS

Cupping therapy, in general, is very safe and has no side-effects. There are a few exceptions, however, and when these are observed the implementation is safe and the benefits are generous. Precaution is necessary when treating patients who may be on anticoagulant drugs, or have an empty stomach, particularly during long fasting periods such as the holy Ramadan month, as fasting temporarily weakens the body's energy.

Do not employ cupping therapy over the eyes, sunburn or burns in general, open wounds or a recent trauma. During pregnancy, avoid cupping to the lower and upper abdomen; the lower back can be cupped until the sixth month of pregnancy, using Light or Medium cupping methods only (see Plates 33 and 34 in the colour plate section).

In patients complaining of lethargy or exhaustion, Empty cupping should be employed for only a very short time (i.e. a maximum of 5 minutes). During the Bleeding cupping application, patients on anticoagulant drugs may bleed more than originally calculated. It is therefore necessary to monitor the bleeding and remove the cup when about 100 mL of blood has been extracted. Such patients also mark or bruise more quickly and the skin takes longer to recover to its normal colour. Cupping (Wet or Dry) is contraindicated for extreme Yin-Xu (fluid deficient) people, in people suspected of haemorrhage of any kind, and on tumours of any form, including tuberculosis. Also, cupping of any kind is contraindicated for people who have suffered a cardiac arrest in the last 6 months. Wet cupping is contraindicated for people suffering from haemophilia or extreme anaemia. Avoid Wet cupping over the large veins such as varicose veins. Cupping therapy is contraindicated in all stages of an acute infectious conditions and diseases.

For sports injuries, please see Chapter 14.

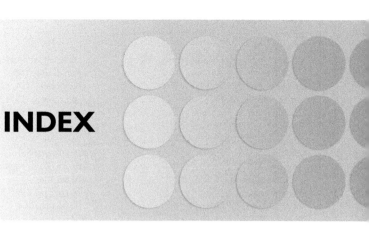

INDEX

Note: Page numbers followed by *f* indicate figures, *b* indicate boxes and *t* indicate tables.

A

abdominal cosmetic cupping, 132, 132*f*
abdominalis muscle, 134*f*
abdominal muscles, myofascial trigger points, 246
abdominal pain, 145–147, 146*f*
 aetiology, 145
 case study, 147*b*, 148*b*
 children's digestive disorders, 146
 cupping points, 148*f*
 gynaecological disorders, 146–147, 147*f*
 pathology, 145
abdominal points, 71, 71*f*
Achilles tendonitis, 215–216
Achilles tendon rupture, 215–216
acne, literature review, 284, 285*f*
acromioclavicular joint arthrosis, 225
active myofascial trigger points, 232
acupuncture, Pinyin, 145
acupuncture points, wet cupping, 109
acute sports injuries, 211
ADD (attention deficiency disorder), 155–156
adductor pollicis muscle, myofascial trigger
  points, 240, 241*f*
ADHD (attention-deficit hyperactivity
  disorder), 155–156
adhesive capsulitis (frozen shoulder), 225
 strong cupping, 97*b*
adults, 120–121
Africa, history of cupping, 1, 2*f*
Aids to Paediatric Nursing, 118–119
alcohol rub method, fire introduction to cup,
  82, 82*f*
Alexander, F Matthias, 75
Alexander technique, 75, 75*f*
allergic rhinitis, 184–185, 185*f*
Al-Qanun (Fi'l-Tibb), 5
Al-Qayyim, 5
amenorrhoea, 192–200, 193*f*
anaemia, 149, 150*f*
 case study, 149*b*
ankle, 215
 sprains, 215, 215*f*
ankylosing spondylitis, 185, 185*f*
appetite, poor *see* poor appetite
applications of cupping, 37
arcuate artery, 125
arm, body toning, 136
aromatherapy, 72
asthma, 150–153, 153*f*
 aetiology, 150–151
 case study, 153*b*

children, 152*f*
 full (excessive) type, 151–153
 lung and kidney-Yin deficiency, 151
 lung Qi and kidney-Yang deficiency, 151
 pathology, 150–151
atrophy syndrome, 154–155, 154*f*
 case study, 155*b*
attention deficiency disorder (ADD),
  155–156
attention-deficit hyperactivity disorder
  (ADHD), 155–156
Avicenna (Ibn-Siwa), 5, 19
axillary artery, 125
azygos vein, 126

B

back pain, 159*f*
 case studies, 158*b*
 lower *see* lower back
back points, children, 119–120
Back-Shu points, children, 119–120
bamboo boiling method, herbal cupping,
  112–113, 113*f*
bamboo cups, 12*f*
basilar artery, 125
basilic vein, 126
Bayfield, Samuel, 4, 144
bed-wetting (nocturnal enuresis),
  159–160
 case study, 160*b*
Bell's palsy, 177–178
Ben Cao Gang Mu She, 2-3
benefits of cupping, 47–64
 blood, 56–58
 lymphatic drainage, 56
 lymphatic system, 48–56
 skin, 47–48
biceps brachii muscle, 134*f*
 myofascial trigger points, 237, 239*f*
bi syndrome, 173–175
 case study, 175*b*
Bladder (BL) channel, Zang-Fu, 52*f*
bladder prolapse, 208
blanket cupping method, 29, 29*b*, 30*f*
BL (Bladder) channel, Zang-Fu, 52*f*
bleeding, 143
bleeding cupping *see* wet cupping
  (Xue Guan Fa)
blinding, evidence-based research, 286

Blood
 benefits of cupping, 56–58
 effects of cupping, 63
 mechanism of cupping, 61–62
 Qi, 58
 stagnation, 58, 194, 195
Blood deficiency, tiredness, 180
Blood injury, 229
body fluids, stagnation, 59
body layers, traditional Lanna medicine, 43
body toning, cosmetic cupping, 133–141, 134*f*
boils/carbuncles, 161–162, 161*f*
 case studies, 162*b*
bone fractures, 214
Bo Shu, 1
brachial artery, 125
brachialis muscle, 134*f*
brachioradialis muscle, 134*f*
breast enhancement, 128–129, 129*f*
breast pain
 during menstruation, 193, 194*f*
 moving cupping, 100*b*
broken veins, 181–182, 181*f*
 case study, 182*b*
bronchitis, 186, 186*f*
bruising, 89
Buddhist medicine, 33–46
 definition, 33–34
 disease causes, 35–36
 element imbalance/disturbance, 35–36
 history of, 33
 principles, 34–35
 treatment approaches, 36
buttock pain, 222–223
 myofascial trigger points, 242
buttocks, body toning, 140, 140*f*

C

calf muscle (gastrocnemius) injuries, 216–217,
  217*f*
CAM *see* complementary and alternative
  medicine (CAM)
Cambodia, 21*f*
carbuncles *see* boils/carbuncles
carpal tunnel syndrome, 186, 187*f*
Causes and Cures (Hildegard of Bingen), 26
cellulite, cosmetic cupping, 130, 131*f*
Central America, 28
cerebral arteries, 125
cervical pain, case studies, 38*b*

cervical spondylosis, literature review, 283, 284*f*
chest, body toning, 135, 135*f*
chest pain, 162–163
  case study, 163*b*
children, 118–122, 119*f*
  abdominal pain, 146
  attitude to, 118
  cup size, 118
  digestive disorders, 146
  patient preparation, 66
  poor appetite, 207, 207*f*
China, 1, 20
chiropracty, 74, 74*f*
chronic fatigue syndrome (encephalomyelitis), 186–187, 188*f*
clavicle, 134*f*
clear complexion, cosmetic cupping, 126–128, 128*f*
Cold Uterus, kidney deficiency, 195
colitis, 187, 188*f*
common carotid artery, 125
common cold, 163–165, 164*f*, 167*f*
  case study, 165*b*
common iliac artery, 125
communicating arteries, 125
complementary and alternative medicine (CAM), 72–78
  Alexander technique, 75, 75*f*
  aromatherapy, 72
  chiropracty, 74, 74*f*
  four-zone cupping therapy map, 73*f*
  kinesiology, 75
  massage, 72–73
  osteopathy, 74–75
  physiotherapy, 76–77, 77*f*
  polarity, 76
  reflexology, 76, 76*f*
  shiatsu, 75–76
complexion, cosmetic cupping, 126–128, 128*f*
Conception Vessel (Ren Mai) channel, Zang-Fu, 55*f*
conjunctivitis, 190, 191*f*
consent, informed, 86, 86*t*
constipation, 165–166
  case study, 166*b*
constitution, weak, 182, 183*f*
cooling *see* ice cupping (cooling)
coracobrachialis muscle, myofascial trigger points, 237, 238*f*
coronary arteries, 125
cosmetic cupping, 123–143
  abdominal cupping, 132, 132*f*
  application, 124
  blood vessel problems, 125–126
  body toning, 133–141, 134*f*
  breast enhancement, 128–129, 129*f*
  cellulite, 130, 131*f*
  clear complexion, 126–128, 128*f*
  contraindications, 143
  cup types, 124, 124*f*
  expectations, 126, 127*f*
  eyes, 127–128
  facelift, 127
  frequency asked questions, 142–143
  frequency of, 143

heavy leg syndrome, 132–133, 133*f*
  pain during, 143
  positioning, 124, 125*f*
  preparation, 123, 124*f*
  weight loss, 130–132, 131*f*
cotton ball method, fire introduction to cup, 79, 80*f*
cough, 166–168, 167*f*
  empty (flash) cupping, 108*b*
cranium, 134*f*
C-reactive protein (CRP), evidence-based research, 254*t*
CRP (C-reactive protein), evidence-based research, 254*t*
cun, 145, 145*f*
cup equipment *see* equipment. *specific types*
Cupping Mark Diagnosis, 45, 46*f*, 90, 90*f*
cupping marks *see* marks of cupping
cupping out the Wind (Vietnam), 30*b*
cupping torch method, fire introduction to cup, 80*f*
cutaneous facial muscle, myofascial trigger points, 233, 233*f*

D
deep veins, 126
dehydration, 142–143
deltoid muscle, 134*f*
  myofascial trigger points, 237, 238*f*
depression, 187–189
  heart patterns, 189
  liver pattern Qi stagnation, 189
  spleen patterns, 189
diaphragm, body toning, 137, 137*f*
diarrhoea, 190, 190*f*
diet, preparation for cupping, 89
digestive organs, effects of cupping, 62*b*
disease causes
  Buddhist medicine, 35–36
  Wind, 43
dislocated shoulder, 225–226
disposable cupping sets, 14, 15*f*
dizziness, 143
draining method *see* moving cupping (Tui Guan Fa); needle cupping; strong cupping; wet cupping (Xue Guan Fa)
dropped eyelid (ptosis), 190, 191*f*
dry cupping
  definition, 36
  lymphatic system, 54*f*, 56
  traditional Lanna medicine, 45
  wet cupping *vs.*, 18
Du Mai (Governing Vessel, DM/GV) channel, Zang-Fu, 54*f*
duration of sessions, 142
dysmenorrhoea, 168–170, 169*f*
  case study, 170*b*

E
Earth element, traditional Lanna medicine, 41–42
ecchymosis, 89
eczema, case study, 177*b*

The Edwin Smith Surgical Papyrus, 27
effects of cupping, 62*b*, 63–64
  blood, 63
  digestive organs, 62*b*
  joints, 62*b*
  muscles, 62*b*
  nervous system, 63
  skin, 62*b*
  Wind element, 63–64
Egypt, 4, 12, 13*f*
elbow injuries, 226–227, 228*f*
elderly, 70, 71*f*
electromagnetic cupping apparatus, 8–9, 9*f*
elements
  imbalance/disturbance, 35–36.
  see also specific elements
emotional problems, empty (flash) cupping, 108*b*
empty (flash) cupping (Shan Gua Fa), 106–107, 107*f*, 108*f*
  application, 107
  cough, 108*b*
  emotional problems, 108*b*
  lung cancer, 108*b*
  suitable conditions, 107
  traditional Lanna medicine, 45
encephalomyelitis (chronic fatigue syndrome), 186–187, 188*f*
enuresis, nocturnal *see* bed-wetting (nocturnal enuresis)
eosinophils, evidence-based research, 254*t*
epilepsy, 191, 192*f*
equipment, 8–15
  bamboo cups, 12, 12*f*
  disposable cupping sets, 14, 15*f*
  electromagnetic cupping apparatus, 8–9, 9*f*
  glass cups, 12–13, 13*f*
  magnetic squeeze rubber cups, 11, 11*f*
  pistol-handle valve cups, 9–11, 10*f*
  portable cupping pumps, 9
  rubber cups, 13, 14*f*
  screw-top cups, 9, 10*f*
  silicone cups, 13, 14*f*
  squeeze rubber top cups, 11, 11*f*
  two-in-one cupping set with electrical stimulation, 14–15, 15*f*
erectile dysfunction, 203, 203*f*
erythrocyte sedimentation rate (ESR)
  definition, 249–250
  evidence-based research, 249*t*, 254*t*
ESR *see* erythrocyte sedimentation rate (ESR)
Europe, regulation, 7
even method *see* light-moving cupping; water cupping (Shui Guan Fa)
evidence-based research, 247–310
  blinding, 286
  haematological parameters, 248
  inflammatory mediators, 251, 252*f*, 253*t*, 254*t*
  literature review, 277–278
  myofascial pain syndrome, 256, 257
excessive (full) type asthma, 151–153
expectations of cupping therapy, 87–90
explanation, patient preparation, 65
extensor, 134*f*
extensor carpi radialis brevis muscle, myofascial trigger points, 240, 240*f*
extensor carpi radialis longus muscle, myofascial trigger points, 240, 240*f*

extensor carpi ulnaris muscle, myofascial trigger points, 240, 240*f*
external oblique muscle, 134*f*
eyes, 190
    cosmetic cupping, 127–128

F
facelift, 127
facial cupping, clear complexion, 126–128, 128*f*
facial oedema, light-moving cupping, 101*b*
facial paralysis, 177–178
    case study, 178*b*
    literature review, 282, 283*f*
facial points, 70, 70*f*
fatigue, case studies, 37*b*
feet
    body toning, 138, 140*f*
    cupping under, 70, 70*f*
female infertility, 193–194, 196*f*
female sexual frigidity, 196–198, 198*f*
    Cold-type frigidity (Kidney-Yang), 197–198
    Hot-type frigidity (Liver-Qi stagnation), 197, 198
femoral artery, 125
ferritin
    definition, 255
    evidence-based research, 252*f*, 254*t*
fever, 170–171
fibrinogen
    definition, 255
    evidence-based research, 252*f*, 254*t*
Fire element
    Buddhist medical principles, 34
    individuals with predominance of, 34
    traditional Lanna medicine, 42
fire introduction to cup, 79–83
    alcohol rub method, 82, 82*f*
    cotton ball method, 79
    cupping torch method, 79–80, 80*f*
    lighter flame method, 82, 83*f*
    paper burning method, 83, 83*f*
    wick method, 80, 81*f*
flash cupping *see* empty (flash) cupping (Shan Gua Fa)
flexor carpi radialis muscle, myofascial trigger points, 240, 241*f*
flexor carpi ulnaris muscle, myofascial trigger points, 240, 241*f*
folk heritage, 17–32
    intellectual position, 22
    lack of written records, 21–22
    women's role, 22–27, 23*f*, 24*f*
food, stagnation, 59
forearm
    body toning, 136, 136*f*
    injuries, 226–227, 228*f*
    myofascial trigger points, 240
    pain, 240
forgetfulness, 200, 200*f*
four-zone cupping therapy, 77–78
    map, 73*f*
frequency asked questions (FAQ), cosmetic cupping, 142–143
frequency of cupping, 121

frozen shoulder *see* adhesive capsulitis (frozen shoulder)
full cupping *see* wet cupping (Xue Guan Fa)
full (excessive) type asthma, 151–153

G
Gall Bladder (GB) channel, Zang-Fu, 54*f*
gastrocnemius muscle, 134*f*
    myofascial trigger points, 245, 246*f*
glass cups, 12–13, 13*f*
gluteus maximus muscle, 134*f*
gluteus medius muscle, 134*f*
Goodheart, George, 75
gout, 201, 201*f*
gracilis muscle, 134*f*
Greece
    history of cupping, 19
    women's role, 23–24
groin pain, 221–222
growing pains, 171, 172*f*
Gua Sha, 60–61, 60*f*, 61*f*
gynaecological disorders, 146–147, 147*f*

H
haematological parameters, evidence-based research, 248, 249*t*
haemoglobin, evidence-based research, 249*t*, 254*t*
hairy skin, 142
hamstrings, 134*f*
    injury, 219–221, 220*f*
A Handbook of Prescriptions for emergencies, 3
hand cupping, 65–66, 66*f*
    cosmetic cupping preparation, 123, 124*f*
hand pain, myofascial trigger points, 240
hangover, 201
hayfever, 184–185, 185*f*
headaches, 201–202, 202*f*
    strong cupping, 97*b*
head and neck cupping, 68, 68*f*
head pain, myofascial trigger points, 232–237
Healing with the Medicine of the Prophet, 5
Heart (HT) channel, Zang-Fu, 51*f*
heart patterns, depression, 189
heavy leg syndrome, cosmetic cupping, 132–133, 133*f*
heavy periods (menorrhalgia), 195–196, 197*f*
hepatic artery, 125
hepatic vein, 126
herbal cupping (Yao Guan Fa), 112–114
    application, 112–114
    bamboo boiling method, 112–113, 113*f*
    herbs in cup method, 114
    suitable conditions, 114
herbal remedies, skin complaints, 176
herpes zoster therapy, literature review, 281–282, 281*f*
hiccups, 202, 203*f*
Hilchot Deol, 69
Hildegard of Bingen, 26
hip injuries, 221–222, 223*f*
hip pain, moving cupping, 100*b*
Hippocrates, 19

Hippocratic Corpus, 27
history of cupping, 1–16
    Buddhist medicine, 33
    early methods, 1–4, 2*f*, 3*f*
    early roots, 18–19
    Greek enlightenment, 19
    Jewish tradition, 4
    medieval records, 25–26, 26*f*
    middle East, 4, 5–6, 6*b*
    present day, 7–8
    Western world, 4
holiday season, 87
hot needle and Moxa cupping, 104–106, 105*f*
    Achilles tendon injuries, 216, 216*f*
    application, 104
    dysmenorrhoea, 169*f*
    female sexual frigidity, 197, 198*f*
    hip and groin injuries, 222
    painful periods, 106*b*
    suitable conditions, 104–106
hyperactivity, 208
hyperhidrosis (night sweating), 206, 206*f*
hypertension, 171–172
    case study, 172*b*
hypochondriac region, body toning, 136, 137*f*

I
Ibn-Siwa (Avicenna), 5, 19
ice cupping (cooling), 116–117, 116*f*
    application, 117
    suitable conditions, 117
ileocolic artery, 125
iliocostalis lumborum muscle, myofascial trigger points, 242, 243*f*
iliotibial band syndrome (ITBS), 218–219, 220*f*
immobility, case studies, 38*b*
immunoglobulin screen, evidence-based research, 254*t*
infertility
    female, 193–194, 196*f*
    male, 204, 204*f*
inflammatory mediators, evidence-based research, 251, 252*f*, 253*t*, 254*t*
influenza, 163–165, 164*f*
informed consent, 86, 86*t*
infraspinatus muscle, myofascial trigger points, 234, 236*f*
innominate artery, 125
insomnia, 202–203
interlobar artery, 125
interlobular arteries, 125
internal oblique muscle, 134*f*
ITBS (iliotibial band syndrome), 218–219, 220*f*

J
Jewish tradition, history of cupping, 4
joints, 69, 69*f*
    effects of cupping, 62*b*

K
Kennedy, Charles, 4
Kidney (K) channel, Zang-Fu, 52*f*

kidney deficiency, 194–195
    Blood stagnation, 194, 195
    Cold Uterus, 195
    kidney-Yang deficiency, 194
    kidney-Yin deficiency, 194
    liver-Qi stagnation, 194, 195
    phlegm-Dampness, 194, 195
Kidney-Yang deficiency, 194
Kidney-Yin deficiency, 194
kinesiology, 75
Kleinman, Arthur, 22
knees
    injuries, 218, 219*f*
    pain, 103*b*
    swollen, 103*b*

L

lacrimation, 190
Lane, James Davis, 4
Large Intestine (LI) channel, Zang-Fu, 49*f*
laryngitis, 173, 173*f*
latent myofascial trigger points, 232
latissimus dorsi muscle, 134*f*
    myofascial trigger points, 237, 237*f*
legs
    body toning, 138, 139*f*
    lower, myofascial trigger points, 242–245
levator scapulae muscle, myofascial trigger
    points, 234, 235*f*
ligaments, 213
light cupping *see* weak (light) cupping
lighter flame method, fire introduction to cup,
    82, 83*f*
light-moving cupping, 100–101
    application, 101
    facial oedema, 101*b*
    poor appetite, 102*b*
    stomach pain, 102*b*
    suitable conditions, 101
lingual artery, 125
lingual vein, 126
literature review, evidence-based research,
    277–278
Lithuania, 20–21
Liver (Liv) channel, Zang-Fu, 54*f*
liver-Qi stagnation, 197, 198
    depression, 189
    dysmenorrhoea, 168
    kidney deficiency, 194, 195
local points, children, 119–120
Lom-Pit (Wind-poison), traditional Lanna
    medicine, 44
longissimus thoracis muscle, myofascial trigger
    points, 242, 243*f*
lower back
    body toning, 140–141, 141*f*
    injuries, 223–225, 224*f*
lower back pain, 157
    medium cupping, 95*b*
    myofascial trigger points, 242
lower body, musculoskeletal pain, 174, 174*f*
lower leg pain, myofascial trigger points,
    242–245
lower limbs, sports injuries, 215–225
lower zone, four-zone cupping therapy, 77–78
lumbago pain, case studies, 40*f*

lumbar artery, 125
lumbar intervertebral disc prolapse, literature
    review, 285, 285*f*, 286*f*
lumbar pain, myofascial trigger points, 242
lung and kidney-Yin deficiency, asthma, 151
lung cancer, empty (flash) cupping, 108*b*
Lung (LU) channel, Zang-Fu, 49*f*
lung Qi and kidney-Yang deficiency, asthma,
    151
lying sideways, 67*f*
lymphatic system, 57*f*
    benefits of cupping, 48–56
    dry cupping, 54*f*, 56
    infections, 48–56
    moving cupping, 54*f*, 56
    waste matter, 56
lymphocyte count, evidence-based research,
    252*f*, 254*t*
lymphoedema, 56
lymphoma, 56

M

magnetic squeeze rubber cups, 11
male infertility, 204, 204*f*
male sexual illness, 203–204
mandible, 134*f*
marks of cupping, 87, 88*f*
    dark, 143
    fading of, 87
    unsightly, 87, 89*f*
Marsden, William, 4
massage, 72–73
massage oil, 88
masseter muscle, myofascial trigger points,
    232, 233*f*
mastitis, 198–199, 199*f*
Mawangdui Medical manuscripts, 20
maxilla muscle, 134*f*
mechanism of cupping, 61–62
medial tibial stress syndrome (MTSS),
    217–218, 218*f*
median/channel cupping, 78
medical models, 19, 20–21
medium cupping, 94, 95*f*, 97*f*
    abdominal pain, 145–146
    application, 94
    buttock pain, 223
    hip and groin injuries, 222
    iliotibial band syndrome, 218–219,
        220*f*
    knee injuries, 218, 219*f*
    lower back injuries, 224
    lower back pain, 95*b*
    quadriceps femoris injuries, 221
    shingles, 95*b*
    shoulder injuries, 226
    shoulder pain, 95*b*
    suitable conditions, 94
menorrhalgia, 195–196, 197*f*
menstruation
    breast pain during, 193, 194*f*
    heavy, 195–196, 197*f*
mental issues, case studies, 37*b*
methods of cupping *see* types of cupping.
    specific methods
middle back, body toning, 133, 141*f*

middle East
    history of cupping, 4, 5–6, 6*b*
    present day, 6
middle zone, four-zone cupping therapy, 77
migraine, 201–202
Minoan civilisation, 19
Mishna Thora, 69
moles, 143
monocytes, evidence-based research, 254*t*
moving cupping (Tui Guan Fa), 98–99, 99*f*
    Achilles tendon injuries, 216
    application, 98
    breast pain, 100*b*
    buttock pain, 223
    calf muscle (gastrocnemius) injuries, 217, 217*f*
    hamstring injury, 220–221
    hip pain, 100*b*
    light *see* light-moving cupping
    lower back injuries, 224–225
    lymphatic system, 54*f*, 56
    shoulder injuries, 226
    suitable conditions, 99
    thigh pain, 100*b*
Moxa cupping *see* hot needle and Moxa cupping
MTSS (medial tibial stress syndrome),
    217–218, 218*f*
multi-functionality of cupping, 64
multiple sclerosis, weak (light) cupping, 94*b*
mumps, 204, 205*f*
muscles
    effects of cupping, 62*b*
    injuries, 214
    strains, 214
    tears, 214.
    see also specific muscles
muscular system, 134*f*
musculoskeletal pain, 173–175
    case study, 175*b*
    lower body, 174, 174*f*
    upper body, 174
Mycenaean civilisation, 19
myofascial pain syndrome, evidence-based
    research, 256, 257
myofascial trigger points, 231–246
    abdominal muscles, 246
    active, 232
    buttock pain, 242
    causes of, 231
    forearm pain, 240
    hand pain, 240
    head pain, 232–237
    latent, 232
    location, 232
    lower back pain, 242
    lower leg pain, 242–245
    lumbar pain, 242
    neck pain, 232–237
    shoulder pain, 232–237
    treatment methods, 231
    upper chest pain, 240–242.
    see also specific muscles

N

neck
    body toning, 133
    stiff, 103*b*

neck pain
  body toning, 135*f*
  myofascial trigger points, 232–237
  needle cupping (draining method), 103*b*
needle cupping, 102–103, 102*f*
  application, 102–103
  knee pain, 103*b*
  neck pain, 103*b*
  stiff neck, 103*b*
  suitable conditions, 103
  swollen knees, 103*b*
nervous system, effects of cupping, 63
neutrophils, evidence-based research, 254*t*
night sweating (hyperhidrosis), 206, 206*f*
nocturnal enuresis *see* bed-wetting (nocturnal
    enuresis)
number of cups, 121–122, 121*f*

O

occipital, 134*f*
oedema, facial, 101*b*
oral suction, 18, 19
osteopathy, 74–75

P

pain
  abdomen *see* abdominal pain
  breasts *see* breast pain
  cervical, 38*b*
  chest *see* chest pain
  groin, 221–222
  growing pains, 171, 172*f*
  hand, 240
  head, 232–237
  knees, 103*b*
  lower back *see* lower back pain
  lumbar pain, 242
  neck *see* neck pain
  periods, hot needle and Moxa cupping, 106*b*
  sacrum, 39*b*
  shoulder *see* shoulder pain
  thighs, 100*b*
  upper back, 153*f*, 156, 157*f*
pain threshold, patient preparation, 65–66
palmaris longus muscle, myofascial trigger
    points, 240, 241*f*
palm cupping, 65–66, 66*f*
Palmer, Daniel David, 74
paper burning method, fire introduction to cup,
    83, 83*f*
paralysis
  face *see* facial paralysis
  strong cupping, 97*b*
patella, 134*f*
pathogen entry, traditional Lanna medicine, 43–44
patient positioning, 66, 67*f*
  importance of, 84–85
  lying sideways, 67*f*
  prone position, 67*f*
  standing, 69, 69*f*
  supine position, 66, 67*f*
  upright sitting, 66, 67*f*
patient preparation, 65–71
  children, 66
  explanation, 65

pain threshold, 65–66
position *see* patient positioning
relaxation, 65
treatment room, 65
pectoralis major muscle, 134*f*
  myofascial trigger points, 240–242, 241*f*
pelvic inflammatory disease (PID), 199, 199*f*
Pericardium (P) channel, Zang-Fu, 53*f*
periods, heavy, 195–196, 197*f*
peroneal brevis muscle, myofascial trigger
    points, 245, 246*f*
peroneal longus muscle, myofascial trigger
    points, 245, 246*f*
peroneus muscle, 134*f*
Perspex cups, cosmetic cupping, 124, 124*f*
phlegm-Dampness, kidney deficiency, 194,
    195
physiotherapy, 76–77, 77*f*
PID (pelvic inflammatory disease), 199, 199*f*
Pinyin acupuncture, 145
piriformis muscle, myofascial trigger points,
    242, 244*f*
pistol-handle valve cups, 9–11, 10*f*
platelet count, evidence-based research, 252*f*,
    254*t*
pneumonia, 25
Poland, 25
polarity, 76
poor appetite, 206–207, 206*f*
  children, 207, 207*f*
  light-moving cupping, 102*b*
poor constitution, 182, 183*f*
poor sleep, weak (light) cupping, 93*b*
popliteal artery, 126
portable cupping pumps, 9
portal vein, 126
positioning
  patient *see* patient positioning
  practitioner, 80*f*
practitioner position, 80*f*
preparation *see* patient preparation
prevention, cupping role, 24–25
procedure of cupping, 79–86
  application of cup, 84–85
  cup cleaning, 85–86
  fire introduction *see* fire introduction
    to cup
  removal of cup, 84–85, 85*f*
  symmetric application, 83–84
professional indemnity insurance, 7
pronator teres, 134*f*
prone position, 67*f*
prostatitis, 204, 205*f*
psoriasis, 208, 209*f*
  wet cupping, 112*b*
ptosis, 190, 191*f*
pulmonary arteries, 126
pulmonary vein, 126

Q

Qi, 58
  blood, 58
  deficiency, tiredness, 179
  low, 143
  mechanism of cupping, 61
  stagnation, 60, 211

quadratus lumborum muscle, myofascial trigger
    points, 242, 244*f*
quadriceps, 134*f*
quadriceps femoris injuries, 221, 222*f*

R

radial artery, 126
RBC (red blood count), evidence-based
    research, 249*t*, 254*t*
rectus femoris, 134*f*
red blood count (RBC), evidence-based
    research, 249*t*, 254*t*
reflexology, 76, 76*f*
regulation of cupping, 7
relaxation, patient preparation, 65
renal arteries, 126
Ren Mai (Conception Vessel, Ren/CV)
    channel, Zang-Fu, 55*f*
repetitive strain injury (RSI), wet cupping,
    111*b*
restlessness, 208, 210*f*
  weak (light) cupping, 93*b*
RF (rheumatoid factor), evidence-based
    research, 249*t*
rheumatoid factor (RF), evidence-based
    research, 249*t*
rhomboid major muscle, myofascial trigger
    points, 237, 238*f*
rhomboid minor muscle, myofascial trigger
    points, 237, 238*f*
Romania, 24*f*
rotator cuff injuries, 226
RSI (repetitive strain injury), wet cupping,
    111*b*
rubber cups, 13, 14*f*
  cosmetic cupping, 124, 124*f*

S

sacral and lower limb zone, four-zone cupping
    therapy, 78
sacral pain, case studies, 39*b*
safeguards, cupping role, 25
safety concerns, 79, 84–86
San Jiao (Triple Warmer) channel, Zang-Fu,
    53*f*
sciatica, 157
  case studies, 40*f*
screw-top cups, 9, 10*f*
semispinalis capitis muscle, myofascial trigger
    points, 233, 233*f*
Sen (channels), traditional Lanna medicine,
    44
sensation, skin, 47
serratus anterior muscle, 134*f*
serratus posterior inferior muscle, myofascial
    trigger points, 242, 242*f*
sexual frigidity, female *see* female sexual
    frigidity
sexual problems, 158, 159*f*
  see also specific diseases/disorders
Shan Gua Fa *see* empty (flash) cupping (Shan
    Gua Fa)
shiatsu, 75–76
shingles, medium cupping, 95*b*
shin splints, 217–218, 218*f*

Shonishin: Japanese Pediatric Acupuncture,
   119–120
shoulder
   body toning, 136, 136*f*
   dislocated, 225–226
   injuries, 225–226, 227*f*
   lesions, 38*b*, 38*f*, 39*b*
shoulder pain
   medium cupping, 95*b*
   myofascial trigger points, 232–237
   strong cupping, 97*b*
Shui Guan Fa *see* water cupping
   (Shui Guan Fa)
Sicily, 23*f*
sickness models, 19
Sigehisa Kuriyama, 27–28
silicon cups, 14*f*
   cosmetic cupping, 124, 124*f*
size of cups, children, 118
skin, 48*f*
   benefits of cupping, 47–48
   effects of cupping, 62*b*
   hairy, 142
   injuries, 213
   sensation, 47
   temperature control, 47
   texture, 142
   Zang-Fu, 47–48
skin complaints, 176.
   see also specific diseases/disorders
Small Intestine (SI) channel, Zang-Fu, 51*f*
sodium hypochlorite, cup cleaning,
   85–86
soleus muscle, 134*f*
   myofascial trigger points, 245, 246*f*
spinal stress fractures, 223
Spleen (SP) channel, Zang-Fu, 50*f*
spleen patterns, depression, 189
splenius capitis muscle, myofascial trigger
   points, 233, 233*f*
splenius cervicis muscle, myofascial trigger
   points, 233, 233*f*
sports injuries, 211–230
   acute stage, 211
   lower limbs, 215–225
   prevalence, 211
   Qi stagnation, 211
   treatment contraindications, 215
   upper limbs, 217.
   see also specific injuries
Sports Medicine: A Comprehensive Approach,
   212
sprains, 213
   ankle, 215, 215*f*
squeeze rubber top cups, 11*f*
stagnation, 59–60
   Blood, 58, 194, 195
   body fluids, 59
   food, 59
   liver-Qi *see* liver-Qi stagnation
   Qi, 60, 189, 211
standing, 69, 69*f*
sternocleidomastoideus, 134*f*
stiff neck, needle cupping (draining method),
   103*b*
stomach, body toning, 137–138, 138*f*
Stomach (ST) channel, Zang-Fu, 50*f*

stomach pain, light-moving cupping, 102*b*
Stone, Randolph, 76
stress fractures, 214
stroke (wind-stroke), 177–178, 178*f*
   case study, 179*b*
strong cupping, 95–97, 96*f*, 97*f*
   adhesive capsulitis, 97*b*
   application, 96
   buttock pain, 223
   frozen shoulder syndrome, 97*b*
   headaches, 97*b*
   hip and groin injuries, 222
   iliotibial band syndrome, 218–219
   paralysis, 97*b*
   shoulder injuries, 226
   shoulder pain, 97*b*
   suitable conditions, 96–97
subclavian artery, 126
superficial vein, 126
supine position, 66, 67*f*
Supplement to Outline of Herbal Pharmacopeia, 3
supraspinatus muscle, myofascial trigger points,
   234, 235*f*
Susen Liang Fang, 2
swollen knees, needle cupping (draining
   method), 103*b*
symmetric application, procedure of cupping,
   83–84
symptoms, element imbalance/disturbance,
   36

T
Taiwan, 8*f*, 28
   folk heritage, 22
   women's role, 23–24
temperature control, skin, 47
tenderness, 88
tendons, 213
   rupture, 213
tensor fascia latae muscle, 134*f*
teres minor muscle, 134*f*
   myofascial trigger points, 234, 236*f*
Thailand, 36
   see also traditional Lanna medicine (TLM)
Thich Phuoc Tan, 25
thighs
   body toning, 138, 139*f*
   pain, 100*b*
thrombosis, venous, 126
Tibb al-A'imma (Islamic Medical Wisdom), 5
Tibet, 36
tibial artery, 126
tibialis anterior muscle, myofascial trigger
   points, 245, 245*f*
tiredness, 179–180
   case study, 180*b*
TLM *see* traditional Lanna medicine (TLM)
tonifying methods *see* empty (flash) cupping
   (Shan Gua Fa); herbal cupping (Yao
   Guan Fa); medium cupping; weak (light)
   cupping
toothache, 209
torticollis (wry neck), 27–28, 210
traditional Lanna medicine (TLM), 41–42
   body layers, 43
   cupping applications, 44–45

   definition, 41
   Earth, 41–42
   elements, 41–42
   see alos individual elements
   Fire, 42
   Lom-Pit (Wind-poison), 44
   pathogen entry, 43–44
   Sen (channels), 44
   Water, 42
   Wind, 42, 43–44
trapezius muscle, 134*f*
   myofascial trigger points, 234, 234*f*
treatable disorders, 144–183, 184–210.
   see also specific disorders
treatment room, patient preparation, 65
triceps, 134*f*
triceps brachii muscle, myofascial trigger
   points, 237, 239*f*
trigeminal neuralgia, 208–209
The Trigger Point Manual, 231
Triple Warmer (San Jiao) channel, Zang-Fu, 53*f*
Tui Guan Fa *see* moving cupping
   (Tui Guan Fa)
Tunisia, 28
Turkey, 91
two-in-one cupping set with electrical
   stimulation, 14–15, 15*f*
types of cupping, 91–117
   decision on, 84–86
   traditional Lanna medicine, 45.
   see also specific types

U
ulcer, venous, 126
ulnar artery, 126
underperformance syndrome, 227–229
United Kingdom (UK), history of cupping, 4
upper back
   body toning, 133, 142*f*
   pain, 153*f*, 156, 157*f*
upper body, musculoskeletal pain, 174
upper chest pain, myofascial trigger points,
   240–242
upper zone, four-zone cupping therapy, 77
upright sitting, 66, 67*f*
uric acid, evidence-based research, 249*t*
USA, regulation, 7
uterus prolapse, 208

V
varicose veins, 181–182, 181*f*
vastus intermedius muscle, 134*f*
vastus lateralis muscle, 134*f*
   myofascial trigger points, 242, 244*f*
vastus medialis muscle, 134*f*
   myofascial trigger points, 245, 245*f*
veins, broken *see* broken veins
venous blood, 126
venous thrombosis, 126
venous ulcer, 126
Vietnam
   cupping out the Wind, 30*b*
   folk heritage, 25
   history of cupping, 20
vulvitis, 200, 200*f*

W

waste matter, lymphatic system, 56
water cupping (Shui Guan Fa), 114–115, 115*f*
   application, 115
   suitable conditions, 115
Water element
   Buddhist medical principles, 34
   individuals with predominance of, 34
   traditional Lanna medicine, 42
WBC (white blood count), evidence-based
      research, 249*t*, 254*t*
weak constitution, 182, 183*f*
weak (light) cupping, 92–93, 97*f*
   abdominal pain, 145–146
   application, 92, 93*f*
   lower back injuries, 224
   multiple sclerosis, 94*b*
   poor sleep, 93*b*
   quadriceps femoris injuries, 221
   restlessness, 93*b*
   suitable conditions, 93
weather effects, 27
weight loss, cosmetic cupping, 130–132, 131*f*
Wei Ke Zen-Zhong, 2–3
Wei Qi, 58–59
Western world, 4
wet cupping (Xue Guan Fa), 109–110, 110*f*,
      111*f*
   acupuncture points, 109
   application, 109–110
   cup removal, 109–110, 111*f*

decision on, 84
definition, 36
dry cupping *vs.*, 18
literature review, 281–282, 281*f*
psoriasis, 112*b*
repetitive strain injury, 111*b*
suitable conditions, 110
traditional Lanna medicine, 45
white blood count (WBC), evidence-based
      research, 249*t*, 254*t*
wick method, fire introduction to cup, 80, 81*f*
Wind element, 27–29
   Buddhist medical principles, 34
   cupping out the Wind (Vietnam), 30*b*
   diagnosis of, 43
   disease causes, 43
   effects of cupping, 63–64
   individuals with predominance of, 34
   traditional Lanna medicine, 42, 43–44
   Wind (and Cold) eliminating treatment, 29*b*
   Yang regions, 28
Wind (and Cold) eliminating treatment, 29*b*
Wind-poison (Lom-Pit), traditional Lanna
      medicine, 44
Wind-stroke *see* stroke (wind-stroke)
women's role, folk heritage, 22–27, 23*f*
wry neck (torticollis), 27–28, 210

X

Xue Guan Fa *see* wet cupping (Xue Guan Fa)

Y

Yang regions, Wind, 28
Yao Guan Fa *see* herbal cupping (Yao Guan Fa)
*The Yellow Emperor's Classic of Internal Medicine
      (Huang Di Nei Jing Su Wen)*, 28–29

Z

Zang-Fu, 47–48
   Bladder (BL) channel, 52*f*
   Du Mai (Governing Vessel, DM/GV)
      channel, 54*f*
   Gall Bladder (GB) channel, 54*f*
   Heart (HT) channel, 51*f*
   Kidney (K) channel, 52*f*
   Large Intestine (LI) channel, 49*f*
   Liver (Liv) channel, 54*f*
   lung (LU) channel, 49*f*
   Pericardium (P) channel, 53*f*
   Ren Mai (Conception Vessel, Ren/CV)
      channel, 55*f*
   San Jiao (Triple Warmer, SJ/TW) channel,
      53*f*
   Small Intestine (SI) channel, 51*f*
   Spleen (SP) channel, 50*f*
   Stomach (ST) channel, 50*f*
Zhao Xueming, 2–3
Zouhou Fang, 1–2
zygomatic arch, 134*f*
zygomatic major muscle, myofascial trigger
      points, 233, 233*f*

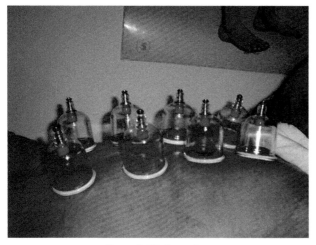

PLATE 1 Weak cupping.

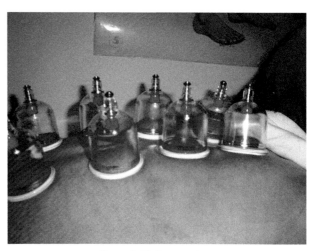

PLATE 2 Medium cupping.

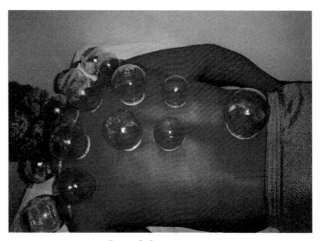

PLATE 3 Strong cupping.

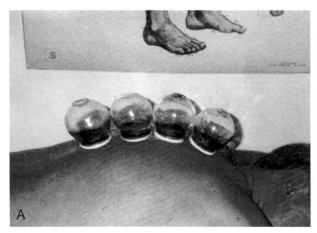

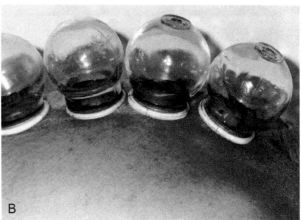

PLATE 4 (A, B) Bleeding cupping.

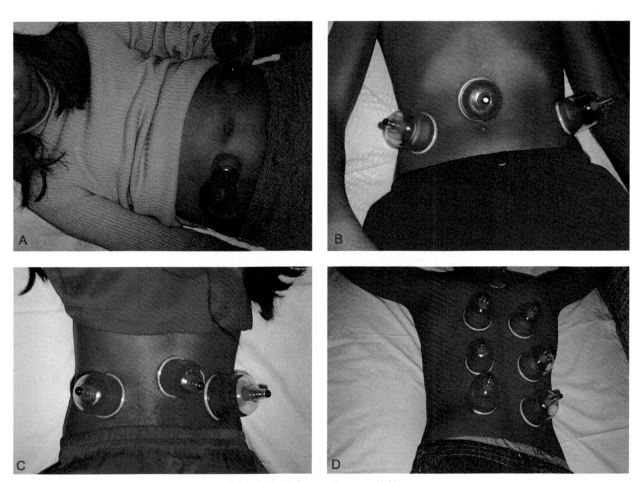

PLATE 5 (A–H) Cupping therapy in children.

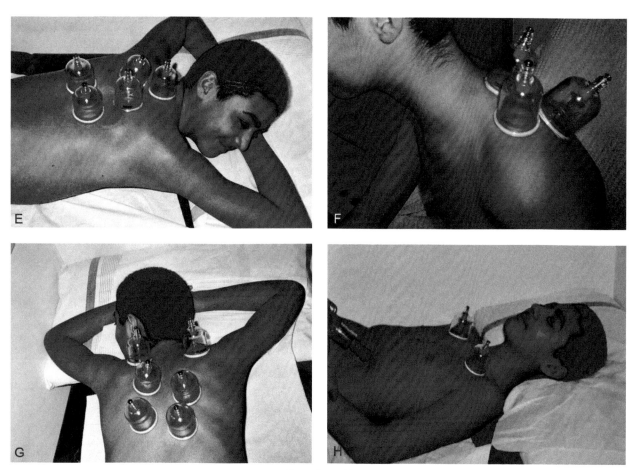

PLATE 5 cont'd

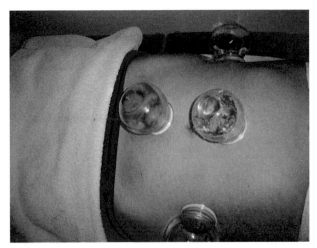

PLATE 6 Anaemia.

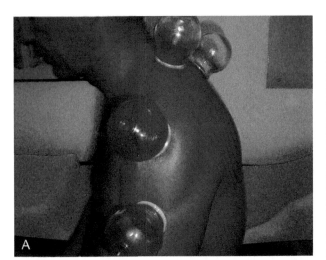

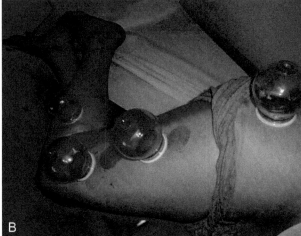

PLATE 7 (A, B) Atrophy syndrome.

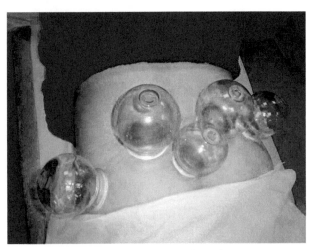

PLATE 8 Back pain and sexual complaints.

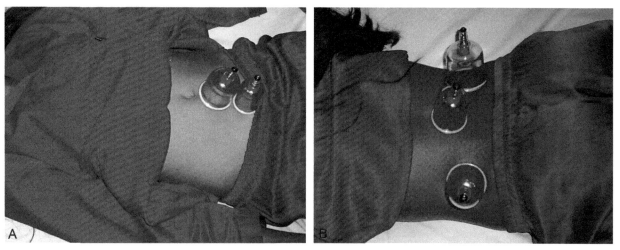

PLATE 9 (A, B) Bed wetting.

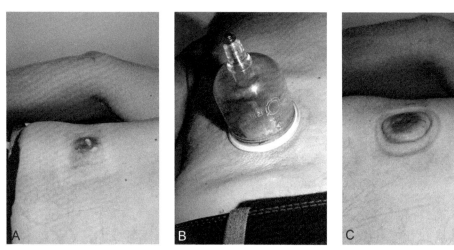

PLATE 10 (A–C) Cupping over a boil.

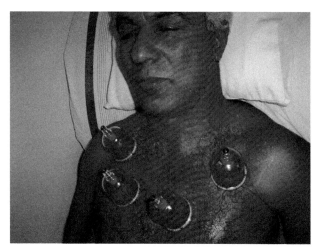

PLATE 11 Chest pain.

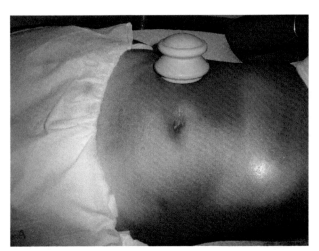

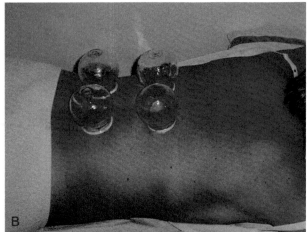

PLATE 12 (A, B) Constipation.

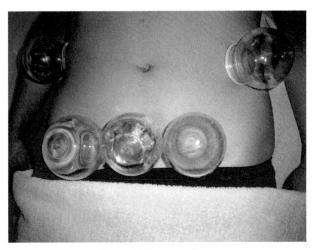

PLATE 13 Dysmenorrhoea.

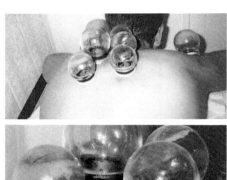

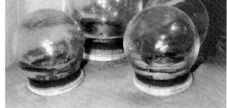

PLATE 14 Fevers.

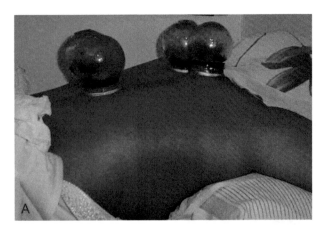

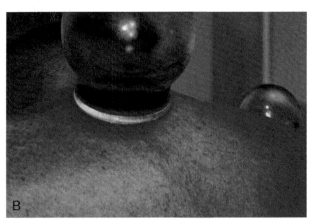

PLATE 15 (A, B) Hypertension.

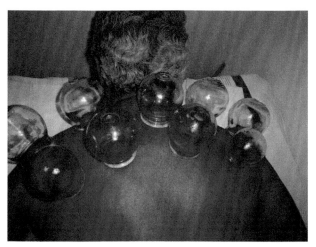

PLATE 16 Musculoskeletal pain, upper body.

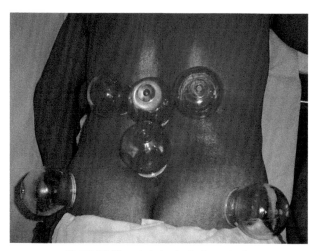

PLATE 17 Musculoskeletal pain, lower back.

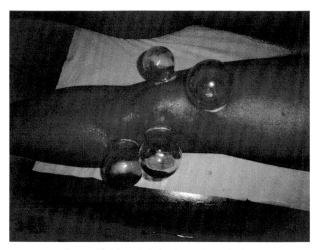

PLATE 18 Musculoskeletal pain, lower limbs.

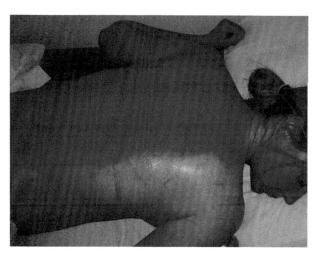

PLATE 19 Skin complaints.

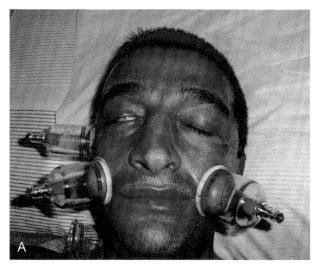

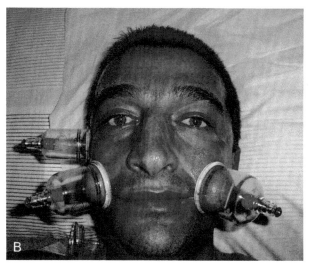

PLATE 20 (A, B) Facial paralysis due to trauma.

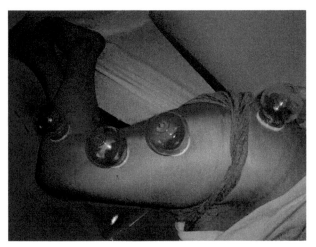

PLATE 21 Wind-stroke.

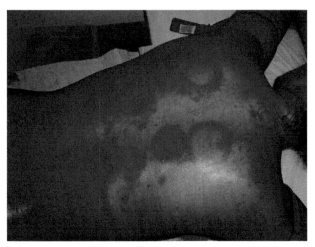

PLATE 22 Tiredness.

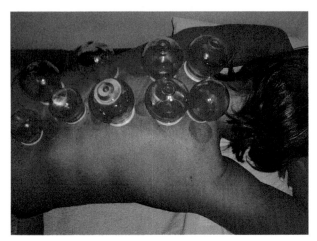

PLATE 23 Depression.

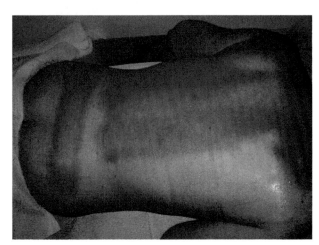

PLATE 24 Hangover.

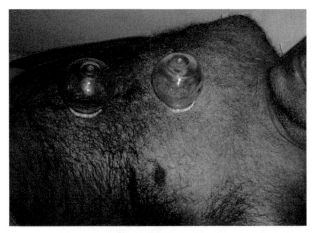

PLATE 25 Hiccups.

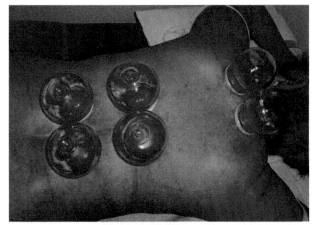

PLATE 26 Insomnia.

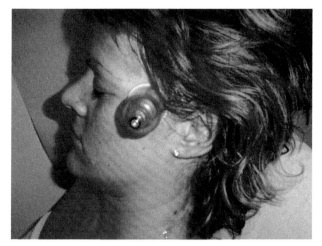

PLATE 27 Lacrimation.

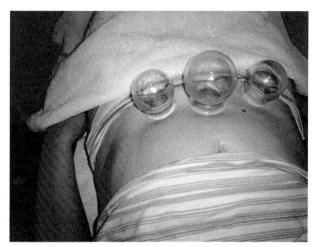

PLATE 28 Bladder prolapse.

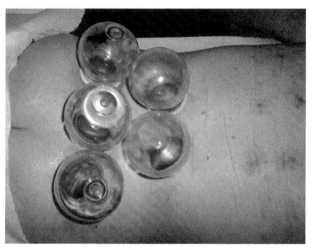

PLATE 29 Prolapse of the uterus.

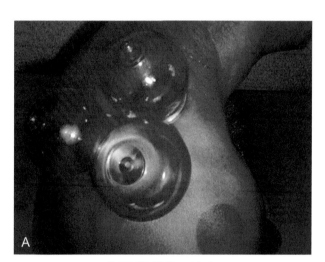

PLATE 30 (A) Spondylosis.

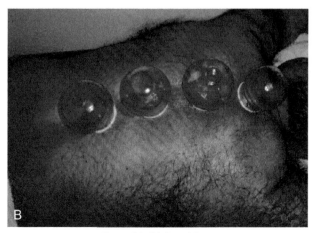

PLATE 30 (B) Spondylosis.

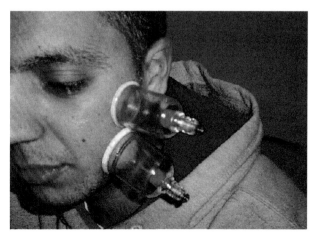

PLATE 31 Toothache.

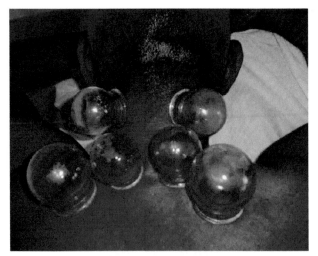

PLATE 32 Torticollis (wry neck).

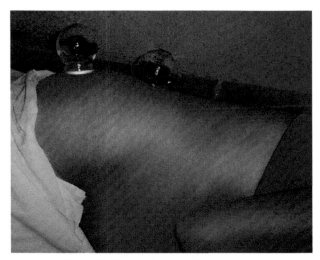

PLATE 33 Cupping therapy during pregnancy.

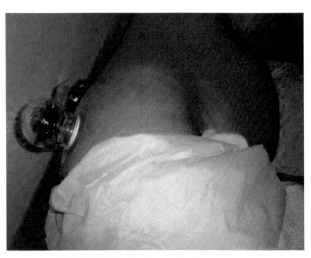

PLATE 34 Cupping therapy during pregnancy.

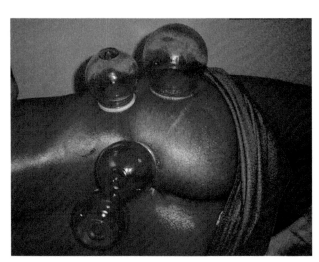

PLATE 35 Buttock pain.

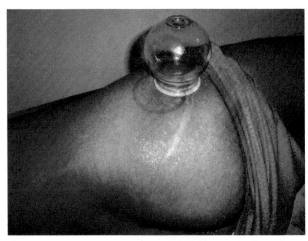

PLATE 36 Moving cupping on the gluteus muscle.

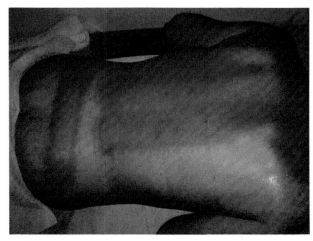

PLATE 37 Vertical moving cupping to the lower back.

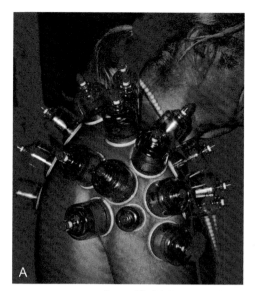
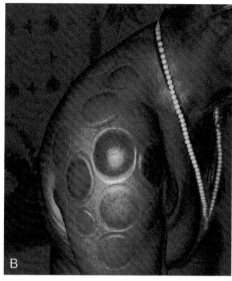

PLATE 38 (A) Treatment of shoulder pain; (B) Result after treatment.

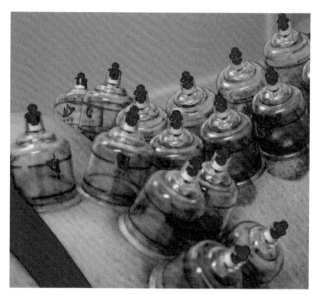

PLATE 39 Treatment of lumbago pain.

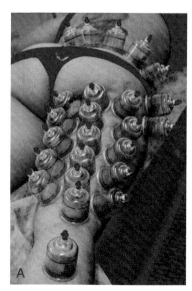
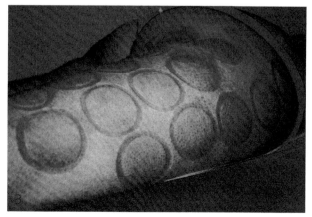

PLATE 40 (A) Treatment of sciatica pain; (B) result after treatment.

Bright Red - Indicates excessive heat in the area and possible inflammation. Flash cupping is generally used. With inflammation and especially in acute injuries bleeding may be indicated. In such a case it's helpful to use cooling balms and liniments to cool the area. We don't usually use ice for this

A

Deep Red to Magenta - Indicates stagnant heat. Cupping and bleeding are indicated. You can then use a drawing liniment or trauma liniment that is cooling to neutral.

B

Purple Blue - Indicates stagnation with the absence of heat. wind is stuck in an area and it is unable to move. Cupping is indicated. heating therapy can be used to disperse the area. With the presence of stagnation, you may want to cup more often and bleeding may be indicated.

C

Dark Blue to Purple Black - Indicates chronic build-up of "poison wind". The blood in the area is toxic and needs to be drained.

D

Dark colouring receding after cup is removed means that the toxins are sinking back into the body and need to be drawn out with more cupping and drawing liniments, balms or poultices.

E

Pale Whitish - Indicates the area is lacking in circulation because of a blockage somewhere around the area. For this condition cupping is not indicated. Stop cupping immediately and apply external warmth. Use hot compresses or a heating balm

F

PLATE 41 Diagnosis through cupping marks: (A) bright red; (B) deep red to magenta; (c) purple-blue; (d) blue to purple-black; (e) dark colouring receding after cup is removed; (f) pale whitish.

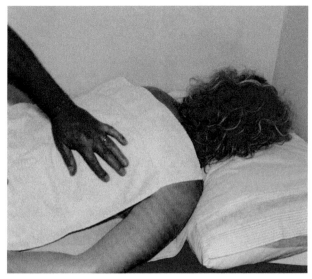

PLATE 42 Preparing the area for cupping with towels.

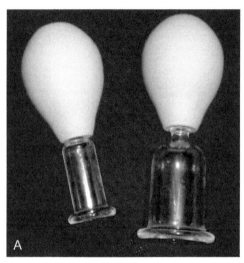

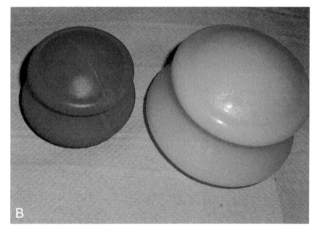

PLATE 43 (A) Clear Perspex or (B) silicon or rubber cups are ideal for cosmetic cupping applications.

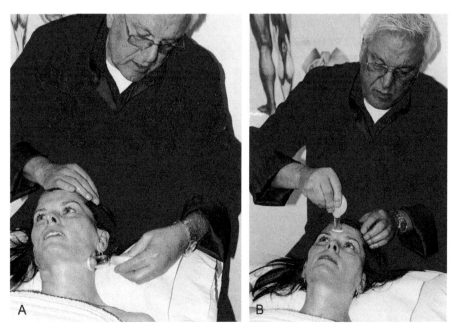

PLATE 44 (A, B) Positioning for cosmetic cupping sessions to the head and neck: Empty, Light or Light-moving cupping techniques are mostly employed.

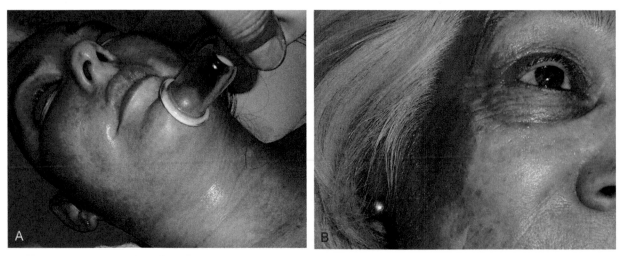

PLATE 45 (A) During treatment the surface of the skin is expected to appear warm with pink/reddish colour. (B) A cupping mark as a result of 3 minutes' cupping to the face.

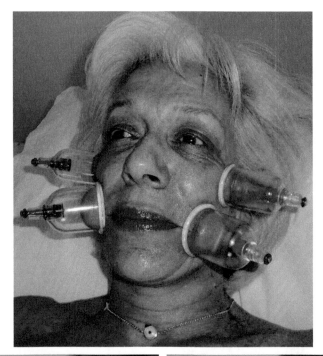

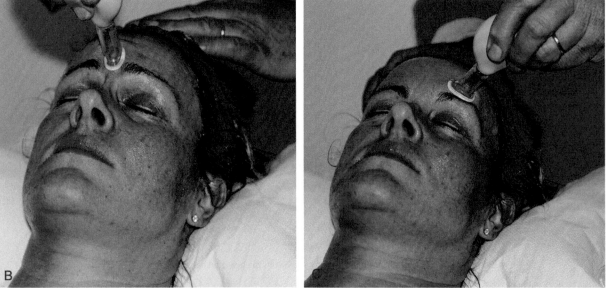

PLATE 46 (A–C) Facial cupping for a clearer complexion.

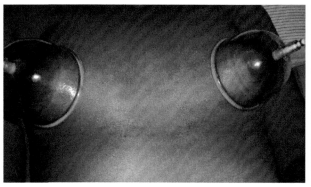
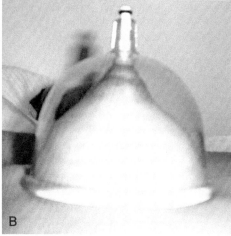

PLATE 47 (A, B) Cupping for breast enhancement.

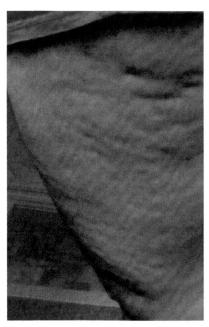
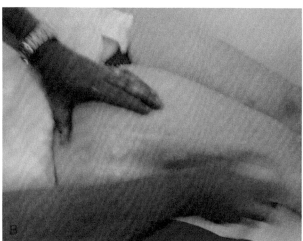

PLATE 48 (A, B) Treating cellulite.

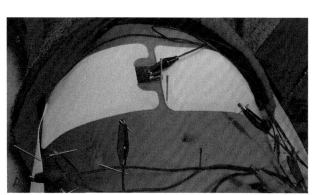
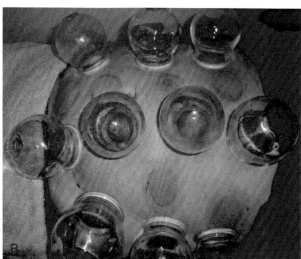

PLATE 49 (A, B) Cupping for weight loss.

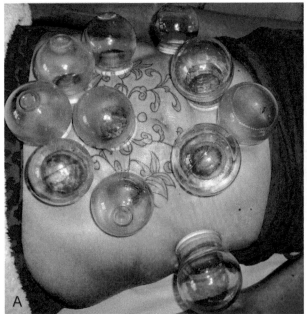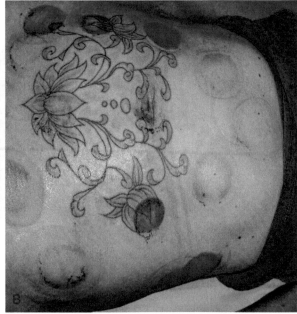

PLATE 50 (A, B) Abdominal cupping.

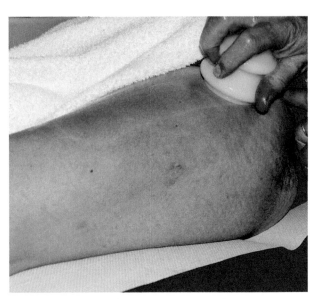

PLATE 51 Cupping for heavy leg syndrome.

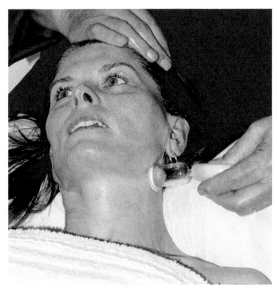

PLATE 52 Cupping the neck.

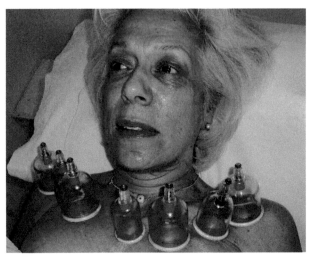

PLATE 53 Cupping the chest.

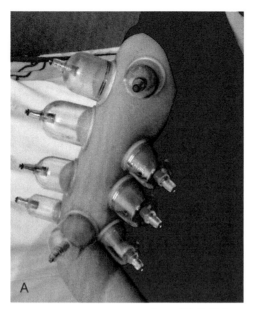
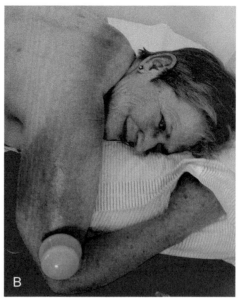

PLATE 54 (A,B) Cupping the shoulder and arm.

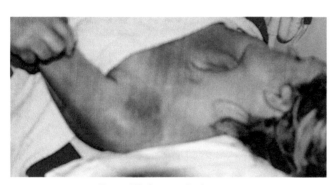

PLATE 55 Cupping the forearm.

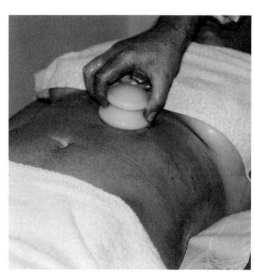

PLATE 56 Cupping the hypochondriac region.

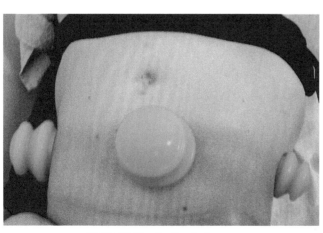

PLATE 57 Cupping the diaphragm.

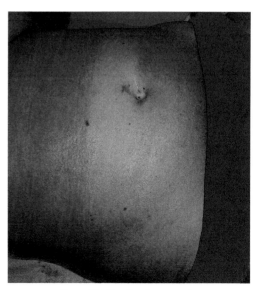

PLATE 58 Cupping the stomach.

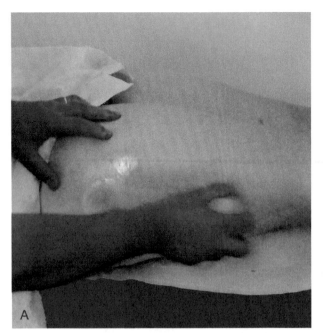
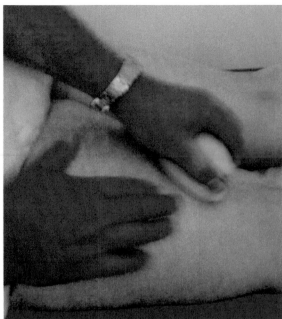

PLATE 59 (A, B) Cupping the thighs.

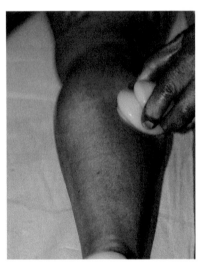

PLATE 60 Cupping the legs.

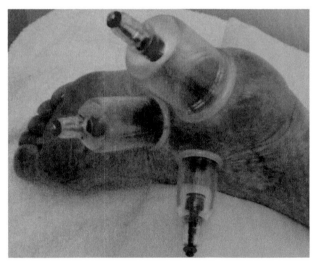

PLATE 61 Cupping the feet.

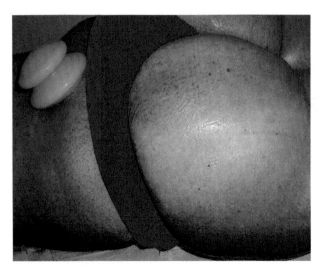
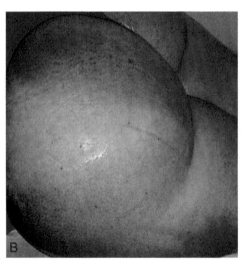

PLATE 62 (A, B) Cupping the buttocks.

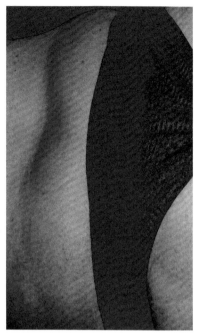

PLATE 63 Cupping the lower back.

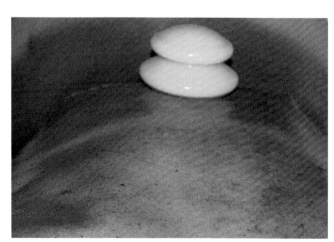

PLATE 64 Cupping the middle back.

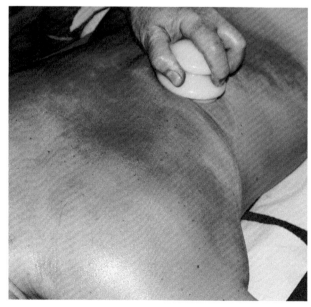

PLATE 65 Cupping the upper back.

Printed and bound by CPI Group (UK) Ltd, Croydon, CR0 4YY

03/10/2024

01040368-0001